ADVANCED NUTRITION
Micronutrients

ADVANCED NUTRITION
Micronutrients

Carolyn D. Berdanier
Professor, Foods and Nutrition
University of Georgia
Athens, Georgia

Illustrations by: Toni Kathryn Adkins

CRC Press
Boca Raton Boston London New York Washington, D.C.

Acquiring Editor: Marsha Baker
Project Editor: Debbie Didier
PrePress: Carlos Esser
Cover Design: Dawn Boyd

Library of Congress Cataloging-in-Publication Data

Berdanier, Carolyn D.
       Advanced nutrition / Carolyn D. Berdanier : Illustrations by Toni
Kathryn Adkins.
           p.   cm. -- (Modern nutrition)
       Includes bibliographical references and index.
       Contents: v. 1. Macronutrients
       ISBN 0-8493-8500-8 (v. 1)
       1. Nutrition. 2. Metabolism.   3. Energy metabolism.   I. Title.
II. Series: Modern nutrition (Boca Raton, Fla.)
QP141.B52 1994
612.3'9—dc20   94-11519
                                                                               CIP

No claim to original U.S. Government works
International Standard Book Number 0-8493-2664-8
Library of Congress Card Number 94-11519
Printed in the United States of America   2 3 4 5 6 7 8 9 0
Printed on acid-free paper

Series Preface for Modern Nutrition

The CRC Series in Modern Nutrition is dedicated to providing the widest possible coverage of topics in nutrition. Nutrition is an interdisciplinary, interprofessional field par excellence. It is noted by its broad range and diversity. We trust the titles and authorship in this series will reflect that range and diversity.

Published for a scholarly audience, the volumes of the CRC Series in Modern Nutrition are designed to explain, review, and explore present knowledge and recent trends, developments, and advances in nutrition. As such, they will also appeal to the educated layman. The format for the series will vary with the needs of the author and the topic, including, but not limited to, edited volumes, monographs, handbooks, and texts.

Contributors from any bona fide area of nutrition, including the controversial, are welcome.

Ira Wolinksy, Ph.D.
Series Editor

Preface

In the first volume of this two-volume book, *Advanced Nutrition: Macronutrients*, the needs for the macronutrients were discussed. The absorption, metabolism, excretion, and function of the various sources of energy as well as detailed discussions of the need for water and energy balance were presented. The needs for the micronutrients, as well as explanations of how these nutrients function in the body, were deferred to this, the second volume.

While most vitamins function at the metabolic level, the discoveries of how some of the vitamins and minerals work at the genomic level are quite exciting. Finally, we have an understanding of the pathophysiology of the plethora of diseases labeled nutrient deficiency disorders. Beriberi, pellagra, anemia, scurvy, embryonic and fetal malformation, rickets, osteoporosis, and a number of subtle (and not so subtle) disorders are finally connected to specific nutrients such that we can now understand why certain symptoms develop when an inadequate intake occurs. We have also come to understand, in part, the genetic diversity of the many species that require these nutrients. Nutrient-gene interactions as well as nutrient-nutrient and nutrient-drug interactions have become major research endeavors by nutrition scientists throughout the world. These scientists are truly hybrids in the world of science. They must have expertise in nutrition, biochemistry, physiology, and genetics, and if they are interested in human nutrition they must also understand human social systems and human medicine or have a physician collaborator.

Nutrition science is not as simple as finding a nutrient and determining its function. Today's science requires a far more complicated approach. The techniques of yesteryear are no longer adequate by themselves. The techniques of other disciplines must be brought to bear as well. The student will make new discoveries by studying the present database and finding the gaps in our knowledge. Nowhere is this as apparent as in the study of the micronutrients. While the animal of primary interest is the human, most research uses animals of other species because of the need to make organ, cell, and subcell measurements that are impossible to perform in the human. For this reason, the scientist needs to be all-inclusive in the study of nutrient needs.

Interspecies comparisons provide ample opportunities to learn how specific nutrients function and interact with other nutrients. After all, nutrition is a composite science requiring skills of integration and comprehension of the whole living system.

Acknowledgments

The author wishes to express her sincere thanks to the faculty and students of the University of Georgia Nutrition Science graduate program for their unfailing encouragement to prepare this volume. Particular appreciation is extended to Art Grider and Mary Ann Johnson for reading the initial drafts of the minerals section. In addition, the author is very grateful to Dr. Donald McCormick of Emory University and Dr. Dennis Medieros of Ohio State University whose meticulous reading of the manuscript provided much-needed revisions. Without their careful evaluation the present book would not have been possible. Needless to say, countless hours were expended by Kathy Adkins White and Tonya Whitfield to prepare the text and illustrations. Their expertise and dedication are much appreciated. Lastly, this text would not have been possible without the contributions of Dr. Mark Failla of the University of North Carolina at Greensboro. His intuitive thinking and excellent organization of the vast body of knowledge about the micronutrients provided the framework for the book. Without this starting point the integration of the various aspects of the micronutrients would have been a daunting task. Thanks Mark!

Author

Carolyn D. Berdanier, Ph.D., is a Professor of Nutrition at the University of Georgia in Athens, Georgia. She received a B.S. degree from The Pennsylvania State University and M.S. and Ph.D. degrees from Rutgers University in Nutrition in 1966. After a post-doctoral fellowship year with Dr. Paul Griminger at Rutgers, she served as a Research Nutritionist with the Human Nutrition Institute which is part of ARS, a unit of the U.S. Department of Agriculture. In 1975 she moved to the University of Nebraska College of Medicine where she continued her research in nutrient gene interactions. In 1977 she moved to the University of Georgia where she served as Head of the Department of Foods and Nutrition. She stepped down from this post ten years later and devoted her full time efforts to research and teaching in her research area. Her research on the diet and genetic components of diabetes and vascular disease has been supported by NIH, USDA, U.S. Department of Commerce, The National Livestock and Meat Board, and the Egg Board. She is a member of the American Institute of Nutrition, the American Society for Clinical Nutrition, The Society for Experimental Biology and Medicine, American Diabetes Association, and several honorary societies in science. She has served on the Editorial Boards of the *FASEB Journal*, *The Journal of Nutrition*, and *Nutrition Research and Biochemistry Archives*. She has also served as a Contributing Editor *for Nutrition Reviews* and Editor of the AIN News Notes. Current research interests include studies on aging, the role of diet in damage to mitochondrial DNA, and the role of specific dietary ingredients in the secondary complications of diabetes.

Table of Contents

Micronutrients, Human Health and Well Being

TABLE OF CONTENTS

I. OVERVIEW

Historically, nutrition science came into being because of the discoveries of the roles of certain nutrients in disease development. Examination of the early medical literature is especially revealing in this respect. The Egyptian papyri, the early Greek writings, the monastic scripts, and even passages of the bible describe the role of food in the prevention or treatment of diseases. For example, ox liver was frequently prescribed for anemia. Those early physicians did not know what ox liver actually did, but they knew that the pale and listless people who came to them for help would improve if they consumed this food item. Later, as humans became more adventurous and left the shores of their homelands to explore the world in ships, other diseases became apparent. Through astute observations, a number of physicians/scientists found that simple diet modifications could prevent or cure these disorders. The British physician, Lind, made the connection between citrus fruit and scurvy. Bonitus and Takaki likewise made the connection between brown rice and beriberi. Through the years these diseases have become uncommon in today's world. They have not disappeared, however, because whenever a population faces a food crisis, be it due to war or crop failure or financial collapse, nutrient deficiencies will appear and have adverse effects on health. They also appear in people who, through ignorance of the importance of consuming a wide variety of foods, select foods that do not provide sufficient amounts of the micronutrients. These people may be of normal weight or even overweight yet they may be inadequately nourished with respect to one or more of the essential vitamins and minerals. As scientists became aware of this problem within an ostensibly well-nourished group of people, they developed techniques that would sensitively detect marginal or inadequate intakes of specific nutrients. This work is ongoing and is the basis for nutrition assessment. Through work with animals that develop analogous deficiency symptoms, these techniques or tests of intake adequacy were related to particular biochemical functions of the individual micronutrients. These then, became the tools for assessment of the nutritional status of humans. The results of these tests also became the basis for the continuing evaluation of nutrient intake and the recommendations for daily intake, presently known as the Recommended Dietary Allowance (RDA), for each of the needed nutrients. Not all of the micronutrients described in this text have an RDA because sometimes there are insufficient data to support

1

such a recommendation. However, for several nutrients there are recommendations of an intake that should be safe and adequate. The RDA table not only is used as a guide for determining diet adequacy, it is also a device for planning food aid, i.e., food stamps, school lunch programs, etc. The table is used as a basis for educating people about food choice and is used by the food industry (in a modified form) for its food packaging labels.

II. ASSESSMENT

Assessment of the nutritional status of populations as well as individuals occurs at several levels. Overall assessment examines birth and death statistics, life span, family size, economic factors, food distribution, food handling and preservation, and food disappearance from the marketplace. These measures or databases are all useful in assessing the likelihood of intake adequacy for large populations and can serve as barometers of diet adequacy and inadequacy. They do not apply to the individual.

More detailed methods are needed for an individual nutritional assessment vis à vis intake adequacy. An individual assessment requires a careful analysis of the foods consumed concomitant with whole-body assessment and then a functional, physiological, and biochemical assessment of organs and tissues. This type of nutritional assessment can be quite detailed and very expensive. Except under research conditions where very specific questions are being addressed, this detailed assessment is usually not needed.

As detailed in Unit 1 of *Advanced Nutrition: Macronutrients*, food surveys, epidemiological studies, and population statistics provide a wealth of information about large groups of people and, as detailed in Unit 2 of that text, assessment of body size and composition can provide, from an anthropometric point of view, information on an individual's health status. Measurements of height, weight, bone density, fat mass, and muscle mass indicate whether the energy and protein needs are being met. Normal growth and development do not occur when macronutrient intake is inadequate. On the other hand, there can be specific tissue or cell failures when one or more of the micronutrient requirements are not met. Rickets, a breakdown in the growth and development of bone, is one such failure. Anemia, a failure to produce functionally adequate red blood cells, is another. Signs and symptoms of each of these as well as other failures are sought when the nutritional status of the individual is determined. One of the most accessible tissues for use in assessing micronutrient status is the blood. Both red cells (erythrocytes) and white cells (leukocytes) can be examined, as can the sera. Red cells are easier to isolate and assess than are white cells because of their larger size and greater number. However, because malnutrition is frequently characterized by anemia, there may be fewer red cells to work with for these analyses. Anemia can be due to inadequate hemoglobin synthesis, inadequate red cell synthesis and maturation, or both. Vitamin A, B_6, folacin, B_{12}, ascorbic acid, iron, copper, and zinc deficiencies can have anemia as a characteristic. Red cells are constantly being replaced; hence, a deficiency in any one of the many components needed for the replacement of the red cell and its chief component, hemoglobin, will result in anemia. Furthermore, in the hierarchy of essential needs for these nutrients, red cell replacement may be relatively low; therefore, anemia can be a fairly sensitive indicator of nutrient status. The body has many red cells and can function, if necessary, with fewer. A 10 or 20% reduction in functional capacity is not incompatible with life. However, optimal function of that body might not be realized.

Erythrocytes at maturity are circular, biconcave disc-like cells having no nucleus. They are about 7.7 μm in diameter. Their principal function is to carry oxygen from the lungs to all the cells of the body and exchange this oxygen for carbon dioxide which is then transported back to the lungs for expiration. The average adult male has 5.5 to 7×10^5 red cells per milliliter of blood whereas the average adult female has 4.5 to 6×10^5 red cells per milliliter whole blood. These red cells contain hemoglobin, a globular protein having the iron-containing heme as an essential component. It is this iron-containing hemoglobin that carries the oxygen or carbon dioxide.

Table 1 Normal Blood Values for Measurements Made to Assess the Presence of Anemia

Measurement	Normal Values	Iron Deficiency Anemia	Chronic Disease	B_{12} or Folic Acid Deficiency
Red blood cells (10^6/ml³)	Males: 4.6–6.2 Females: 4.2–5.4	Low	Low	Low
Hemoglobin (g/dl)	Males: 14–18 Females: 12–16	Low	Low	Low
Hematocrit (vol %)	Males: 40–54 Females: 37–47	Low	Low	Low
Serum iron	60–280 µg/dl	Low	Low	Normal
TIBC[a]	250–425 µg/dl	High	Low	Normal
Ferritin	60	Less than 12	Normal	Normal
Percent saturation	90-100%	Low	Normal to high	Normal
Hypochromia	No	Yes	Slight	None
Microcytes	Few	Many	Slight	Few
Macrocytes	Few	Few	None	Many
RDW (RBC size)		High	Normal to low	Very high
Red cell folate	>360 nmol/l	Normal	315–358	<315
Serum folate	>13.5 mg/ml	Normal	Normal	Low (<6.7 mg/ml)
Serum B_{12}	200–900 pg/ml	Normal	Normal	Low
MCV[b]	82–92 µl³	Less than 80	Normal	Greater than 80 to 100

[a] Indirect measure of serum transferrin; iron binding capacity.
[b] Mean cell volume. When volume increases, the size of the red cell has increased (↑ % of megaloblasts).

The life span of the red cell is about 120 days; thus, the half life is 60 days. That is, it would take 4 months to replace every red cell in the body or 2 months to replace 50% of them. Anemia results when there is a failure to replace these cells. Table 1 summarizes the features of the various forms of anemia. Normal values for these measurements are also shown.

Red cells are synthesized in the red marrow (Figure 1) of bone. The reticular cells give rise to daughter cells called hemocytoblasts. These in turn divide into basophilic erythroblasts. These erythroblasts are large, nucleated cells with a red cytoplasm and traces of hemoglobin. As development proceeds, the hemoglobin concentration increases. The cell proceeds from the basophilic erythroblast to the megaloblast and from there to the mature normoblast. The mature normoblast resembles the mature erythrocyte in size and hemoglobin content but still has a nucleus. This is lost in the final stage of red cell development when the normoblast divides and becomes the mature erythrocyte. Almost all of the latter stages of red cell development can be found in normal blood. Megaloblasts, normoblasts, and mature red cells are found in varying amounts. In persons with pernicious anemia there will be far more immature cells than normal cells because erythropoiesis is not occurring normally. Only vitamin B_{12} deficiency (due to inadequate uptake) results in pernicious anemia.

However, both B_{12} and folacin are needed for red cell replication and development. Hence, both vitamin deficiencies are characterized by megalobastic anemia. B_6 deficiency will result in microcytic anemia. This is characterized by a reduction in hemoglobin synthesis as well as red cell production. Hence the red cells are fewer in number and smaller in size. Serum iron may be increased under these conditions and as soon as B_6 is provided this excess iron is incorporated into the hemoglobin structure and erythropoiesis is restored to normal.

Microcytic anemia may also be observed when either copper or iron intake is inadequate. In this situation the serum iron level (<75 µg/dl) is below normal rather than elevated, as is the case with B_6 deficiency. Zinc deficiency likewise can affect both red cell production and hemoglobin synthesis. The effect of zinc is an indirect one due to its role in protein synthesis and gene expression. Zinc deficiency in part mimics iron deficiency.

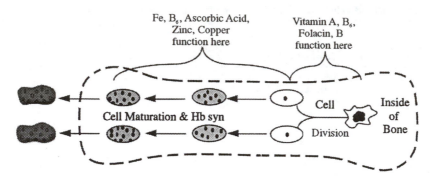

Figure 1   Red cell formation and maturation.

The laboratory tests for anemia as well as for other nutrition related disorders assume that the deficiency condition is a simple one. That is, that the deficiency is due to the inadequate intake of one nutrient or nutrient class. Rarely does that occur. Because intake adequacy is an attribute of the food supply, a single deficiency is unlikely. Rather, the deficient state may develop as a response to a nutrient-nutrient interaction whether it be a macronutrient-micronutrient, mineral-mineral, mineral-vitamin, or vitamin-vitamin interaction effect. Shown in Table 2 is a compilation of interacting nutrients with notations as to where these interactions take place. With many of the mineral-mineral interactions it is the effect of one on the other with respect to absorption by the enterocyte.

Assessment of micronutrient status also includes the determination of the concentration of nutrients in the serum or plasma. These indicate how much of that nutrient is being transported. These levels do not give an indication of the stores, but if the diet intake has been assessed the investigator can make some assumptions about the nutrient with regard to whether it is moving towards a tissue reservoir or away from it. With most of the water-soluble vitamins, tissue reservoirs are negligible. That is, very small amounts of these vitamins are stored for future use. With the other micronutrients such is not the case. The fat-soluble vitamins can be stored as detailed in Unit 4 and the minerals likewise as detailed in Units 6 and 7. Table 3 gives the normal blood levels of micronutrients in addition to those values presented in Table 1.

Urine analysis can also provide information about micronutrient status. The excretion of some minerals and vitamin metabolites can provide an indication of intake and use. Described in Units 3 and 4 are the various metabolites one could expect to find in well-nourished healthy individuals. Not all of the minerals (see Units 6 and 7) will be found in urine because of differences in absorption efficiency. Those that are well absorbed, i.e., sodium, potassium, and chloride, can be found in the urine while most of the others will be found in the feces as unabsorbed ions or salts. Fecal analysis is rarely used in nutritional status assessments. Normal values for nutrients in the urine are presented in Table 4. In some instances, the assessment of status is performed by providing a load of either the nutrient or another nutrient that requires a certain vitamin for its metabolism. For example, a load dose of ascorbic acid might be given followed by a 24-hr urine collection, which in turn is used to determine the amount of ascorbic acid excreted. Knowing the urinary ascorbic acid level before and after the load allows for the calculation of percent recovery and this in turn reflects tissue saturation or status. With folacin, a load of histidine is administered as a challenge and FIGLU (formiminoglutamic acid) is measured in the urine excreted over 8 hours, following the load. Histidine is metabolized to formininoglutamate which reacts with tetrahydrofolate to generate N^5formiminotetrahydrofolate that can then serve in 1-carbon transfers. One-carbon transfer is essential to purine synthesis (see Units 2 and 5). Inadequate folacin status will result in more FIGLU excretion because there is an inadequate supply of the vitamin to transfer the formimino group. The same principle is applied to the evaluation of B_{12} status. However, in this instance the substance used is valine, not histidine, and the metabolite (methylmalonic acid) will rise in concentration when B_{12} intake is low. This is because B_{12} participates as a coenzyme in the synthesis of succinyl

Table 2 Micronutrient Interactions

	Calcium	Phosphorus	Potassium	Sodium	Magnesium	Zinc	Iron	Copper	Iodine	Fluorine	Vitamin A	Vitamin D	Vitamin E	B12	Vitamin K	Riboflavin	Niacin	Thiamin	Ascorbic acid	B6	Folacin
Calcium	X	↑a	↓a	↓a↑m	↑m↓a						↑a	↑a, m				↑m		↑m	↑m		
Phosphorus	↑a	X	↑m	↑m	↓a							↑a								↑↓m	
Potassium	↑↓m	↑a	X	↑a	↑a, ↑m							↑a								↑↓m	
Sodium	↑↓m	↑a		X	↑a, ↑m							↑m								↑m	
Magnesium	↓a	↑m		↓a, ↑m	X							↑a					↑m	↑m		↑m	
Zinc						X		↓a, ↑m			↑m	↑a							↑m	↓a	↑m
Iron	↑m	↓a				↓a	X	↓a, ↑m	↑m		↑m		↑m	↑m		↑m	↑m		↑a	↑m	
Copper						↓a	↓a, ↑m	X				↓a		↑a		↑m	↑m				
Iodine									X												
Fluorine	↓a									X							↑m				
Cobalt																					
Chromium					↓a	↓a	↓a														
Manganese							↓a, ↑m	↓a													
Molybdenum								↑m													
Selenium																					

Note: ↑ increase; ↓ decrease; a, absorption; m, metabolism.

Table 3   Normal Values for Micronutrients in Blood

Ascorbic acid, plasma	0.6–1.6 mg/dl	Phosphorus	3.4–4.5 mg/dl
Calcium, serum	4.5–5.3 meq/l	Potassium	3.5–5.0 meq/l
β-Carotene, serum	40–200 µg/dl	Riboflavin, red cell	>14.9 µg/dl cells
Chloride, serum	95–103 meq/l	Folate, plasma	>6 ng/ml
Lead, whole blood	0–50 µg/dl	Pantothenic acid, plasma	≥6 µg/dl
Magnesium, serum	1.5–2.5 meq/l	Pantothenic acid, whole blood	≥80 µg/dl
Sodium, plasma	136–142 meq/l	Biotin, whole blood	>25 ng/ml
Sulfate, serum	0.2–1.3 meq/l	B_{12}, plasma	>150 pg/ml
Vitamin A, serum	15–60 µg/dl	Vitamin D 25(OH)–D_3, plasma	>10 ng/ml
Retinol, plasma	>20 µg/dl	α-Tocopherol, plasma	>0.80 mg/dl

Note: For more information on blood analysis see: NHANES Manual for Nutrition Assessment, CDC, Atlanta, GA (contact Elaine Gunter); ICNND Manual for Nutrition Surveys, 2nd ed., 1963, U.S. Government Printing Office, Washington, D.C.; Sauberlich et al., 1974, *Laboratory Tests for the Assessment of Nutritional Status,* CRC Press, Boca Raton, FL.

Table 4   Normal Values for Micronutrients in Urine

Calcium, mg/24 hr	100–250
Chloride, meq/24 hr	110–250
Copper, µg/24 hr	0–100
Lead, µg/24 hr	<100
Phosphorus, g/24 hr	0.9–1.3
Potassium, meq/24 hr	25–100
Sodium, meq/24 hr	130–260
Zinc, mg/24 hr	0.15–1.2
Creatinine, mg/kg body weight	15–25
Riboflavin, µg/g creatinine	>80
Niacin metabolite,[a] µg/g creatinine	>1.6
Pyridoxine, µg/g creatinine	≥20
Biotin, µg/24 hr	>25
Pantothenic acid, mg/24 hr	≥1
Folate, FIGLU[b] after histidine load	<5 mg/8 hr
B_{12}, methylmalonic acid after a valine load	≤2 mg/24 hr

Note: For more information on urine analyses see: ICNNO, 1963, *Manual for Nutrition Surveys,* 2nd ed., U.S. Government Printing Office, Washington, D.C.; Sauberlich et al., 1974, *Laboratory Tests for the Assessment of Nutritional Status,* CRC Press, Boca Raton, FL; NHANES Manual for Nutrition Assessment, CDC, Atlanta, GA; Gibson, R.S., 1990, *Principles of Nutrition Assessment,* Oxford University Press, New York.

[a] N^1-methylnicotinamide.
[b] Formiminoglutamic acid.

CoA from methylmalonyl CoA. This reaction is part of the degradation of propionate. Thus, in the deficient state one would be able to find methylmalonic acid in the urine after a valine load since a catabolite of valine is propionate.

Evaluation of status should include a physical examination of the subject. As mentioned, this includes body weight, height, and composition. It also includes a careful clinical evaluation of the hair, joints, nails, skin, muscle, nervous system, and endocrine system. Questions about appetite, physical activity, and emotional state can also be included. Shown in Table 5 are features that are usually included in a clinical evaluation. Decreased appetite, for example, can suggest thiamin or zinc deficiency as well as protein-energy malnutrition. This probably would result in weight loss — particularly of the fat mass and muscle mass. Subjects that are pale likely are anemic and could

Table 5   Clinical Evaluation of Nutritional Status

Feature
Body weight for height, age, gender
Appetite
Skin: color, texture, general appearance
Hair: appearance, texture, strength
Mouth, teeth, and tongue: carries, gum health, color
Neck: shape, strength
Abdomen: liver size, absence of tenderness
Extremities: absence of edema, bone and joint strength and flexibility, muscle strength
Neurologic signs: tetany, tingling, poor or exaggerated reflex activity, decreased mental clarity, disorientation, impaired balance

be malnourished with respect to folacin, B_{12}, or iron. This finding would be confirmed with blood analysis, as described. Vitamin A deficiency could be observed through the skin lesion, follicular hyperkeratosis. This is a rough texture found on the legs and arms, particularly on the backs of the upper arm. A generalized dermatitis would suggest inadequate essential fatty acid, zinc, or B-vitamin intake, whereas numerous bruises would suggest inadequate vitamin C or K status. Hair texture is a clue to inadequate protein synthesis, which in turn is related not only to protein intake but also to energy intake and secondarily to those vitamins and minerals essential to protein synthesis.

A shiny, smooth tongue, bleeding gums, and cracks in the corners of the mouth typify riboflavin deficiency, but can also suggest ascorbic acid deficiency. An enlarged thyroid gland suggests an iodine deficiency. An enlarged liver could be due to general malnutrition but could also be due to exposure to toxins that in turn result in an inability to use the energy and protein and micronutrients consumed. Bone malformation typifies vitamin D inadequacy, but can also be due to inadequate intake of vitamin C or the minerals needed for bone. Neurologic symptoms of tetany could be due to calcium and/or magnesium inadequacy or to B_6 deficiency. Thiamin and niacin deficiency can result in loss of foot or hand reflexive responses and can also be characterized by disorientation and/or dementia. All of these clinical impressions must be confirmed with biochemical/physiological assessments before a diagnosis of malnutrition can be accepted. Of course, reversal of symptoms with appropriate supplementation supports the diagnosis of inadequate nutrient intake.

III. FACTORS AFFECTING MICRONUTRIENT NEEDS

The scientists providing the recommendation for micronutrient requirements and their associated recommended dietary allowances assume that the consumer is healthy with no inherent metabolic or physiologic problems. This is not always true. People afflicted with one of the many malabsorption diseases, for example, need larger intakes of vitamins and minerals to compensate for their disabilities. The details of these absorption problems are described in each of the micronutrient sections. In addition to these influences on micronutrient intake and use, there are a number of drugs used to treat illnesses that also interfere with nutrient use. Some of these are listed in Table 6.

There are many more drugs that influence nutrient need than can be shown in this table. However, a large database describing and quantifying these interactions is not available. In many instances, the influence of the chronic use of a given drug on the need for one or more nutrients has not been studied. In other instances, data are available only from acute studies. This is an area of research that has not been widely addressed.

Lastly, micronutrients, especially the vitamins, can themselves be drugs when taken to excess. Detailed in Units 3 and 4 are the consequences of vitamin toxicity. Not all vitamins will be toxic when consumed in excess, but with some this can be a problem that needs recognition.

Table 6   Drugs That Influence Vitamin Use

Drug Class	Nutrient Affected
Diuretics	
Spironolactone	Vitamin A
Thiazide	Potassium
Bile acid sequestrant	
Cholestyramine	Vitamin A, Vitamin B_{12}, folacin
Colestipol	Vitamin A, Vitamin K, Vitamin D
Laxative	
Phenolphthalein	Vitamin A, Vitamin D, Vitamin K, potassium
Anticonvulsant	
Phenytoin	Vitamin D, Vitamin K, folacin
Anticoagulant	
Coumarin, decoumarol	Vitamin K
Warfarin	
Immunosuppressant	
Cyclosporin	Vitamin K
Antibacterial	
Isoniazid	Niacin, B_6
Sulfasalazine	Folacin
p-Aminosalicylic acid	Vitamin B_{12}
Neomycin	Vitamin B_{12}
Tetracycline	Calcium, magnesium, iron, zinc
Anti-inflammatant	
Phenylbutazone	Niacin
Chelating agents	
EDTA	Calcium, magnesium, lead
Penicillamine	Copper, Vitamin B_6
Thiosemicarbazide	Vitamin B_6
Anticholinergic	
L-DOPA	Vitamin B_6
Antihypertensive	
Hydralazine	Vitamin B_6
Antimalarial	
Pyrimethamine	Folacin
Antineoplastic	
Methotrexate	Folacin
Antihistamine	
Ametidine	Vitamin B_{12}
Theophylline	Protein
Antacids	
Aluminum hydroxide	Folate, phosphate
Magnesium hydroxide	Phosphate
Sodium bicarbonate	Folacin
Other	
Ethanol	Niacin, folacin, thiamin
Mineral oil	Vitamin A, β-carotene

Integration of the Functional Aspects of Vitamins and Minerals

TABLE OF CONTENTS

I. OVERVIEW

At the turn of the century, scientists seeking to understand the role of diet in health maintenance began to use rats in their research on nutrient needs. When these animals were fed diets consisting of purified proteins, fats, and carbohydrates, they died. It was soon found that specific minerals and additional factors, termed accessory food factors by Hopkins, were present in an unrefined diet and were necessary to sustain life. The minerals and these "accessory factors" were needed in very small amounts. Because it was thought that the "accessory factors" all contained nitrogen, they were called amines. Casimir Funk, an early nutrition scientist, coined the term "vitamines" to indicate that these amines were vital to the survival of the animal. Later, after it was discovered that not all vitamins contained amines, the final "e" was dropped from the word.

Vitamins are a large group of potent organic compounds necessary in minute amounts in the diet. They are usually divided into two classes based on their solubility characteristics. The water-soluble vitamins are soluble in water and usually function as coenzymes in the metabolism of protein, fats, and carbohydrates. The fat-soluble vitamins are not usually soluble in water but are soluble in one or more solvents such as alcohol, ether, or chloroform.

Each of the vitamins has a specific chemical structure and many can be synthesized rather inexpensively. Thus, multivitamin supplements can be purchased in drugstores for a modest price. While specific vitamins can cure specific deficiency diseases, as indicated in Unit 1 and detailed in the sections on each of the vitamins, the use of supplements by people consuming a wide variety of raw and cooked foods may be unnecessary.

Before the vitamins were chemically isolated and described, scientists began naming the compounds. In some instances, different research groups were studying the same compound and unwittingly gave different names to the same vitamin. This contributed confusion to the identity of vitamins. Frequently, the name chosen described the food source or the deficiency symptom. Thus, for years thiamin was known as the antiberiberi factor, vitamin K was known as the coagulation factor, and vitamin E as the wheat germ factor or the antisterility factor. As nutrition scientists began publishing their findings, it became important to establish a uniform nomenclature and one based on the alphabet was devised. Compounds having vitamin activity were alphabetized in order of their discovery. Now, however, information about the vitamins has expanded to such an extent that this nomenclature system is outmoded. Chemically descriptive terms are now being used that more correctly identify the vitamin in question. Nonetheless, alphabetical designations are still being used and the reader will encounter some of these in this text.

As scientists learned more about the vitamins they began to reclassify them according to function rather than solubility. Thus, we have vitamins that serve as membrane stabilizers, as coenzymes, or that have antioxidant properties and/or that act at the genomic level. Some vitamins fall into more than one category. For example, ascorbic acid serves as a general antioxidant, as a redox agent (as a substrate being oxidized to dehydroascorbic acid), and yet also acts at the levels of transcription and translation for the protein, procollagen. Vitamin A is another one that is multifunctional. It has a direct role in the visual cycle, is an antioxidant, stimulates the RNA transcription for the retinoic acid receptor, and when bound to this receptor serves as a transcription factor for the transcription of numerous mRNAs. As the reader progresses through the units and sections devoted to the individual vitamins, this multifunctionality will be described.

Similarly, as the roles for each of the minerals were elucidated, the minerals likewise were subdivided into two groups based not on solubility characteristics but on the magnitude of need. Thus, we have the macrominerals and the microminerals. The human need for the former is much greater per day than the need for the latter. Just as some vitamins can serve as coenzymes in intermediary metabolism, minerals serve as cofactors in many of these same reactions. Vitamins and minerals both have active roles in the formation and maintenance of the body's structure as well as its function. Minerals and vitamins are essential to the regulation of metabolism and, as well, are important components for the expression of many specific genes.

II. THE ROLE OF MICRONUTRIENTS IN GENE EXPRESSION

Among the many functions that vitamins and minerals serve in the body, one stands out in its primacy. That is, the service in gene expression. Almost every micronutrient is involved either directly as part of a cis- or trans-acting factor in RNA transcription, or as an important coenzyme in the synthesis of the purine and pyrimidine bases, or as a coenzyme in intermediary metabolism which provides substrates and energy for the support of cell replication, cell growth, DNA replication, RNA transcription, RNA translation, and protein synthesis. Figure 1 illustrates the process of gene expression and Table 1 itemizes specific effects of vitamins and minerals on this process. Some of these effects are direct, some are indirect. Many of the symptoms of vitamin deficiencies can be traced to this involvement in gene expression. Gene products and cell types with very short half-lives will be among the first to be affected by the absence of a given micronutrient. Hence, skin lesions are a frequent feature of the deficient state because epithelial cells have an average half-life of 7 days. Red blood cells have an average half-life of 60 days and many nutrient deficiencies are characterized by anemia. Similarly, vitamin- and mineral-dependent gene products (enzymes, receptors, transporters) also will be affected should that particular nutrient be in short supply. Conversely, we have instances of diversity within a population such that one individual's nutrient intake is fully adequate while another individual in the same population, consuming that same amount of that same nutrient, is in the deficient state. This contrast is due to individual genetic

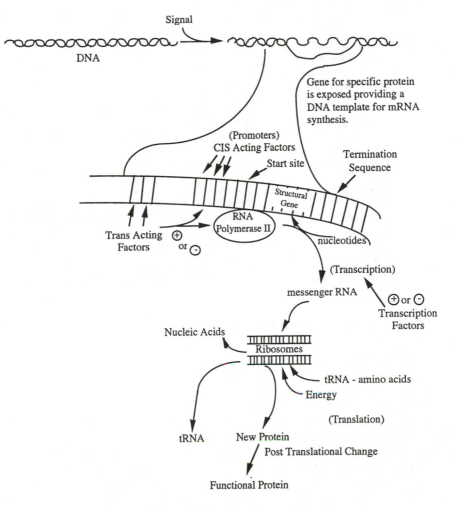

Figure 1 Overview of gene expression.

variability and can be found in every species and strain of living creatures. The explanation for this variability, not only in nutrient needs and tolerances but also in such characteristics as skin color, height, weight, or any of the myriad characteristics that distinguish one species from another and one individual from another, is in the genetic material, DNA.

The mammalian genome contains 4×10^9 base pairs (bp) and exists as a double-stranded helix with the purine and pyrimidine bases arranged in a preordained sequence and held together by phosphate and ribose groups. There is far more DNA in each cell than is used. In contrast to the DNA found in single-cell organisms (prokaryotes), eukaryotic genes contain interrupting sequences that are noncoding. That is, at intervals along a structural gene there are series of bases that do not participate in the expression of that gene. These are called introns. Exons are those base sequences that provide the coding of the genes. The introns do base pair when mRNA is transcribed, but the parts of the message transcribed by these introns are removed by splicing during nuclear RNA editing prior to export. Each mammalian cell has a complete genome in its nucleus but not all of this is transcribed. This central molecule of life consists of many discrete sequences which encode or dictate the amino acid sequence of every protein in the body, which in turn dictates the functional

Table 1 Specific Nutrient Effects on Gene Expression

Nutrient	Gene	Effect
Retinoic acid	Retinoic acid receptor and other proteins	↑ Transcription
Vitamin B$_6$	Steroid hormone receptor	↓ Transcription
Ascorbic acid	Procollagen	↑ Transcription ↑ Translation
Vitamin K	Prothrombin	↑ Post-translational carboxylation of glutamic acid residues
Potassium	Aldosterone synthetase	↑ Transcription
Zinc	Zinc fingers	Allows binding of cis or trans factors to specific DNA binding sites
Iron	Ferritin	When bound to ferritin mRNA allows translation to proceed
Folacin	DNA, RNA	Purine and pyrimidine synthesis
B$_{12}$	DNA, RNA	Purine and pyrimidine synthesis
Thiamin	All genes	As part of TPP it plays a role in bioenergetics
Riboflavin	All genes	As part of FAD it plays a role in producing ATP
Niacin	All genes	As part of NAD it plays a role in producing ATP
B$_6$	All genes	Purine and pyrimidine synthesis
Vitamin D	Calcium binding proteins	↑ Transcription
Vitamin E	All genes	Protects against free radical damage to DNA

attributes of each organelle, cell type, tissue, and organ. These proteins serve as structural elements, enzymes, transporters, receptors, messengers, and central integrators of the use of all the other nutrients needed by living creatures.

Gene expression is a highly controlled process. Its regulation includes transcription control, RNA processing control, RNA transport control, translational control, mRNA stability control, and post-translation control. Each of these control points have nutritionally mediated aspects. In most of the genes studied to date, more nutrients affect transcription than translation or post-translation processing. There are some exceptions, as shown in Table 1 and described later in this text. Transcription control is exerted by that portion of the DNA called the promoter region plus transcription factors that bind either to this region or to an upstream region that in turn affects the activity of either cis-acting factors or the polymerase activity. RNA polymerase II binds to the promoter region just upstream of the start codon for the gene. The promoter region is located in the 5′ flanking region upstream from the structural gene on the same strand of DNA. Cis-responsive elements are located about −40 to −200 bp from the start site. Some promoters, i.e., TATA, GC, and CCAAT boxes, are common to many genes transcribed by RNA polymerase II. These sequences interact with transcription factors that in turn form preinitiation complexes. The mechanisms of such transcriptional regulation have recently been reviewed by Semenza and by Johnson et al. Trans-acting factors are usually proteins produced by other genes which influence transcription. Trans-acting factors can be proteins or peptide hormones or steroid hormone-receptor protein complexes, or vitamin-receptor protein complexes, or minerals, or mineral-protein complexes. The mechanism for binding hormone receptors to specific regions of DNA has been reviewed and described by Freedman and Luisi (see Supplemental Readings list).

The promoter region contains the start site for RNA synthesis. RNA polymerase II binds to this specific DNA sequence and, under the influence of the various transcription factors, RNA transcription is initiated. The RNA polymerase II opens up a local region of the DNA double helix so that the gene to be transcribed is exposed. One of the two DNA strands acts as the template for complementary base pairing with incoming ribonucleotide triphosphate molecules. The nucleotides are joined until the polymerase encounters a special sequence in the DNA called the termination sequence. At this point, transcription is complete. Following this process the newly formed RNA is edited and processed. This processing removes nearly 95% of the bases. The resultant shortened

RNA then migrates out of the nucleus and becomes associated with ribosomes whereupon translation takes place.

This outline of transcription has omitted a number of important details with respect to transcription control. For example, the regulation of transcription is exerted by a group of proteins that determine which region of the DNA is to be transcribed. Cells contain a variety of sequence-specific DNA binding proteins. Nutrients can bind to these proteins and have their effect in this way. These proteins are of low abundance and they function by binding to specific regions on the DNA. The regions are variable in size but are usually between 8 and 15 nucleotides. Depending on the binding protein and the nutrient bound to it, transcription is either enhanced or inhibited and indeed cell types may differ because of these proteins. Since all cells contain the same DNA, gene expression in discrete cell types is controlled at this point simply by the binding of these very specific DNA binding proteins. Thus, genes for the synthesis of insulin, for example, could be turned on in the pancreatic β cell, but not in the myocyte, simply because the β cell has the needed specific DNA binding proteins that the myocyte lacks. At some point in differentiation, the myocyte failed to acquire sufficient amounts of these regulatory factors and thus can not synthesize and release insulin.

In many instances, specific DNA binding proteins contain zinc and as such are referred to as zinc fingers. Gene expression is regulated by the formation of these zinc fingers, yet they comprise only a part of this regulation. Most genes are regulated by a combination of regulatory factors. In some, a group of DNA binding proteins interact to control the activation or inhibition of transcription. Not all of these proteins are of equal power in all instances. There may be a "master" regulatory protein that serves to coordinate the binding of several "lesser" proteins. This is important for the coordinate expression of genes in a single pathway, as happens, for example, in the expression of the genes that encode the multienzyme complex, fatty acid synthetase.

Mutations in genes that encode any one of these transcription factors could result in disease. Mutations in genes encoding transcription factors often have pleiotropic effects because these factors regulate a number of different genes. So, too, are the effects of nutrients which are required components of these transcription factors. An example is the series of genes which encode the enzymes needed for the conversion of a fibroblast to a myocyte. The mammalian skeletal muscle cell is very large and multinucleated. It is formed by the fusion of myoblasts (myocyte precursor cells) and contains characteristic structural proteins as well as a number of other proteins that function in energy metabolism and nerve-muscle signaling. When muscle is being synthesized all of these proteins must be synthesized at the same time. In proliferating myoblasts very few of these proteins are present, yet, as these myoblasts fuse, the messenger RNAs for these proteins increase as does the synthesis of the proteins. This indicates that the expression of the genes for muscle protein synthesis is responding to a single regulatory DNA binding protein. This protein (Myo D1) has been isolated and identified and occurs only in muscle cells. Should this protein be inserted in some other cell type such as a skin cell or an adipocyte, for example, the same expression will occur. That is, the skin or fat cell will look like a muscle cell. It will take on the characteristics of a myoblast and become a myocyte.

Of interest is the fact that although all of the genes needed for synthesis in the myocyte and its master controller are present, synthesis will not occur or will occur at a very limited rate if one or more of the essential amino acids needed for this synthesis are absent or deficient in the diet. Here is an example of a gene-nutrient interaction that has control properties with respect to muscle protein synthesis and this interaction ultimately affects the overall process of growth. Turning this situation around, if the master regulator Myo D1 is aberrant, or if one or more of the genes which encode the enzymes needed for protein synthesis in the myocyte have mutated such that the enzyme in question is nonfunctional or only partly functional, muscle development will cease or be retarded. In either instance, abnormal growth will result.

As mentioned, transcription is regulated by both the nearby upstream promoter region and the distant enhancer elements. The upstream enhancer element can include a TATA box and extends for about 100 bp. Enhancer fragments further upstream can bind multiple proteins which, in turn, can influence transcription. These factors are proteins and are labeled JUN, AP2, ATF, CREB, SP1, OTF1, CTF, NF1, SRE, and others.

One well-studied group of DNA binding proteins are those which bind steroid hormones. These are called the steroid receptors and bind to specific base sequences called steroid response elements (SREs). Steroids that enhance (or inhibit) transcription act by binding to one of these specific proteins which, in turn, binds to DNA. These complexes thus explain how cells respond to a steroid hormone stimulus. The proteins consist of about 100 amino acids and zinc. As mentioned, they recognize a specific DNA sequence. For some members of this family of proteins, the transcription-enhancing domain is localized at the amino terminus of the polypeptide chain. At the carboxy terminus is the binding site for the steroid hormone. Steroid hormones, via binding to their cognate receptors and to the hormone response element on the DNA, also enhance the transcription of mitochondrial genes. The recognition of this function of steroid hormones provides a further explanation of how these hormones function in energy balance. Enhanced mitochondrial gene expression should result in an increased mitochondrial function, i.e., enhanced activity of oxidative phosphorylation. In turn, this would result in increased ATP production which is needed for cell function and tissue growth. Although this action of specific steroid hormones has been shown to occur in mitochondria, we do not know whether vitamins A and D act in this way.

Post-transcriptional regulation of gene expression is the next stage of control. As mentioned above, newly formed mRNA is edited prior to leaving the nucleus. RNA transcription can be terminated prematurely with the result of a smaller than expected gene product. A single mRNA can be translated into several different gene products, usually peptides. These proteins or peptides may have comparable or opposing functions depending on the products in question. As described, messenger RNA is edited and processed such that only 5% of this RNA leaves the nucleus. The 95% which remains is degraded and the purine and pyrimidine bases are reused or are subject to further degradation. The RNA that leaves the nucleus does so through pores in the nuclear membrane. This is an active process, the details of which are not well understood.

Not all of the mRNA that exits the nucleus is immediately translated into protein. Translation can be blocked by specific proteins that bind at sites near the 5′ end of the molecule. This binding exerts negative translational control on gene expression. The mRNA has been made but the protein is not made. An example of this is seen in the regulation of the synthesis of ferritin by iron. Ferritin mRNA is not translated unless iron is bound to a response element that is part of the message. This allows for a rapid shift in ferritin synthesis when iron is present and an equally rapid shift away from ferritin synthesis when iron is in short supply. When iron is present, the iron response element folds away from the start site for translation making it available for use. When iron is absent, this start site is covered up by the iron response element which serves as a negative control element. Several mRNAs are subject to translational control by nutrients in this fashion.

The mRNAs have a very short half-life when compared to DNA and the other RNAs. If mRNA half-life is shortened or prolonged, gene expression is affected. Many of the very unstable mRNAs have half-lives in terms of minutes — among these are those which code for short-lived regulatory proteins such as the protooncogenes, fos and myc. This instability is probably due to an A- and U-rich 3′ untranslated region. Stability of mRNA can be affected by steroid hormones, nutritional state, and drugs.

Once the mRNA has migrated from the nucleus to the cytoplasm and attaches to ribosomes, translation is ready to begin. All of the amino acids needed for the protein being synthesized must be present and attached to a transfer RNA (tRNA). These tRNA-amino acids dock on the mRNA again, using base pairing, and the amino acids are joined to one another via the peptide bond. The newly synthesized protein is released as it is made on the ribosome and changes to its conformation and structure occur. These changes depend on the constituent amino acids and their sequence.

Post-translational modification includes a wide variety of changes. For example, nuclear-encoded proteins needed for the mitochondrial metabolism are synthesized with a leader sequence that allows them to migrate into the mitochondria. This leader is then removed as the oxidative phosphorylation system is assembled. Another example is prothrombin, which is assembled with a large number of glutamic acid residues. In the presence of vitamin K these residues are carboxylated, and this post-translational change results in a dramatic increase in the calcium binding capacity of the resultant protein. Unless prothrombin can bind calcium, it cannot function in the clotting process. This is another example of how a nutrient can affect gene expression: in this instance the expression of functional prothrombin. The site of the nutritional effect is that of post-translational protein modification.

III. SYNTHESIS OF PURINES AND PYRIMIDINES

The purines and pyrimidines are the bases that comprise DNA and RNA. They are synthesized *de novo* and this synthesis requires, both directly and indirectly, a number of vitamins and minerals. The purines are adenine and guanine while the pyrimidines are cytosine, uracil, and thymine. Uracil is used for RNA synthesis whereas thymine is used mainly for DNA synthesis. The purines form glycosidic bonds to ribose via the N(9) atoms, whereas the pyrimidines do this using their N(1) atoms. The inosine monophosphate synthesis (IMP) pathway, shown in Figure 2, is the pathway for adenine and guanine triphosphate synthesis. Also shown in Figure 2 are the minerals and vitamins needed at each step in the pathway. Lipoic acid is a cofactor but not a vitamin for the normal individual. Similarly, choline and inositol are not usually considered as vitamins yet these two compounds are also involved in intermediary metabolism. Where ATP is involved in a reaction step, all of the vitamins which serve as coenzymes in intermediary metabolism are needed. This includes niacin, thiamin, riboflavin, pantothenic acid, biotin, folacin, vitamin B_{12}, and vitamin B_6. Also needed are the minerals of importance to the redox reactions of oxidative phosphorylation (OXPHOS), i.e., iron, copper and, of course, the iodine containing hormone, thyroxine, which regulates OXPHOS, and the selenium-containing enzyme (5'-deiodinase) that converts thyroxine to its active form, triiodothyronine. Figure 3 illustrates the involvement of the vitamins and minerals in intermediary metabolism. The pyrimidine pathway (Figure 4) is simpler than the purine synthesis pathway. However, one can see where micronutrients are involved here as well. Transamination and one-carbon transfer — reactions requiring pyridoxine and folacin and of course all those minerals and vitamins needed as coenzymes for intermediary metabolism — are once again called into play so that sufficient energy is available to support the synthetic pathway. The involvement of the vitamins in the provision of energy and substrates for not only DNA and RNA synthesis but also for the synthesis of other macromolecules important to life is outlined in Figure 3.

IV. MICRONUTRIENTS AS STABILIZERS

Although vitamins and minerals serve in gene expression as just described, and as coenzymes and cofactors in the many reactions of intermediary metabolism, certain of the micronutrients have a unique role as stabilizers. They function in assuring that cells and tissues continue as intact structures and that these cells continue to reproduce themselves faithfully. This role for the micronutrients is that of protection from insult by free radicals or peroxides. Peroxides are a normal product of metabolism. They are useful agents in the defense against pathogens. However, peroxides are very reactive substances. They can damage the membranes that are the physical barriers to the cells and the organelles within the cell. They can react with DNA. The DNA, enclosed within the

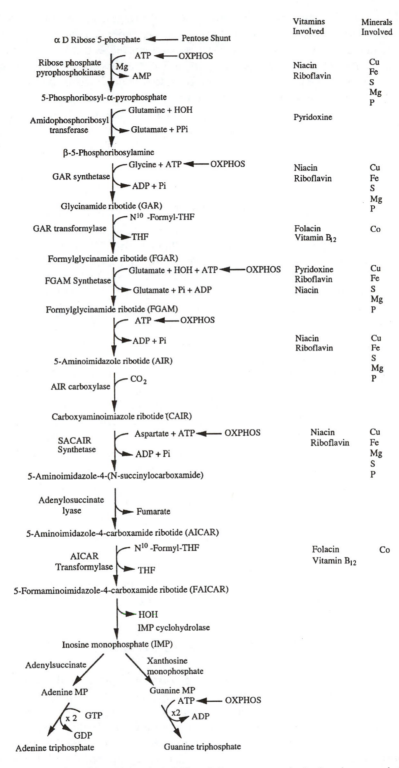

Figure 2 Purine synthesis. In this pathway the addition of ribose occurs prior to ring closure and phosphorylation.

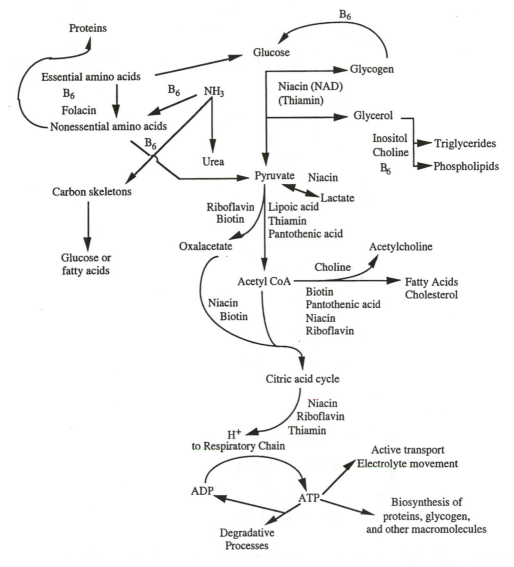

Figure 3 Involvement of the vitamins and other organic nutrients in intermediary metabolism.

nucleus, can repair itself. Occasionally, there is a missense repair and very occasionally this results in a mutation which is random. That is, the damage and subsequent missense repair can occur anywhere in the nuclear DNA and the resultant gene product could be one of more than a million products encoded by the nuclear genome. In addition, this damage might occur in only a few cells out of the many million within a given tissue or organ. Widespread damage from a single exposure is certainly possible, but probably not very frequent. Rather, slight but continued and possible cumulative damage is more likely. Whether degenerative diseases such as cardiovascular disease could be due to free radical damage to lipid-carrying proteins and/or to vascular tissue has yet to be documented. This is a very active area of nutrition research. Peroxide or free radical damage to the nuclear genome is not as serious on an individual genomic basis as damage to the mitochondrial genome. This genome encodes only 13 products but these products are important components of the mitochondrial respiratory chain and ATP synthesis. The mitochondrial DNA does not have the repair capacity of the nuclear genome. In fact, its repair capacity is quite limited. When added to the fact that the mitochondria consume about 90% of all the oxygen associated with the cell, the

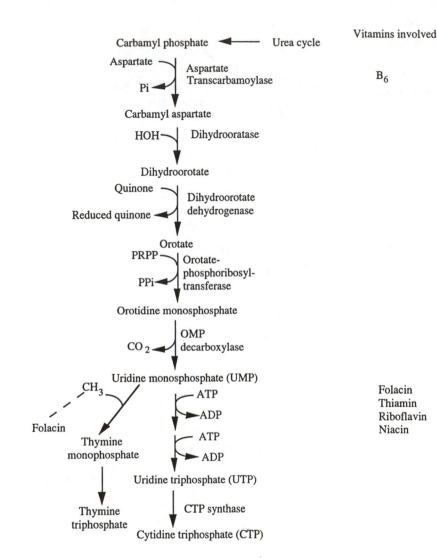

Figure 4   Pyrimidine synthesis. In this pathway the pyrimidine ring is formed before it is attached to ribose and phosphorylated.

potential for free radical damage is quite large. Fortunately, each cell has many hundreds to thousands of mitochondria so the loss of a few has little impact on the overall health and well-being of the cell or organ or whole animal. Nonetheless, should wholesale destruction of the genome occur, the results could be quite devastating. This rarely occurs.

Fortunately, there is a very active antioxidant system in place that protects against such damage. This is described in the sections devoted to vitamin E and selenium. Some of the vitamins and minerals play an important role in this system. Vitamin E quenches free radicals as they form via the conversion of tocopherol to the tocopheroxyl radical, which is then converted to its quinone. Vitamin K serves as an H^+/e^- donor/acceptor in its role to facilitate the carboxylation of the peptide glutamyl residues of certain proteins to their epoxide form. Vitamin C and vitamin A are both good H^+/e^- donor/acceptors in the suppression of free radical formation. Of course, indirectly, all those vitamins that serve as coenzymes are involved as well. Shown in Figure 5 is the free radical suppression system. Note the importance of selenium. In Unit 3, which discusses the antioxidant function of vitamin E, it is pointed out that there is a complementary role for selenium (see Unit 7).

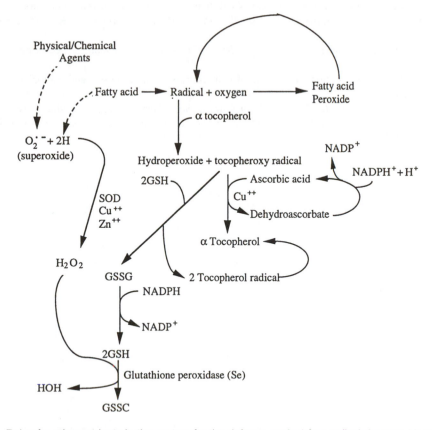

Figure 5 Roles for micronutrients in the system for the defense against free radical damage. Various agents can react with fatty acids to produce peroxides and superoxides. These very reactive materials are suppressed by the system above.

Some of the antioxidant role for vitamin E could be met if there was a sufficient intake of selenium. This mineral is important to the glutathione peroxidase enzyme which, as can be seen in Figure 5, is an important component of the free radical suppression system. Selenium plays a role in both the synthesis of this enzyme and as a required cofactor. As will be discussed in the units on minerals, several of these have roles in gene expression and these roles have overall importance to the physiological function of the body.

SUPPLEMENTAL READINGS

Atchison, M.L. 1988. Enhancers: mechanisms of action and cell specificity, *Annu. Rev. Cell Biol.,* 4:127.

Berdanier, C.D. and Hargrove, J.L., Eds. 1993. *Nutrition and Gene Expression,* CRC Press, Boca Raton, FL, 579 pgs.

Chien, K.R. 1993. Molecular advances in cardiovascular biology, *Science,* 260:916-917.

Combs, G.F. Jr. 1992. *The Vitamins,* Academic Press, New York, 528 pgs.

Demonacos, C.V., Karayanni, N., Hatzoglou, E., Tsiriyrotes, C., Spandidos, D.A., and Sekerio, C.E. 1996. Mitochondrial genes as sites of primary action of steroid hormones, *Steroids,* 61:226-232.

Derman, E. 1982. Transcriptional control in the production of liver specific mRNAs, *Cell,* 23:731-740.

Evans, R.M. 1988. The steroid and thyroid hormone superfamily, *Science,* 240:889-891.

Freedman, L.P. and Luisi, B.F. 1993. On the mechanism of DNA binding by nuclear hormone receptors: a structural and functional perspective, *J. Cell. Biochem.,* 51:140-150.

Johnson, P.F., Sterneck, E., and Williams, S.C. 1993. Activation domains of transcriptional regulatory proteins, *J. Nutr. Biochem.,* 4:386-398.

Jump, D.B., Lepar, G.J., and MacDonald, O.A. 1993. Retinoic acid regulation of gene expression in adipocytes. In Berdanier, C.D. and Hargrove, J.L., Eds., *Nutrition and Gene Expression,* CRC Press, Boca Raton, FL, pp. 431-454.

Maniatis, T., Goodbourn, S., and Fischer, J.A. 1987. Regulation of inducible and tissue specific gene expression, *Science,* 236:1237.

Semenza, G.L. 1994. Transcriptional regulation of gene expression: mechanisms and pathophysiology, *Hum. Mutat.,* 3:180-199.

Vogt, J.G. and Vogt, D. 1990. *Biochemistry,* John Wiley & Sons, New York, pg. 771-986; 1086-1178.

Yamamoto, K. 1985. Steroid receptor regulated transcription of specific genes and gene networks, *Annu. Rev. Genet.,* 19:209.

Fat-Soluble Vitamins

TABLE OF CONTENTS

There are four vitamins that are soluble only in fat solvents and not in water. As such, these vitamins are found in lipid extracts of tissues and foods. They are named alphabetically in the order of their discovery.

I. VITAMIN A

Vitamin A was the first vitamin identified as an essential micronutrient needed by humans. Although it has been recognized as a chemical entity for about 60 years, foods rich in this vitamin have long been prescribed as treatment for night blindness. Ancient Egyptian physicians recommended the consumption of ox or chicken liver for people unable to see at night. In India it was recognized that inadequate diets were related to night blindness and, in France, that diets consisting of sugar, starch, olive oil, and wheat gluten fed to animals resulted in ulcerated corneas. Mori, in Japan, reported on the curative power of cod-liver oil in the treatment of conjunctivitis and, later, Hopkins in the U.S., reported on the importance of whole milk in such treatments. During the 1920s, Osborne and Mendel at Yale and McCollum's group in Wisconsin identified a substance in cod-liver oil, egg yolk, and butterfat that cured night blindness and which was essential for normal growth. They called this substance "fat soluble A."

Table 1 Nomenclature of Major Compounds in the Vitamin A Group

Recommended Name	Synonyms
Retinol	Vitamin A alcohol
Retinal	Vitamin A aldehyde, retinene, retinaldehyde
Retinoic acid	Vitamin A acid
3-Dehydroretinol	Vitamin A_2 (alcohol)
3-Dehydroretinal	Vitamin A_2 aldehyde; retinene$_2$
3-Dehydroretinoic acid	Vitamin A_2 acid
Anhydroretinol	Anhydrovitamin A
Retro Retinol	Rehydrovitamin A
5,6-Epoxyretinol	5,6-Epoxyvitamin A alcohol
Retinyl palmitate	Vitamin A palmitate
Retinyl acetate	Vitamin A acetate
Retinyl β-glucuronide	Vitamin A acid β-glucuronide
11-*cis*-Retinaldehyde	11-*cis* or Neo b vitamin A aldehyde
4-Ketoretinol	4-Keto vitamin A alcohol
Retinyl phosphate	Vitamin A phosphate
β-Carotene	Provitamin A
α-Carotene	Provitamin A
γ-Carotene	Provitamin A

A. Structure and Nomenclature

Vitamin A is not a single compound. It exists in several forms and is found in a variety of foods such as liver and highly colored vegetables. The IUPAC-IUB Commission on Biochemical Nomenclature has proposed the following rules for naming the compounds having vitamin A activity. The parent substance, all-*trans* vitamin A alcohol, is designated "all-*trans* retinol." Derivatives of this compound are named accordingly. In Table 1 are listed the major vitamin A compounds.

In foods of animal origin the vitamin usually occurs as the alcohol (retinol). However, it can also occur as an aldehyde (retinal) or as an acid (retinoic acid). In foods of plant origin, the precursor to the vitamin is associated with the plant pigments and is a member of the carotene family of compounds. These latter compounds can be converted to vitamin A in the animal body and are known as provitamins. Of the carotenes, β-carotene is the most potent.

Figure 1 gives the structure of vitamin A as all-*trans* retinol. Some of the biologically important compounds having vitamin A activity are shown in Figure 2.

Note that all of these compounds have a β-ionone ring to which an isoprenoid chain is attached. This structure is essential if a compound is to have vitamin activity. If any substitutions to the chain or ring occur, then the activity of the compound as vitamin A is reduced. For example, substitution of methyl groups for the hydrogen on carbon 15 of the side chain results in a derivative that has

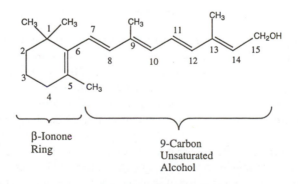

Figure 1 Structure of all-*trans* retinol.

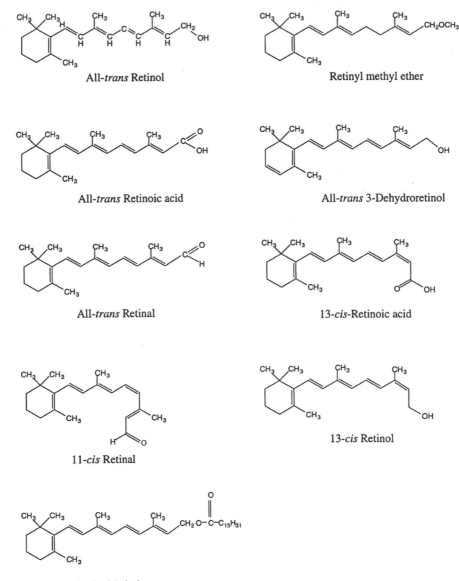

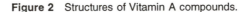

Figure 2 Structures of Vitamin A compounds.

no vitamin activity. However, the preparation of a methyl ester or other esters at carbon 15 results in a very stable compound with full vitamin activity. In addition to improving the chemical stability of the compound, these ester forms confer an improved solubility in food oils. These vitamin ester forms are frequently used in food products for vitamin enrichment.

If the side chain is lengthened or shortened, vitamin activity is lost. Activity is also reduced if the unsaturated bonds are converted to saturated bonds or if the side chain is isomerized. Oxidation of the β-ionone ring and/or removal of its methyl groups likewise reduces vitamin activity. Some of these substituted or isomerized forms are potent therapeutic agents. For example, 13-*cis* retinoic acid has been used in the treatment of certain kinds of cancer. Other analogs, notably the fluoro and chloro derivatives, have been synthesized with the hope of providing chemotherapeutic agents for the treatment of certain skin diseases and cancer.

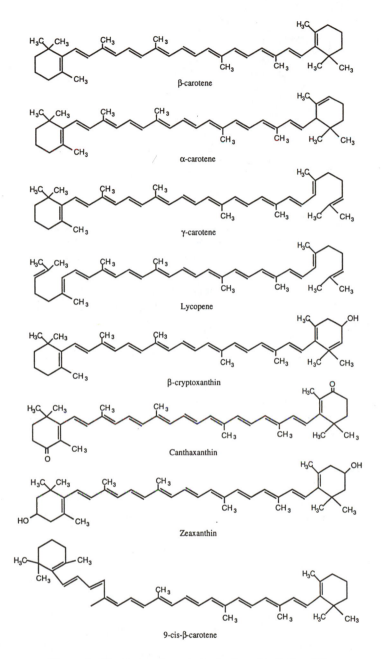

Figure 3 Structures of carotenes having vitamin A activity.

The provitamin A group consists of members of the carotene family. Shown in Figure 3 are the structures of some of these compounds. Also shown are structures of related compounds that, although highly colored, have little potential as a precursor of retinol. More than 600 members of the carotenoid family of pigments exist. However, only 50 or so can be converted (or degraded) into components that have vitamin activity. All these compounds have many conjugated double bonds and thus each can form a variety of geometric isomers. β-Carotene, for example, can assume a cis or a trans configuration at each of its double bonds and in theory could have 272 isomeric forms. The asymmetric carotene, α-carotene, can, in theory, appear in 512 forms. The vitamin A

Table 2   Carotenoids With Vitamin A Activity

Compound	Relative Potency
β-Carotene[a]	100
α-Carotene	53
γ-Carotene	43
Cryptoxanthin	57
Lycopene	0
Zeaxanthin	0
Xanthophyll	0

[a] Reference compound for subsequent compounds. Note that β-carotene compared to all-*trans* retinol is only half as active.

activity of the provitamin members of the carotene family is variable. Theoretically, β-carotene should provide two molecules of retinol. However, in living systems this does not always happen. The β-carotene content of food varies with the growing conditions and the post-harvest storage of the food. In addition, the digestibility of the food affects the availability of the vitamin. Even when fully available, β-carotene and other provitamin A compounds may not be absorbed efficiently and, further, the enzymes responsible for cleaving the β-carotene into two equal parts may not be active. In general, the β-carotene molecule will provide about 50% of its quantity as vitamin A. During its cleavage by the enzyme β-carotenoid 15,15′-dioxygenase, there is some oxidative conversion of the cleavage product to retinal and some oxidation to retinoic acid. This retinoic acid is rapidly excreted in the urine. Other carotenes are less potent than β-carotene, due not only to a decrease in their absorption, but also to their chemical structures, which do not meet the requirements described above for vitamin activity. These compounds are listed in Table 2. Note that some of these compounds, i.e., xanthophylls and lycopenes, have no vitamin activity even though they are highly colored and are related chemically to β-carotene.

B. Chemical Properties

Through the careful work of Karrer and associates, the structures of both β-carotene and all-*trans* retinol were determined. It was only after this work was completed that it was realized that β-carotene was a precursor for retinol.

With the structures now known, the next step was the crystallization of the compounds. This was accomplished for vitamin A from fish liver by Holmes and Corbet. Ten years later, in 1947, Arens and van Drop and also Isler et al. were able to synthesize pure all-*trans* retinol. The chemical synthesis of β-carotene was achieved shortly thereafter. With the crystallization, structure identification, and synthesis came the understanding of the physical and chemical properties of these compounds and the development of techniques to measure their presence in food. All-*trans* retinol is a nearly colorless oil and is soluble in such fat solvents as ether, ethanol, chloroform, and methanol. While fairly stable to the moderate heat needed to cook foods, it is unstable to very high heat, to light, and to oxidation by oxidizing agents. Alpha-tocopherol or its acetate (vitamin E), through its role as an antioxidant, prevents some of the destruction of retinol.

The above properties of vitamin A allow for the removal of the vitamin from foods by fat-solvent extraction and its subsequent determination using agents such as antimony trichloride (the Carr-Price reaction), which produce a blue color. The intensity of the color is directly proportional to the amount of retinol in the material being analyzed. More recently, the development of high resolution (high pressure) chromatography (HPLC) has made possible the separation and quantification of each of the vitamers A. This technique is very sensitive and can detect microgram amounts of the vitamers. β-Carotene is also soluble in fat solvents such as acetone or ethanol. It is bright yellow in color and it, too, is stable to moderate heat but unstable to light or oxidation.

HPLC is used to separate and quantitate the members of the large carotenoid family. Several isomers and derivatives (Figure 2) of retinol have been identified. The isomerization of all-*trans* retinol to a mixture of its isomers is enhanced by high temperatures, ultraviolet light, and iodine or iron. While the isomerization of all-*trans* retinol to 11-*cis* retinol is an important *in vivo* reaction for the maintenance of the visual cycle, the production of isomers outside of the body through the application of high heat, light, and oxidizing agents results in a loss in biological activity of the original compounds. For example, retinyl acetate, if irradiated in hexane, forms an asymmetrical dimer (kitol) which has less than 1% of its original activity. This dimer has been isolated from whale-liver oil and some investigators have suggested that, in this species, the kitol could serve as a storage form of the vitamin. However, whether the kitol found in the whale liver was produced enzymatically or was consumed by the whale as a contaminant of its food supply has not been determined. In any event, for most species, vitamin A is stored in the liver not as a kitol but as an ester with a fatty acid (usually palmitate) in a lipid-protein complex.

Retinal, the aldehyde, combines with various amines to form Schiff bases. This reaction is important to the formation of rhodopsin within the visual cycle (see Figure 4). If mineral oil is present with retinal and the amine, the retinal may first form a hemiacetal which then reacts with a variety of amines to form the Schiff base. All-*trans* retinal also reacts with both the sulfhydryl and amino groups of cysteine or the amino group of tryptophan to form a five-membered thiazolidine ring. The formation of the thiazolidine ring is enhanced if formaldehyde is present. The resulting compound has a red color which is bleached upon exposure to light. This reaction, similar to the bleaching of rhodopsin (the visual pigment in the eye) with light exposure, does not utilize the same amino acid that is used in rhodopsin. In the latter, retinal binds to the epsilon amino group of lysine rather than the amino group of tryptophan or cysteine. Bleaching occurs when the energy transmitted by the light causes a shift in the electrons within the N-retinyl lysine. The same principle is involved in the loss of color with light exposure of N-retinyl cysteine and N-retinyl tryptophan. Interestingly, the many retinyl-amino acid complexes possible in the laboratory apparently do not form in the body. This is probably due to the limited amounts of both the free vitamin and the free amino acids. Both are usually bound or complexed to some other compound and are not readily available for this reaction.

In nature, vitamin A and carotene are bound to proteins, particularly the lipoproteins. Indeed, the vitamin is stored as an ester in those tissues (notably the liver) which synthesize lipoprotein. Usually, retinol is covalently bound to palmitic acid as well as being associated with a protein. The vitamin also complexes with other proteins as part of its mechanism of action at the subcellular level.

Retinol and its derivatives are soluble in nonpolar solvents, but not in water. However, retinol or retinyl esters can be made miscible in water with the use of detergents such as Tween 80™ (polyoxyethylene sorbitan monooleate). The resulting aqueous micellar suspension allows for the preparation of aqueous multivitamin supplements that are then useful for infants, small children, or persons unable to swallow a capsule. Studies of the absorption of vitamin A in this form, compared to the absorption of vitamins dissolved in an oil, have shown that this form of the vitamin is readily absorbed. This is particularly important for those persons having a fat absorption problem as in pancreatitis, celiac disease, idiopathic steatorrhea, biliary disease, or short gut syndrome.

Aqueous preparations are also useful to the food processor wishing to fortify or enrich a particular food product. Some food formulations would not be compatible with an oil-based vitamin A preparation, whereas an aqueous preparation combines very well with the ingredients in the food.

C. Biopotency

The varying potencies of the different vitamin A compounds have, in the past, contributed confusion to the literature. This has been resolved by the establishment of a standard definition for vitamin A. One international unit (IU) of vitamin A is defined as the activity of 0.3 µg of all-*trans*

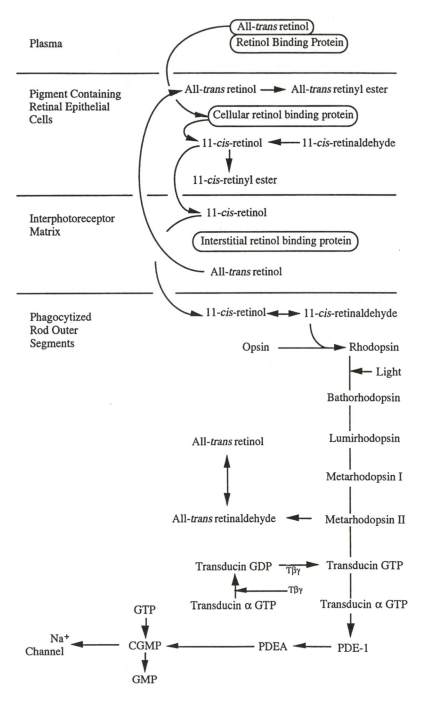

Figure 4 The visual cycle.

retinol. Because β-carotene must be converted to retinol to be active, and because this conversion is not 100% efficient, 1 μg of all-*trans* β-carotene is equivalent to 0.167 μg of all-*trans* retinol. For other members of the carotene family, appropriate (as per Table 2) correction factors must be applied to determine the vitamin A activity in terms of retinol equivalents (RE). In general, however, 1 mg of retinol is roughly equivalent to 6 mg β-carotene and 12 mg of mixed dietary carotenes. The use

Table 3   Retinol Equivalents (RE) for Humans

Compound	μg/IU	IU/μg	RE/μg
All-*trans* retinol	0.300	3.33	1.00
All-*trans* retinyl acetate	0.344	2.91	—
All-*trans* retinyl palmitate	0.549	1.82	—
All-*trans* β-carotene	1.800	0.56	0.167
Mixed carotenoids	3.600	0.28	0.083

From Olson, J.A., *Handbook of Vitamins*, 2nd ed., Machlin, L.J., Ed., Marcel Dekker, New York, 1990. With permission.

of the term retinol equivalents allows for the calculation of the vitamin A activity found in a variety of foods, each containing one or more vitamin A compounds. For example, if 100 g of a given food contained 100 mg of α-carotene, which has 53% of the potency of β-carotene, the retinol equivalence would be $100 \times 0.53 \times 0.167$ or 8.851. Thus, this food would provide 8.851 retinol equivalents or 29.5 IU of vitamin A (8.851/0.3) per 100 g. Most tables of food composition give the vitamin A content in terms of IU; however, the reader should be aware of how these units are derived and realize that corrections must be made to allow for availability and efficiency of conversion of the provitamin to the active vitamin form, all-*trans* retinol. Table 3 lists the retinol equivalents (REs) for major vitamin A sources.

D. Sources

Vitamin A and its carotene precursors are present in a variety of foods. Red meat, liver, whole milk, cheese, butter, and fortified margarine are but a few of the foods containing retinol. Carotene-rich foods include the highly colored fruits and vegetables such as squash, carrots, rich green vegetables (peas, beans, etc.), yellow fruits (peaches, apricots), and vegetable oils.

E. Metabolism of Vitamin A

1. Absorption

The availability of the vitamin depends largely on the form ingested and on the presence and activity of the system responsible for its uptake. Figure 5 schematically shows the route of retinol absorption. It is generally accepted that all-*trans* retinol is the preferred form for absorption. Retinal and retinoic acid are less well absorbed although both will disappear from the intestinal contents at a rate commensurate with an active transport system. Absorption requires the presence of food lipid and bile salts. Carotenoids are absorbed less efficiently, via diffusion. There is no active carrier for carotene within the luminal cell. Carotene is oxidatively cleaved to retinal, which is reduced to retinol and to small amounts of longer-chain β-apocarotenoids. Both central and exocentric cleavages are known to occur. The cleavage enzymes are very unstable and are rapidly inactivated. Two enzymes are involved in central cleavage; the first, β-carotene-15,15'-dioxygenase, catalyzes the cleavage of the central double bond to yield two molecules of retinal. The second, retinal reductase, catalyzes the reduction of retinal to retinol. This reaction is shown in Figure 6. The conversion of β-carotene to Vitamin A is not 100% efficient; thus, 2 mol of retinol are not obtained from 1 mol of β-carotene.

In order for the first enzyme to work, the β-carotene must be solubilized. This means that bile salts and some lipid must be present. Oxygen is also required since this is a dioxygenase type of reaction. Carotene dioxygenase is present in the soluble cell fraction and has been isolated from rat, hog, and rabbit intestinal tissue and characterized. The enzyme of the second reaction, retinal reductase, is also a soluble mucosal cell enzyme. It requires the presence of either NADPH or NADH as a donor of reducing equivalents. It is not particularly specific for the resulting retinal as

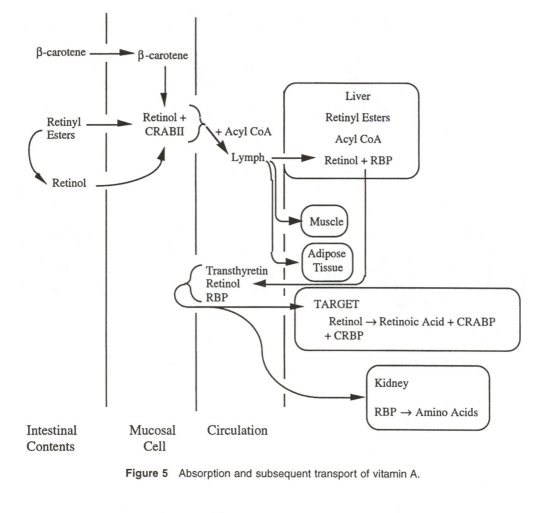

Figure 5   Absorption and subsequent transport of vitamin A.

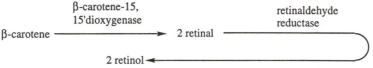

Figure 6   Central cleavage of β-carotene.

it will catalyze the reduction of several short- and medium-chain aliphatic aldehydes in addition to retinal.

There are two pathways for retinol esterification. In the first, an acyl CoA-independent reaction is used. This involves a complex between retinol and Type II cellular retinol binding protein (CRBP II). As retinol intake increases there is a corresponding increase in the activity of the enzyme (acyl CoA retinol acyl transferase), which catalyzes the formation of this complex. Cellular retinol binding protein (CRBP II) is found only in the cytosol of the intestinal mucosal cell and, interestingly, its synthesis is influenced by the intake of particular fatty acids. Suruga et al. have shown that unsaturated fatty acids, particularly linoleic and α-linolenic acid, enhance CRBP II mRNA transcription. These fatty acids also enhance S14 and retinoic acid receptor (RAR) transcription in the adipocyte. Thus, it would appear that vitamin A uptake by the mucosal cell is dependent on dietary fat, not only because of its influence on absorption but also because of its role in enhancing the synthesis of the mucosal cell CRBP II.

The second pathway is an acyl CoA-dependent pathway whereby retinol is bound to any protein, not just the specific CRBP II mentioned above. In both pathways, the retinol is protein-bound prior to ester formation. As mentioned in Section I.A, the esterification of retinol results in a more lipophilic material readily soluble in the lipids of the cell. This, in turn, facilitates its movement into the cell and its metabolic function as well as its storage.

Retinoic acid, like retinal and retinol, is rapidly absorbed by the mucosal cells. However, it is also rapidly excreted (rather than stored, as are the other vitamin forms) in the urine; thus, this form is not as useful as the alcohol or aldehyde forms as a dietary ingredient.

In food, all-*trans* retinol is usually esterified to long-chain fatty acids. Palmitic acid is the most common of these fatty acids. The ester is hydrolyzed in the intestine by a specific esterase which, in some species, is activated by the bile salt, sodium taurocholate. After the ester has been hydrolyzed, the resulting retinol is actively transported (carrier mediated) into the mucosal cell where it is then reesterified to a long-chain fatty acid (palmitic acid) and incorporated into lymph chylomicrons. The absorption of vitamin A thus follows the same route as the long-chain fatty acids of the dietary triacylglycerides, cholesterol, and cholesterol esters. The chylomicrons are absorbed by the lacteals of the lymphatic system and enter the circulation where the thoracic duct joins the circulatory system at the vena cava. Once in the vascular compartment, the triacylglyceride of the retinol-containing chylomicron is removed, leaving the protein carrier, retinol, and cholesterol. Whereas the triacylglycerides are removed from the chylomicrons primarily by the extrahepatic tissues, retinol is removed primarily by the liver. In the liver, hydrolysis and reesterification occur once again as the vitamin enters the hepatocyte and is stored within the cell, associated with droplets of lipid. Interestingly, retinoic acid is absorbed not via the lymphatic system but by the portal system, and does not accumulate in the liver. Retinoic acid, because it is not stored, represents only a very small percentage of the body's vitamin A content.

As mentioned previously, β-carotene is converted to retinol in the mucosal cells of the intestine. Dietary retinal may also be converted to retinol and all forms of the vitamin are transported to the liver as part of the chylomicrons.

2. Transport

It has become apparent that a specific protein is needed for subsequent transport of retinol from the liver to the peripheral target tissues. This protein, called retinol binding protein (RBP), was first isolated by Kanai et al. in 1968. RBP is synthesized in the liver (Figure 5). It is a single polypeptide chain (21,000 Da) and possesses a single binding site for retinol. The mobilization of vitamin A from the liver requires this protein. It binds, on a one-to-one basis, to one molecule of retinol. The usual level of binding protein in plasma is about 40 to 50 µg/ml. However, the level of this protein is responsive to nutritional status. In protein-malnourished children it is depressed while in vitamin A-deficient individuals it is elevated. Patients with renal disease have elevated levels of RBP and may be at risk of developing vitamin A toxicity if vitamin A intake is above normal.

In the patient with renal disease, the increase in the binding protein is probably due to the decreased capacity of the kidney to remove the protein. The kidney is the main catabolic site for RBP. Where protein intakes are low, binding protein levels are also low, thus explaining the simultaneous observations of symptoms of protein and retinol deficiency in malnourished children. This association is due to the inability of the liver in the protein-malnourished child to synthesize the retinol binding protein, thus the child is unable to utilize the hepatic vitamin stores. Once protein is restored to the diet, symptoms of both deficiency syndromes will disappear. If dietary retinol (or its precursors) is lacking, serum RBP levels will fall while hepatic levels rise. Within minutes after retinol is given to a deficient individual, these changes are reversed: serum levels rise while hepatic levels fall. These observations provide clear evidence of the importance of this binding protein in the utilization of retinol. Compounds which influence the levels of this binding protein influence

Table 4   Retinol Binding Proteins

Acronym	Protein	Molecular Weight (Da)	Location	Function
RBP	Retinol binding protein	21,000	Plasma	Transports all-*trans* retinol from intestinal absorption site to target tissues
CRBP	Cellular retinol binding protein	14,600	Cells of target tissue	Transports all-*trans* retinol from plasma membrane to organelles within the cell
CRBP II	Cellular retinol binding protein Type II	16,000	Absorptive cells of small intestine	Transports all-*trans* retinol from absorptive sites on plasma membrane of mucosal cells
CRABP	Cellular retinoic acid binding protein	14,600	Cells of target tissue	Transports all-*trans* retinoic acid to the nucleus
CRALBP	Cellular retinal binding protein	33,000	Specific cells in the eye	Transports 11-*cis* retinal and 11-*cis* retinol as part of the visual cycle
IRBP	Interphotoreceptor or interstitial retinol binding protein	144,000	Retina	Transports all-*trans* retinol and 11-*cis* retinal in the retina extracellular space
RAR	Nuclear retinoic acid receptor, 3 main forms (α, β, γ)		All cells α — Liver β — Brain γ — Liver, kidney, lung	Binds retinoic acid and regions of DNA having the GGTCA sequence
RXR	Nuclear retinoic acid receptors, multiple forms			

the mobilization and excretion of retinol. Estrogens increase the level of this protein whereas cadmium poisoning, because it increases excretion, reduces the level of this protein. In plasma, vitamin A circulates bound to the retinol binding protein which, in turn, forms a protein-protein complex with transthyretin, a tetramer that also binds thyroxine in a 1:1 complex. Because this complex contains the vitamin and thyroxine there is an association of thyroid status and vitamin A status.

Once the RBP complex arrives at the target tissue, it must then bind to its receptor site on the cell membrane. Receptors for retinol and retinoic acid have been identified on the cell membranes of a variety of cells. The retinol is then released from the serum binding protein and transferred into the cell, where it is then bound to intracellular binding proteins. Of interest are the observations that these binding proteins, while similar to the binding protein in the serum, are highly specific for the different vitamin A forms. The CRBP is the cellular retinol binding protein (14,600 Da) while CRABP is the cellular retinoic acid binding protein (14,600 Da), CRALBP is the retinal binding protein (33,000 Da), and IRBP is the interphotoreceptor or interstitial retinol binding protein (144,000 Da). The latter is found only in the extracellular space of the retina. As described earlier, CRBP II is the retinol binding protein found in the mucosal cells of the small intestine. The presence of these binding proteins in different tissues is highly variable. Shown in Table 4 are the features and functions of these binding proteins.

While the bulk transport of the various vitamers A occurs via the chylomicrons which are released into the lymph, there seems to be no specific protein within the chylomicron that has a special affinity for this vitamin. However, once the chylomicron remnants (the remains of the chylomicrons which have lost some of their lipids to the muscle and the adipose tissue) are taken up by the liver, the special binding proteins have their effects. The chylomicron remnant retains most of its original vitamin A content as vitamin A esters. These esters are stored in the hepatocyte or are released into the circulation bound to RBP following hydrolysis.

3. Degradation and Excretion

The early Nobel Prize-winning work of Wald et al., which showed that retinol must be converted to retinal before the vitamin can function in vision, led the way for other workers to investigate the further metabolism of the various active forms. Since vitamin A not only maintains the visual cycle but is also necessary for growth, epithelial cell differentiation, skeletal tissue development, spermatogenesis, and the development and maintenance of the placenta, and because each of these functions requires a specific form of the vitamin, it appears that each of these tissues has specific structural requirements. Retinal involvement in vision has been demonstrated, and it appears that retinol but not retinal or retinoic acid is required for the support of reproduction, and that all of the three forms will support growth and cell differentiation. That the three forms are interchangeable in the latter function suggests that retinoic acid is the active form for this function. Both retinol and retinal can be converted to retinoic acid but the reverse reactions are not possible, and only in specific tissues such as the retina are retinol and retinal interconvertible. From studies using radioactively labeled retinal, retinol, and retinoic acid, it is apparent that retinoic acid is the common metabolic intermediate of the vitamin A group. Once retinol is mobilized from hepatic stores, transported to its target tissue via the retinol binding protein, and transferred to its intracellular active site via the intracellular retinol binding proteins, it is then utilized either as retinol or retinal or converted to retinoic acid. Studies of the excretion patterns of labeled retinol and retinoic acid revealed that retinol was used more slowly than retinoic acid. Label from retinoic acid was almost completely recovered within 48 hr of administration, whereas more than 7 days were required to recover even half of the label from the retinol.

The use of retinoic acid, isotopically labeled in several different locations, allowed Roberts and DeLuca to determine the metabolic pathway of retinoic acid. The label from retinoic acid was recovered as $^{14}CO_2$ from the expired air as well as from ^{14}C-labeled decarboxylated metabolites and the β-ionone ring lacking part of its isoprenoid side chain. The structures of all the metabolites which appear in the urine and feces are not known.

F. Functions of Vitamin A

1. Protein Synthesis

Some of the earliest reports of retinol deficiency included observations of the changes in epithelial cells of animals fed vitamin A-deficient diets. Normal columnar epithelial cells were replaced by squamous keratinizing epithelium. These changes were reversed when vitamin A was restored to the diet. Epithelial cells, particularly those lining the gastrointestinal tract, have very short half-lives (in the order of 3 to 7 days) and as such are replaced frequently. Thus, in vitamin A deficiency, changes in these cells as well as in other cells having a rapid turnover time, indicate that the vitamin functions at the level of protein synthesis and cellular differentiation. Studies of protein synthesis by mucosal cells from deficient and control animals indicated that the vitamin is involved directly in protein synthesis both at the transcriptional and translational level. Such a role for retinol is supported by observations of an alteration in messenger RNA synthesis in vitamin A-deficient animals.

Table 5 lists a number of cellular proteins that have retinoic acid as an influence on their synthesis or activation. Also listed are gene products that require either a cis- or trans-acting retinoic acid-containing transcription factor. Retinol is converted to retinoic acid which regulates cell function by binding to intracellular retinoic acid receptors. Two distinct families of nuclear receptors have been identified. Each of these families, called RAR and RXR, have multiple forms and both are structurally similar to the receptor that binds the steroid and thyroid hormones. These receptors function as ligand-activated transcription factors (see Table 4) that regulate mRNA transcription.

Table 5   Gene Products Influenced by Retinoic Acid

**Proteins That Have Their Synthesis Increased or Decreased Due
to RA-Receptor Effect on the Transcription of Their mRNA**

Growth hormone	Neuronal cell
Transforming growth factor β2	Calcium binding protein,
Transglutaminase	Calbindin
Phosphoenolpyruvate carboxykinase	Ornithine decarboxylase
Gsα	Osteocalcin
Alcohol dehydrogenase	Insulin
t-Plasminogen activator	
Glycerophosphate dehydrogenase	

**Retinoic Acid Receptor Binding Proteins That Function
in mRNA Transcription**

$1,25\text{-}(OH)_2D_3$ receptors
Retinoic acid receptors β
cfos[a]
Progesterone receptors[a]
Zif 268 transcription factor
AP-2 transcription factor
MSH Receptors
Interleukin 6-receptors[a]
Interleukin 2-receptors
EGF receptors (corneal endothelium)
EGF receptors (corneal epithelium)[a]
Peroxisomal proliferator-activated receptors

[a] The activity of these proteins are suppressed when the RA-receptor
is bound to them.

They bind to regions of DNA that have a GGTCA sequence. In some instances, these factors stimulate transcription and in other instances they suppress the process. There is also an interaction of vitamin A with other vitamins. For example, the synthesis of the calcium binding protein, calbindin, is usually regulated by vitamin D. This protein, found in the intestinal mucosal cells and the kidney, is also found in the brain. In the brain its synthesis is regulated by retinoic acid rather than vitamin D. In vitamin A-deficient brain cells, additions of retinoic acid increased the mRNA for calbindin and calbindin synthesis. Additions of vitamin D were without effect. The retinoic acid receptor contains zinc finger protein sequence motifs which mediate its binding to DNA. The carboxyl terminal of the receptor functions in this ligand binding. Retinoic acid binding to nuclear receptors sets in motion a sequence of events that culminates in a change in transcription of the cis-linked gene. That is, proteins are synthesized, and these proteins bind to regions of the promoter adjacent to the start site of the DNA that is to be transcribed. Such binding either activates or suppresses transcription and, as a result, there are corresponding increases or decreases in the mRNA coding for specific proteins. This, in turn, leads to changes in cell function. Table 6 lists a number of enzymes that have been reported to be affected by the deficient state. In each of these instances it could be assumed that the reason for the change in activity could be explained by the effect of vitamin A on the synthesis of these enzymes. Where there is an increase (or decrease) it is likely that transcription, and hence synthesis, is influenced (or kept within normal bounds) when vitamin A intake is adequate.

Recently, several investigators have reported on the need for retinoic acid by the insulin-secreting β cells of the pancreas. The mechanism of action of retinoic acid in this cell type is far from clear. Insulin release is a process that depends on the glucokinase sensing system which, in turn, depends on an optimal supply of ATP. If there is an ATP shortfall the insulin release mechanism will falter and diabetes mellitus may develop. An ATP shortfall can be the result of one or more mutations

Table 6   Enzymes That Are Affected by Vitamin A Deficiency

Enzyme	Reaction	Effect
ATPase	ATP $\leftrightarrow$ ADP + Pi	Increase
Arginase	L-Arginine $\rightarrow$ ornithine + urea	Increase
Xanthine oxidase	Hypoxanthine $\rightarrow\rightarrow$ uric acid	Increase
Alanine amino transferase	L-Alanine α-ketoglutarate$\rightarrow$ pyruvate + L-glutamate	No change
Aspartate amino transferase	L-Aspartate + α-ketoglutarate $\rightarrow$ oxaloacetate + L-glutamate	No change
Vitamin A palmitate hydrolase	Vitamin A palmitate $\rightarrow$ vitamin A + palmitic acid	No change
Vitamin A ester synthetase	Vitamin A + fatty acid $\rightarrow$ ester	No change
$\Delta^{5,3}$ β-Hydroxysteroid dehydrogenase	Removal of H$^+$ group from progesterone, glucocorticoid, estrogen, testosterone	
11β-Steroid hydroxylase	Synthesis of steroid hormones	Decrease
ATP sulfurylase	ATP + SO$_4$ $\rightarrow$ adenyl sulfate + PPi^{-3}	Decrease
Sulfotransferase	Transfers sulfuryl groups to -O and -N of suitable groups. Synthesis of mucopolysaccharides	
L-γ-Gulonolactone oxidase	L-Gulonolactone $\rightarrow$ L-ascorbic acid	Decrease
p-Hydroxyphenol pyruvate oxidase	p-Hydroxyphenyl pyruvate $\rightarrow$ homogentisic acid	Decrease

in the genes encoding the components of OXPHOS and diabetes mellitus can be observed in persons or animals having a mutation in the mitochondrial genome. Many years ago, vitamin A-deficient rats were found to have reduced OXPHOS activity, but it is only recently that vitamin A (as retinoic acid) has been suggested to play a role in OXPHOS gene expression, thereby linking this vitamin to OXPHOS, insulin release, and diabetes mellitus.

There is another aspect of vitamin A nutriture that is of importance when the function of this vitamin is considered. This concerns the structure and function of the nuclear retinoic acid binding protein, the RA receptor. Should this receptor not be synthesized, as can occur in the absence of retinoic acid, the whole cascade of events dependent on the binding of the RA-receptor complex will not occur. Further, should the receptor itself be aberrant in amino acid sequence, both its capacity to bind RA and its affinity for specific regions of the DNA will be affected. In this instance it is easy to understand how cellular differentiation would be affected. Indeed, several investigators have suggested that this could explain the occurrence of congenital defects in a number of species where early embryonic development of the spinal column and the heart might be due to abnormal RA-receptor binding, with the subsequent result of defective differentiation, organ formation, and organ function.

This role for the vitamin, although lacking biochemical mechanistic detail, was among the first functions recognized by early investigators. An excellent paper on retinoid signaling and the generation of cellular diversity in the embryonic mouse spinal cord has recently been published, as has a paper on retinoid signaling in the developing mammal (see articles by Chien et al., Soprano et al., Dutz and Sandell, and the review by DeLuca).

2. Reproduction and Growth

The role of vitamin A in the growth process is related to its function in RNA synthesis as described above. Animals fed vitamin A-deficient diets do not eat well, and their poor growth may stem from their inadequate intakes of not only vitamin A but also the other essential nutrients. As mentioned previously, vitamin A is responsible for the maintenance of the integrity of the epithelial tissues. Since the taste buds are specialized epithelial cells, feeding a deficient diet probably results in a change in the structure and function of these taste buds, resulting in a loss in appetite. As well, other epithelial cells are also affected, particularly those cells which secrete lubricating and digestive fluids in the mouth, stomach, and intestinal tract. The lack of lubrication due to atrophy of these important cells would certainly affect food intake and, hence, result in poor growth. In addition, reduction in food intake itself imposes a stress on the growing animal, and stress, with its attendant hormonal responses such as an increase in thyroid hormone release and an increase in adrenal activity, would have profound influences on protein turnover and energy utilization and, of course, growth.

As mentioned, the role of the vitamin in reproduction relates to its role in RNA and protein synthesis. Ornithine decarboxylase, an enzyme that closely correlates to cell division and tissue growth, has recently been identified as a protooncogene. Ornithine decarboxylase (ODC) is the first rate-limiting enzyme in the biosynthesis of polyamines which are essential for cell growth. Retinoic acid suppresses the transcription of ODC mRNA and by doing so serves as a "brake" on uncontrolled cell growth. This function of retinoic acid on ODC transcription is counterbalanced by retinoic acid-estrogen receptor binding. The latter enhances ODC mRNA transcription. Not only would the growth of a fertilized ova be affected in this manner, but also, through its effects on protein synthesis, vitamin A could affect the synthesis of enzymes needed to produce the steroid hormones which regulate and orchestrate the reproduction process. Several of the enzymes listed in Table 6 are involved in the synthesis of these hormones. Of the enzymes listed, three (ATPase, arginase, and xanthine oxidase) relate primarily to energy or protein wastage, as would be expected to increase in a deficient animal. The transferase and the enzymes of retinol metabolism are unchanged, while enzymes for the synthesis of mucopolysaccharides are decreased.

Observations of increases in the phospholipid content of a variety of cellular and subcellular membranes in vitamin A-deficient rats suggest that enzymes of lipid metabolism are also affected. Cholesterol absorption is increased in the deficient rat and this increase may in turn affect phospholipid synthesis and membrane phospholipid content since mammalian membranes consist largely of cholesterol and phospholipids. Changes in membrane composition conceivably could explain the increased susceptibility of deficient animals to infection, but equally likely is the reduction in the protective effect of a normal intact epithelium which acts as a physical barrier to the pathogenic organisms, and the reduction in the synthesis of antibodies and antibody-forming cells in the spleen of vitamin A-deficient animals.

The secondary characteristics of vitamin A deficiency are probably related to the role of the vitamin in protein synthesis, as described above. The primary characteristics of decreased adaptation to darkness, poor growth, reduced reproductive capacity, xerophthalmia, keratomalacia, and anemia are all related.

3. Vision

Of the various functions vitamin A serves, its role in the maintenance of adaptation to darkness was the first to be fully described on a molecular basis. When animals are deprived of vitamin A, the amount of rhodopsin declines. This is followed by decreases in the amount of the protein, opsin. Rhodopsin is present in the rod cells of the retinas of most animals. The synthesis of rhodopsin and its subsequent bleaching was elucidated by Wald and others. The process is shown in Figure 4. All-*trans* retinol is transported to the retina cell, transferred into the cell, and converted to all-*trans* retinal. All-*trans* retinal is isomerized to the active vitamin, 11-*cis* retinal, which combines with opsin to form rhodopsin. Rhodopsin is an asymmetric protein with a molecular weight of about 38,000 Da. It has both a hydrophilic and a hydrophobic region with a folded length of about 70 Å. It spans the membrane of the retina via seven helical segments that cross back and forth and comprises about 60% of the membrane protein. The light-sensitive portion of the molecule resides in its hydrophobic region. When rhodopsin is exposed to light it changes its shape. The primary photochemical event is the very rapid isomerization of 11-*cis* retinal to a highly strained form, bathorhodopsin. Note that the alcohol (retinol) and the aldehyde (retinal) are interchangeable with respect to the maintenance of the visual function.

Retinoic acid is ineffective primarily because there are no enzymes in the eye to convert the retinoic acid to the active 11-*cis* retinal needed for the formation of rhodopsin.

The formation of iodopsin in the cones involves 11-*cis* retinol and the photochemical isomerization of the 11-*cis* isomer triggers the visual process. In the rhodopsin breakdown process, an electrical potential arises and generates an electrical impulse which is transmitted via the optic nerve to the brain. That 11-*cis* retinal is also involved in color vision (the responsibility of the cones) has been suggested; however, the mechanism of this involvement has not been fully explored. Three major cone pigments have been identified that have absorption maxima of 450, 525, and 550 nm, respectively. Whether these are single pigments or a mixture and whether one or more contain 11-*cis* retinal has not been determined.

G. Hypervitaminosis A

Because the vitamin is stored in the liver, it is possible to develop a toxic condition when very high (10 times normal intake) levels of the vitamin are consumed. As early as 1934, reports appeared in the literature of vitamin A intoxication in humans, rats, and chicks. In chicks, the most obvious clinical signs are a reduced growth rate, an encrustation of the eyelids, and a reddening of the corners of the mouth. In rats, bone fractures are observed. These bone fractures may be related to the unusual brittleness of the bone in hypervitaminosis. In humans, hypervitaminosis A is characterized by increased intracranial pressure resulting in headaches, blurring of vision, and in young children, a bulging fontanel. Hair loss and skin lesions, anorexia, weight loss, nausea, vomiting, vague abdominal pain, and irritability are common symptoms. In experimental animals, excess vitamin A intake during gestation results in congenital malformations in the young. Because of the limitation in the conversion of β-carotene to retinol, vitamin A intoxication is less likely with large intakes of carotene; however, reports of yellowing of the skin of persons consuming large amounts of carrot juice have appeared. This yellowing is likely due to the deposition of carotene and associated pigments in the subcutaneous fat.

H. Recommended Dietary Allowances

Adult requirements for retinol have been estimated using a variety of techniques. Individuals vary in their needs for the vitamin. Reports in the literature indicate that requirements may be increased by fever, infection, cold, hyperthyroidism, chemical toxicants, and excessive exposure to sunlight. In addition, the genetic heritage of the individual introduces an additional measure of variability in the needs of population groups.

To determine an individual's vitamin A requirement, that individual must first be deprived of all dietary sources of the vitamin until the first signs of deficiency appear. Because the liver stores the vitamin, this depletion period may be as long as two years for the human. Once depleted, graded amounts of the vitamin are restored to the diet until signs of the deficiency disappear. When a steady state is achieved, that level of intake is the requirement. Obviously, such a procedure is not practical for large numbers of people. Because of the time and expense involved in determining requirements, recommended intakes are used. These are shown in Table 7. These are estimates of the requirements of large population groups based on detailed studies (as per above) of a small group of subjects. The recommendation is usually twice the determined requirement so as to allow for variability in need. As more data are collected on human subjects, the safety factor may be reduced and the recommended intake changed. Table 7 gives the U.S. recommended dietary allowances for humans in retinol equivalents.

II. VITAMIN D

A. Overview

Just as night blindness has been recognized for centuries as a disease treatable by diet (vitamin A), the classical disease of vitamin D deficiency, rickets, has been evident since ancient

Table 7   Recommended Dietary Allowances (RDA)
          for Vitamin A

Group	Age	RDA (Retinol Equivalents)
Infants	Birth–6 months	375
	7–12 months	375
Children	1–3	400
	4–6	500
	7–10	700
Males	11–14	1000
	15–18	1000
	19–24	1000
	25–50	1000
	51+	1000
Females	11–14	800
	15–18	800
	19–24	800
	25–50	800
	51+	800
Pregnancy		800
Lactation	1st 6 months	1300
	2nd 6 months	1200

times. Historians do not agree as to when the first symptoms of vitamin D deficiency were evident. Some suggest that the stooped appearance of the Neanderthal Man (ca. 50,000 B.C.) was due to an inadequate vitamin D intake rather than being characteristic of a low evolutionary status. Evidence of rickets in skeletons from humans of the Neolithic Age, the first settlers of Greenland, and the ancient Egyptians, Greeks, and Romans has been reported.

The first detailed descriptions of the disease are found in the writings of Dr. Daniel Whistler of Leiden, Netherlands and Professor Francis Glisson in the mid-1600s. Beyond these descriptions and the acceptance of rickets as a disease entity, little progress was made until the late 1800s when it was suggested that the lack of sunlight and "perhaps" poor diet were related to the appearance of bone malformation. It was frequently reported that infants born in the spring and dying the following winter did not have any symptoms of rickets, whereas infants born in the fall and dying the next spring had rickets. Funk, in 1914, suggested that rickets was a nutrient deficiency disorder. This was verified by the brilliant work of Sir Edward Mellanby. Mellanby constructed a grain diet which produced rickets in puppies. When he gave cod-liver oil, the disease did not develop. At that time, Mellanby did not know that there were two fat-soluble vitamins (A and D) in cod-liver oil, and he thought that he was studying the antirachitic properties of vitamin A. Not until the two vitamins were separated and identified was it realized that Mellanby's antirachitic factor was vitamin D. The recognition of vitamin D as a separate entity from vitamin A came from the work of McCollum and associates in 1922. In a landmark paper, McCollum reported the results of his work on the characterization of vitamin A. He described the vulnerability of the vitamin to oxidation and the fact that the antirachitic factor remained even after the cod-liver oil was aerated and heated and the antixerophthalmic factor (vitamin A) was destroyed.

Although the importance of sunlight had long been recognized in the prevention and treatment of rickets, the relationship of ultraviolet light to the dietary intake of vitamin D was not appreciated until Steenbeck, and also Goldblatt et al., demonstrated that ultraviolet light gave antirachitic properties to sterol-containing foods if these foods were incorporated into diets previously shown to produce rickets. From this point on, the research concerning vitamin D, as it was so-named by McCollum and associates, became largely chemical in nature. It has only been within the last decade or so that work on vitamin D has elucidated its mechanism of action.

Table 8   D Vitamers Are Produced from Provitamin Forms When These Precursor Forms Are Exposed to Ultraviolet Light. These Are Not Active Until They Are Hydroxylated at Carbons 1 and 25

Precursor	D Vitamer
Ergosterol	D_2 (Ergocalciferol)
7-Dehydrocholesterol	D_3 (Cholecalciferol)
22,23-Dehydroergosterol	D_4
7-Dehydrositosterol	D_5
7-Dehydrostigmasterol	D_6
7-Dehydrocompesterol	D_7

B. Structure and Nomenclature

Like vitamin A, vitamin D is not a single compound. The D vitamins listed in Table 8 are a family of 9,10-secosteroids which differ only in the structures of their side chains. Figure 7 shows some of these different structures. There is no D_1 because when the vitamins were originally isolated and identified, the compound identified as D_1 turned out to be a mixture of the other D vitamins rather than a separate entity.

Since the other D vitamins were already described and named, the D_1 designation was deleted from the list. All the D vitamin forms are related structurally to four-ring called compounds cyclopentanoperhydrophenanthrenes, from which they were derived by a photochemical reaction. The official nomenclature proposed for vitamin D by IUPAC-IUB Commission on Biochemical Nomenclature relates the vitamin to its steroid nucleus. Each carbon is numbered using the same system as is used for other sterols such as cholesterol. This is illustrated in Figure 8. The numbering system of the four-ring cholesterol structure is retained even though the compound loses its B ring during its conversion to the vitamin.

The chief structural prerequisite of compounds serving as D provitamins is the sterol structure which has an opened B ring that contains a $D_{5,6}$ conjugated double bond. No vitamin activity is possessed by the compound until the B ring is opened.

This occurs as a result of exposure to ultraviolet light. In addition, vitamin activity is dependent on the presence of a hydroxyl group at carbon 3 and upon the presence of conjugated double bonds at the 10-19, 5-6, and 7-8 positions. If the location of these double bonds is shifted, vitamin activity is substantially reduced. A side chain of a length at least equivalent to that of cholesterol is also a prerequisite for vitamin activity. If the side chain is replaced by a hydroxyl group, for example, the vitamin activity is lost. The potency of the various D vitamins is determined by the side chain. D_5, for example, with its branched 10-carbon side chain, is much less active with respect to the calcification of bone cartilage than is D_3 with its 9-membered side chain.

Of the compounds shown in Figure 7, the most common form is that of D_2, ergocalciferol, so-called because its parent compound is ergosterol. Ergosterol can readily be prepared from plant materials and, thus, serves as a commercially important source of the vitamin. Vitamin D_3, cholecalciferol, is the most important member of the D family because it is the only form which can be generated *in vivo*. Cholesterol, from which cholecalciferol takes its name, serves as the precursor. The 7-dehydrocholesterol at the skin's surface is acted upon by ultraviolet light and is converted to vitamin D_3. Here, then, is the connection between diet, sunshine, and rickets sought many years ago when rickets was prevalent in young children. In the absence of sunshine this conversion does not take place. Recall the dress patterns of the people of the eighteenth and nineteenth century. Children (as well as adults) wore many layers of clothing that shielded the skin from ultraviolet light. This practice severely restricted vitamin D synthesis.

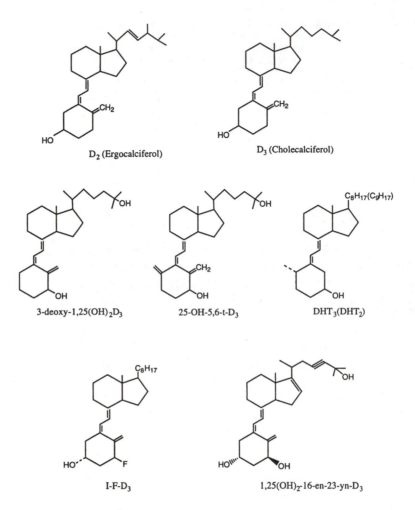

Figure 7   Compounds with vitamin D activity. Not all of these compounds have identical activity.

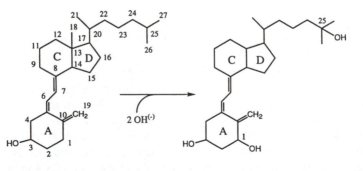

Figure 8   Chemical structure of vitamin D showing carbon numbers of the basic structure. The rings are labeled A, C, and D after the ring letters of cholesterol. When activated, a hydroxyl group is added at carbons 1 and 25 to form 1,25-dihydroxycalciferol.

Table 9   Physical Characteristics of Vitamins D_2 and D_3

Vitamin	Number Double Bonds	Melting Point	UV Absorption Maximum	Molar Extinction Coefficient	Optical Rotation
D_2	4	121°C	265 nm	19,400	$\alpha \frac{20}{D} + 106°$
D_3	3	83–85°C	264–265	18,300	$\alpha \frac{20}{D} + 84.8°$

Most mammals can convert both D_2 and D_3 to the active principles (1,25-dihydroxyergocalciferol and 1,25-dihydroxycholecalciferol) which are responsible for D's biological function. Birds seem unable to make this conversion using D_2 or the resulting hydroxylation product. It is also possible that the conversion product is either rapidly degraded and/or excreted. Thus, birds must be supplied with D_3 rather than D_2 as the vitamin of choice. It has been estimated that for birds, D_2 has only one-tenth the biological activity of D_3 on a molar basis.

C. Physical and Chemical Properties

The history of vitamin D would not be complete without mentioning the careful work of a Frenchman, Charles Tanret, who isolated and characterized a sterol from fungus-infected rye which he called ergosterol. The melting point, optical rotation, and elemental composition of ergosterol reported by Tanret in 1889 were identical to those reported by Windaus more than 30 years later. Windaus and associates were able to elucidate the structures of ergosterol and ergocalciferol. However, their complete structures were not verifiable until the techniques of X-ray analysis and infrared spectroscopy were developed.

The precursors and the vitamins are sterols which are members of the nonsaponifiable lipid class. At room temperature, they are white to yellowish solids with relatively low melting points. The various structural and physical characteristics of D_2 and D_3 are listed in Table 9. Under normal conditions, D_3 is more stable than D_2; however, both compounds undergo oxidation when exposed to air for periods of 24 to 72 hr. When protected from air and moisture and stored under refrigeration, oxidation of the vitamin can be minimized. In acid solutions, the D vitamins are unstable. However, in alkaline solutions they are stable. All the D vitamins are moderately soluble in fats, oils, and ethanol, and very soluble in fat solvents such as chloroform, methanol, and ether. All of the vitamers are unstable to light. In the dry form the vitamers are more stable than when in solution. Stability in solution can be enhanced by the presence of such antioxidants as α-tocopherol and vitamin A.

Although the D vitamins are not soluble in water, they, like the A vitamins, can be made miscible with water through the use of detergents or surfactants. However, because of the vitamins' vulnerability to oxidation, such solutions are very unstable. This is due to the wide dispersion of the vitamin molecules in water which has oxygen dissolved in it. Some protection against this oxidation can be provided if α-tocopherol (vitamin E) is added to the solution. Other chemical alterations can result in decreased vitamin potency as well. Saturation of any of the double bonds or the substitution of a chloride, bromide, or mercaptan residue for the hydroxyl group attached to carbon 3 results in a loss of vitamin activity.

D. Biopotency

The comparative potency of the D vitamers depends on several factors: (1) the species consuming the vitamers; and (2) the particular function assessed. With respect to species specificity, in mammalian species both the D_2 and D_3 are equivalent and both would be given a value of 100 if rickets prevention was used as the functional criterion. However, should these two vitamers be compared in chicks as preventers of rickets, D_2 would be given a value of perhaps 10 while D_3 would be 100. In this instance it is clear that species differ in their use of these two vitamers. A related sterol, dihydrotachysterol, a product of irradiated ergosterol, would have only 5 to 10% of the activity of ergocalciferol. In contrast, the activated forms of D_3 (25-hydroxy and 1,25-dihydroxycholecalciferol) are far more potent (2 to 5 times and 5 to 10 times, respectively) than their parent vitamer, D_3. The synthetic analog of D_3, 1α-hydroxycholecalciferol, likewise has 5 to 10 times the potency of cholecalciferol. There are other vitamin D analogs that have selective biological activity and may have use as therapeutic agents. The analog 3-deoxy-1,25-dihydroxycholecalciferol is far more active as an agent to promote intestinal calcium uptake than as an agent to promote bone calcium mobilization. This is also true for the analog, 25-hydroxy-5,6-cholecalciferol.

The reverse effects, increased bone calcium mobilization rather than increased intestinal calcium absorption, have been shown for analogs having a longer carbon chain at carbon 20 and/or having a fluorine attached at carbon 3 (see Figure 7). Cell differentiation, another vitamin D function, is markedly enhanced by the addition of a hydroxyl group at carbon 3, an unsaturation between carbons 16 and 17, and a triple bond between carbons 22 and 23. This analog has greater activity with respect to cell differentiation than for intestinal calcium uptake and bone calcium mobilization.

E. Methods of Assay

Because mammals require so little vitamin D and because so few foods contain the vitamin, methods for its determination have to be sensitive, reliable, and accurate. A wide variety of assays have been developed that are capable of quantifying fairly well the amount of vitamin D in a test substance. These assays can be divided roughly into two groups: chemical and biological. Biological assays, with few exceptions, are usually more sensitive than chemical assays because so little of the vitamin is required by animals. The smallest amount of vitamin detectable by the biological methods is 120 ng or 0.3 nmol, whereas with the chemical methods the smallest amount detectable is approximately 9 times that or 2.6 nmol. The exception to this comparison is the technique which utilizes high pressure liquid chromatography followed by ultraviolet absorption analysis. This technique can measure as little as 5 ng or 1/24th that of the bioassay techniques. Gas chromatography is also very sensitive, especially if the chromatograph is equipped with an electron capture detector. Using this technique, as little as 50 pg of the vitamin can be detected. This degree of sensitivity is needed for the detection of tissue vitamin levels since, aside from vitamin B_{12}, vitamin D is the most potent of the vitamins. Only small amounts are needed and so only small amounts will be found in those tissues requiring the vitamin.

Table 10 summarizes the main methods that have been used for the detection of biological levels of vitamin D. Under the chemical assay techniques, note that a variety of color reactions can be used in vitamin D quantification. These color reactions are possible because the vitamin contains several rings which can react with a variety of compounds in solution and produce a color. The intensity of the color is directly related to the quantity of the vitamin in solution.

While these colorimetric methods are relatively easy to perform, they have several drawbacks. First, and most important, the color reaction is possible because of the ring structure; many sterols have this same ring structure but few have vitamin activity. Thus, colorimetric methods are not specific enough to permit true vitamin quantification in a mixture. The second drawback is that there must be sufficient vitamin in the test substance to react with the color reagent to produce a measurable color change. This requires instrumentation that is able to measure these changes. In general, this degree of sensitivity is missing in most instruments designed to measure colorimetric changes.

The ring structure of vitamin D, although common to many different sterols, can be utilized very well in assay techniques where the sterols are first separated and then assayed. The vitamin D sterol ring structure has a characteristic ultraviolet absorption spectra. At 264 to 265 nm, the intensity of the light absorbed is directly proportional to the quantity of vitamin D present. Sterols can be separated from the lipid component of a sample by saponification. The nonsaponifiable lipids (the sterols) can be further separated by digitonin precipitation. Vitamin D and its related

Table 10   Summary of Methods Used in Determining Vitamin D Content of Tissues and Foods

Method	Sensitivity[a] (nmoles)	Usual Working Range (nmoles)	Comments
	Chemical Methods		
Colorimetric[b]			
Aniline-HCl	No values given	No values given	Devised in 1925.
Antimony chloride	3.2	3.2–6.5	Used primarily to assess pharmaceutical preparations.
Trifluoroacetic acid	2.6	1–80	
Ultraviolet absorption	2.6	2.6–52	A solution with 5.47 nmol of vitamin D will have an absorbance of 0.10 at 264 nm.
Ultraviolet fluorescence	2.6	2.6–26	Based on the property of acetic anhydride-sulfuric acid induced fluorescence of the vitamin.
Gas chromatography	0.1 pmol	0.01–10	Based on use of an electron capture detector.
High pressure liquid chromatography	0.01	0.05–100	
Gas chromatography-mass spectrometry	0.01	0.01–50	Equipment not widely available due to expense. Can separate and quantify individual vitamers in a mixture.
	Biological Methods		
Rat line test	0.03	0.03–0.07	Time consuming — requires 7 days of feeding after rats become rachitic.
Chick test	0.13	0.006–15	Requires 21 days of feeding.
Intestinal Ca^{2+} absorption	*In vivo* 0.33	0.125–25 µg	Requires 1 day.
	In vitro 0.66	250–1000	Requires 1 day.
Bone Ca^{2+} mobilization	0.32	0.125–25 µg	Requires 1 day.
Body growth	0.06	50–1250	Requires 21–28 days.
Immunoassay of calcium-binding protein	0.0025	1 ng	Requires 1 day.

[a] Defined as the least amount of vitamin detectable by the method.
[b] Other color reagents have also been used.

sterols will not precipitate, whereas cholesterol and the other four-ring sterols will. If the remaining supernatant containing the vitamin D components is then fractionated using chromatographic techniques, the resulting fractions can be assayed according to the amount of ultraviolet light absorbed.

The ultraviolet light absorption characteristic can also be used to determine the extent of conversion of provitamin D to D_2 or D_3. Ergosterol or cholesterol can be irradiated until the resultant compound exhibits the typical absorption spectra characteristic of the vitamin. Of course, just as ultraviolet light is needed for this conversion, one must remember that light in excess will destroy the vitamin and its usefulness will be lost.

There are a number of chemical assay techniques useful for the determination of vitamin D activity in biological samples and a number of biological assay techniques which can be used. The advantages of the bioassay are those of sensitivity and specificity. The disadvantages are those of time, expense, and accuracy. The basis of the bioassay is the idea that the physiological effect is quantifiable and, theoretically, the magnitude of the vitamin effect is in direct proportion to the amount of vitamin D in the test substance. For many years, the standard bioassay for vitamin D was the rat line test first devised by McCollum in 1922. This test consists of depleting rats of their vitamin D stores and then treating them with graded amounts of the test substance for one week.

The rats are then killed, the bones of the forepaws excised and cleaned of adhering tissue, sliced longitudinally, and placed in a solution of silver nitrate. The silver nitrate is absorbed by the areas of the bone where calcium has recently been deposited. These regions will turn black upon exposure to light. The resultant black line is then measured and compared to lines obtained from rats fed known amounts of vitamin D. Thus, the line test is based on the activity of the vitamin in promoting calcium uptake by the bone. While this is probably a good method to estimate vitamin activity in a given substance, it has the pitfall of not distinguishing between the various D forms. The user of this method also must assume that bone calcium deposition is the vitamin's most important function; this is not always true.

Use of the line test to assess vitamin content of human foods is probably acceptable since rats and humans can use all forms of D similarly. However, use of the rat line test to assess the D content of feeds for chickens would present problems due to the fact that the chickens do not use D_2 and D_3 equally well. As pointed out earlier, chickens need D_3 in their diets rather than D_2. Other bioassays listed in Table 10 also are based on a physiological/metabolic parameter which assumes that the quantity of the vitamin in a test substance is proportional to the activity of the system being assessed. Tests such as the intestinal calcium uptake test, the bone calcium mobilization test, the body growth test, and the calcium binding protein assay all have been devised and published. They all have the advantage of assessing the biological potency of the vitamin D contained in the test substance and all are sensitive to quantities of D likely to be present in biological (as opposed to pharmacological) preparations.

F. International Units (IU)

It was from the use of the bioassay techniques that the definition of the international unit (IU) was developed. One IU was defined as the smallest amount of vitamin required to elicit a physiological response, i.e., the calcification of bone. As it was used in this context, with the rat as the reference animal, 1 mg of vitamin D was equivalent to 40,000 IU of the vitamin. In 1931, the World Health Organization of the League of Nations adopted as their international standard of reference for vitamin D the activity of 1 mg of a reference solution of irradiated ergosterol. At the time this definition was developed, researchers were not aware of the different D vitamins nor were they aware of the species specificity for the vitamin form. Later, as knowledge about the vitamin increased, the definition was changed such that the present definition developed by Nelson in 1949 uses cholecalciferol, D_3, as the reference standard — 1.0 g of a cottonseed oil solution of D_3 contains 10 mg of the vitamin or 400 USP units. Thus, the potency of the different D vitamins are related to the most important biologic compounds in the D family.

G. Metabolism of Vitamin D

1. Absorption

Prior to the understanding and elucidation of the conversion of cholesterol to cholecalciferol and then to its activation as 1,25-dihydroxycholecalciferol, considerable attention was given to the mechanisms for the intestinal absorption of vitamin D. It was found that dietary vitamin D was absorbed with the food fats and was dependent on the presence of the bile salts. Any disease which resulted in an impairment of fat absorption likewise resulted in an impairment of vitamin D absorption. Absorption of the vitamin is a passive process which is influenced by the composition of the gut contents. Vitamin D is absorbed with the long-chain fatty acids and is present in the chylomicrons of the lymphatic system. Absorption takes place primarily in the jejunum and ileum. This has a protective effect on vitamin D stores since the bile, released into the duodenum, is the chief excretory pathway of the vitamin; reabsorption in times of vitamin need can protect the body from undue loss. However, in times of vitamin excess, this reabsorptive mechanism may be a detriment rather than a benefit. The vitamin is absorbed in either the hydroxylated or the nonhydroxylated form.

While many of the other essential nutrients are absorbed via an active transport system, there is little reason to believe that absorption of vitamin D is by any mechanism other than passive diffusion. The body, if exposed to sunlight, can convert the 7-dehydrocholesterol at the skin's surface to cholecalciferol, and this compound is then metabolized: first in the liver to 25-hydroxycholecalciferol and further in the kidney producing the active principle, 1,25-dihydroxycholecalciferol. Because the body, under the right conditions, can synthesize *in toto* its vitamin D needs, and because it needs so little of the vitamin, there appears to be little reason for the body to develop an active transport system for its absorption. However, in the person with renal disease, the synthesis of 1,25-dihydroxycholecalciferol is impaired and, in this individual, intestinal uptake of the active form is quite important. Oral supplements can be used to ensure adequate vitamin D status.

Because the body can completely synthesize dehydrocholesterol and convert it to D_2 or D_3, and then hydroxylate it to form the active form, an argument against its essentiality as a nutrient can be developed. In point of fact, because the active form is synthesized in the kidney and from there distributed by the blood to all parts of the body, this active form meets the definition of a hormone, and the kidney, the site of synthesis, meets the definition of an endocrine organ. Thus, whether vitamin D is a nutrient or a hormone is dependent on the degree of exposure to ultraviolet light. Lacking exposure, vitamin D must be provided in the diet and thus is an essential nutrient.

2. Transport

Once absorbed, vitamin D is transported in nonesterified form bound to a specific vitamin D binding protein. This protein (DBP) is nearly identical to the α-2-globulins and albumins with respect to its electrophoretic mobility. All of the forms of vitamin D (25-hydroxy-D_3, 24,25-dihydroxy-D_3, and 1,25-dihydroxy-D_3) are carried by this protein which is a globulin with a molecular weight of 58,000 Da. Its binding affinity varies with the vitamin form. DNA sequence analysis of DBP shows homology with a fetoprotein and serum albumin. DBP also has a high affinity for actin, but the physiological significance for this cross reactivity is unknown. The transcription of the DBP is promoted by a vitamin D-receptor protein transcription factor. Thus, there is a complete loop of a transport protein needed for vitamin D, and which in turn is dependent on vitamin D for its synthesis.

3. Metabolism

Once absorbed or synthesized at the body surface, vitamin D is transported via DBP to the liver. Here it is hydroxylated via the enzyme vitamin D hydroxylase at carbon 25 to form 25-hydroxycholecalciferol. Figure 9 illustrates the pathway from cholesterol to 1,25-dihydroxycholecalciferol. With the first hydroxylation a number of products are formed, but the most important of these is 25-hydroxycholecalciferol. The biological function of each of these metabolites is not known completely. As mentioned, the hydroxylation occurs in the liver and is catalyzed by a cytochrome P-450-dependent mixed-function monooxygenase. This enzyme has been found in both mitochondrial and microsomal compartments. It is a two-component system which involves flavoprotein and a cytochrome P-450 and is regulated by the concentration of ionized calcium in serum. The hydroxylation reaction can be inhibited if D_3 analogs having modified side chains are infused into an animal fed a rachitic diet and a D_3 supplement.

25-Hydroxy-D_3 is then bound to DBP and transported from the liver to the kidney where a second hydroxyl group is added at carbon 1. This hydroxylation occurs in the kidney proximal tubule mitochondria and is catalyzed by the enzyme 25-OH-D_3-1α-hydroxylase. This enzyme has

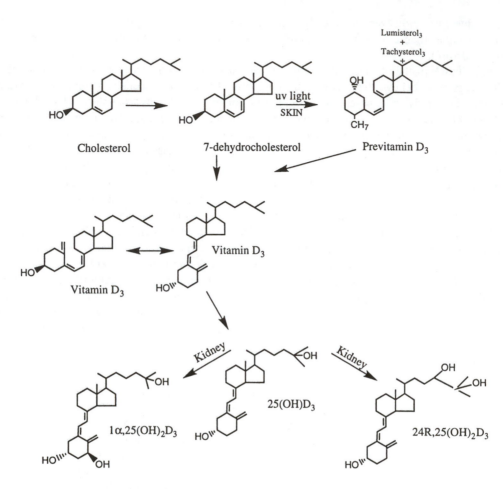

Figure 9 Synthesis of active 1,25-dihydroxycholecalciferol using cholesterol as the initial substrate. Several isomers can result when previtamin D or 7-dehydrocholesterol is converted to D₃, cholecalciferol.

been characterized as a three-component enzyme involving cytochrome P-450, an iron-sulfur protein (ferredoxin), and ferredoxin reductase. The reductant is $NADPH_2$. Considerable evidence has shown that 1,25-dihydroxycholecalciferol is the active principle that stimulates bone mineralization, intestinal calcium uptake, and calcium mobilization. Because this product is so active in the regulation of calcium homeostasis, its synthesis must be closely regulated. Indeed, product feedback regulation exists with respect to the activity of this enzyme and control is also exercised at the level of its mRNA transcription. In both instances, the level of 1,25-dihydroxycholecalciferol (the product) negatively affects 1α-hydroxylase activity and suppresses mRNA transcription of the hydroxylase gene product. In addition, control of the hydroxylase enzyme is exerted by the parathyroid hormone, PTH. When plasma calcium levels fall, PTH is released and this hormone stimulates 1α-hydroxylase activity while decreasing the activity of 25-hydroxylase. In turn, PTH release is down-regulated by rising levels of 1,25-dihydroxycholecalciferol and its analog, 24,25-dihydroxycholecalciferol. Insulin, growth hormone, estrogen, and prolactin are additional hormones that stimulate the activity of the 1α-hydroxylase. The mechanisms that explain these stimulatory effects are less well known and are probably related to their effects on bone mineralization as well as on other calcium-using processes.

Just as several metabolites are formed in the 25-hydroxylase reaction, a number of products also result with the second hydroxylation. Some of these transformations are shown in Figure 10. Also shown are the degradative products found primarily in the feces. These products appear in

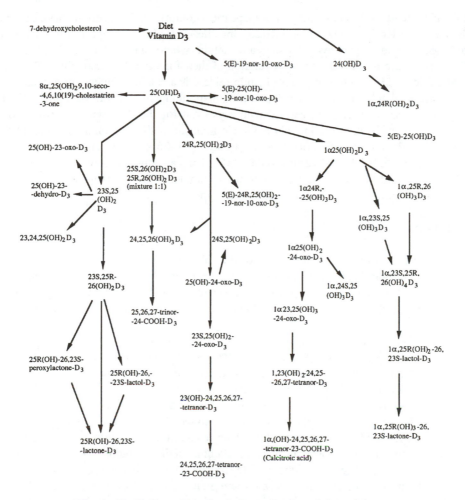

Figure 10   Pathways for vitamin D_3 synthesis and degradation.

the feces because of biliary transport from the liver to the small intestine and subsequent degradation by enteric flora.

D_3 is subject to other metabolic reactions as well (Figure 10). Whether these metabolites have specific functions with respect to mineral metabolism is not fully understood. Instead of 1,25-dihydroxy-D_3, 24,25-dihydroxy-D_3 may be formed and may serve to enhance bone mineralization and embryonic development, and to suppress parathyroid hormone release. 24,25-Dihydroxy-D_3 arises by hydroxylation of 25-hydroxy-D_3. When 25-OH-D_3-1α-hydroxylase activity is suppressed, 24,25-hydroxylation is stimulated. This hydroxylase is substrate inducible through the mechanism of increased enzyme protein synthesis and has been found in kidney, intestine, and cartilage. 24,25-Dihydroxy-D_3 may represent a "spillover" metabolite of D_3. That is, a metabolite is formed when excess 25-hydroxy-D_3 is present in the body. Other D_3 metabolites such as 25-hydroxy-D_3-26,23-lactone also can be regarded as spillover metabolites, since measurable quantities are observed under conditions of excess intake. While 24,25-dihydroxy-D_3 does function in the bone mineralization process, it is not as active in this respect as is 1,25-dihydroxy-D_3.

The question of whether a hydroxy group at carbon 25 is a requirement for vitamin activity has been posed since several D_3 metabolites lack this structural element. Studies utilizing fluoro-substituted D_3 showed conclusively that while maximal activity is shown by the 1,25-D_3 compound, vitamin activity can also be shown by compounds lacking this structure. In part, the structural requisite for vitamin activity may relate to the role the 25-hydroxy substituents play in determining the molecular shape of the compound. This shape must conform to the receptor shape of the cellular membranes in order for the D_3 to be utilized. Specific intracellular receptors for 1,25-dihydroxy-D_3 have been found in parathyroid, pancreatic, pituitary, and placental tissues. All these tissues have been shown to require D_3 for the regulation of their function. For example, in D_3 deficiency, pancreatic release of insulin is impaired. Insulin release is a calcium-dependent process which, by inference, means that there must be a calcium-binding protein whose synthesis requires the vitamin.

As can be seen in Figure 10, several pathways exist for the degradation of the active 1,25-dihydroxycholecalciferol. These include oxidative removal of the side chain, additional hydroxylation at carbon 24, the formation of a lactone (1,25 $OH_2 D_2$-26,23-lactone), and additional hydroxylation at carbon 26. While 25-hydroxycholecalciferol can accumulate in the heart, lungs, kidneys, and liver, 1,25 dihydroxycholecalciferol does not accumulate. The active form is not stored appreciably but is found in almost every cell and tissue type.

4. Function

Until the recognition of the central role of the calcium ion in cellular metabolic regulation, it was thought that vitamin D's only function was to facilitate the deposition of calcium and phosphorus in bone. This concept developed when it was recognized that the bowed legs of rickets was due to inadequate mineralization in the absence of adequate vitamin D intake or exposure to sunlight.

Studies of calcium absorption *in vivo* by the intestine revealed that D-deficient rats absorb less calcium than D-sufficient rats and that rats fed very high levels (10,000 IU/day) absorbed more calcium than did normally fed rats. These observations of the effects of the vitamin on calcium uptake led to work designed to determine the mechanism of this effect. It was soon discovered that vitamin D (1,25-dihydroxy-D_3) served to stimulate the synthesis of a specific gut cell protein that was responsible for calcium uptake. This protein, called the intestinal calcium binding protein (calbindin), was isolated from the intestine and later from brain, bone, kidney, uterus, parotid gland, parathyroid glands, and skin. Several different calcium binding proteins have been found but not all of these binding proteins are vitamin D dependent. That is, once formed, their activity with respect to calcium binding is unaffected by vitamin deficiency. Most, however, are dependent on vitamin D for their synthesis. Thus, these calcium-binding proteins are molecular expressions of the hormonal action of the vitamin.

As animals age, the levels of the calcium-binding protein fall. Yet, when calcium intake levels fall, the synthesis and activity of the binding proteins rise. This mechanism explains how individuals can adapt to low calcium diets. Interestingly, calcium deprivation stimulates the conversion of cholecalciferol to 25-hydroxycholecalciferol in the liver and to 1,25-dihydroxycholecalciferol in the kidney. Aging, however, seems to affect this regulatory mechanism. As humans age, they are less able to absorb calcium and may develop osteomalacia, a condition analogous to rickets in children and characterized by demineralization of the bone. In patients with osteomalacia, intestinal absorption of calcium is decreased, but when 1,25-dihydroxy-D_3 is administered, calcium absorption is increased. It would appear, therefore, that one of the consequences of aging is an impaired conversion of 25-hydroxy-D_3 to 1,25-dihydroxy-D_3, and since less of the latter is available, less calcium binding protein is synthesized. Measures of calcium-binding protein in aging rats, using an immunoassay technique, have shown that this is indeed the case.

Vitamin D also increases intestinal absorption of calcium by mechanisms apart from the synthesis of calcium-binding protein. It does this as part of its general tropic effect as a steroid on a variety of cellular reactions. Vitamin D causes a change in membrane permeability to calcium at the brush border, perhaps through a change in the lipid (fatty acid) component of the membrane. It stimulates the $Ca^{2+}Mg^{2+}$ ATPase on the membrane of the cell wall, increases Krebs cycle activity, increases the conversion of ATP to cAMP, and increases the activity of the alkaline phosphatase enzyme. All these effects in the intestinal cell are independent of the vitamin's effect on calcium-binding protein synthesis.

In addition to its role in calcium absorption, vitamin D serves to induce the uptake of phosphate and magnesium by the brush border of the intestine. The effect on phosphate uptake is independent of its effect on calcium absorption and is due to an effect of the vitamin on the synthesis of a sodium-dependent membrane carrier for phosphate. The effect of vitamin D on magnesium absorption is incidental to its effect on calcium absorption, since the calcium-binding protein has a weak affinity for magnesium. Thus, if synthesis of the calcium-binding protein results in an increase in calcium uptake, it also results in a significant increase in magnesium uptake.

a. Regulation of Serum Calcium Levels

Serum calcium levels are closely regulated in the body so as to maintain optimal muscle contractility and cellular function. Several hormones are involved in this regulation: 1,25-dihydroxy-D_3 produced by the kidney, parathyroid hormone released by the parathyroid gland, and thyrocalcitonin released by the thyroid C cells. Each has a specific function with respect to serum calcium levels and all three are interdependent. Vitamin D_3 increases blood calcium by increasing intestinal calcium uptake and decreases blood calcium by increasing calcium deposition in the bone. In the relative absence of vitamin D, parathyroid hormone increases serum calcium levels by increasing the activity of the kidney 1α-25-hydroxylase with the result of increasing blood levels of 1,25-dihydroxy-D_3 and through enhancing bone mineral mobilization and phosphate diuresis. Parathyroid hormone in the presence of vitamin D has the reverse action on bone. When both hormones (parathormone and 1,25-D_3) are present, bone mineralization is stimulated. Even though the parathyroid hormone stimulates the production of 1,25-dihydroxy-D_3, D_3 does not stimulate parathyroid hormone release. Thyrocalcitonin serves to lower blood calcium levels through stimulating bone calcium uptake, and its effect is independent of parathyroid hormone yet is dependent on the availability of calcium from the intestine. If serum calcium levels are elevated through a calcium infusion, thyrocalcitonin will be released and stimulate bone calcium uptake even in animals lacking both parathyroid hormone and D_3.

b. Mode of Action at the Genomic Level

The process of vitamin D (1,25-dihydroxycholecalciferol)-receptor binding to specific DNA sequences follows the classic model for steroid hormone action. Like vitamin A, vitamin D binds to a receptor protein (vitamin D receptor protein, VDR) in the nucleus. This receptor protein is a member of the steroid hormone receptor superfamily. The receptor protein then acquires an affinity for specific DNA sequences located upstream from the promoter sequence of the target gene. These specific DNA sequences are called response elements. The receptor protein consists of a structure in which two zinc atoms are coordinated in two finger-like domains. The N-terminal finger confers specificity to the binding while the second finger stabilizes the complex. When bound, transcription of the cognate protein mRNA is activated. Several response elements have been identified, with each being specific for a specific gene product. As shown in Figure 11, the response elements have in common imperfect direct repeats of six base pair half elements separated by a three-base-pair spacer. Affinity of the nuclear receptor protein for vitamin D is modified by phosphorylation. Two sites of phosphorylation have been found and both are on serine residues. One site is located in the DNA binding region at serine 51 between two zinc-finger DNA binding motifs, and if phosphorylated by protein kinase C (or a related enzyme) DNA binding is reduced. The second site is located in the hormone-binding N-terminal region at serine 208. It has the opposite effect. When phosphorylated, probably by casein kinase II or a related enzyme, transcription is activated.

The vitamin-protein receptor complex that binds to the DNA consists of three distinct elements: 1,25-dihydroxycholecalciferol (the hormone ligand), the vitamin receptor, and one of the retinoid

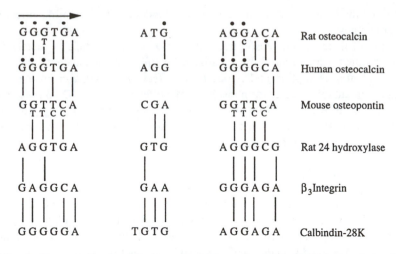

Figure 11   Vitamin D response elements for osteocalcin, osteopontin, D_3-24-hydroxylase, β_3 integrin, and calbindin 28K. Circles above bases indicate guanine residues that have been shown by methylation interference experiments to be protected upon protein binding to the vitamin D responsive element. The small letters below the large ones indicate points at which base substitutions have been found and which abolish responsiveness to vitamin D. (Adapted form Whitfield, G.K. et al., *J. Nutr.*, 125, 1690, 1995. With permission.)

X receptors (RXRα). Here is an instance where, once again, a vitamin D-vitamin A interaction occurs. The 9-*cis* retinoic acid can attenuate the induction of the transcriptional activation that occurs when the vitamin D-receptor complex binds to the vitamin D responsive element. Perhaps 9-*cis* retinoic acid has this effect because when it binds to the retinoid X receptor, it blocks or partially occludes the binding site of the vitamin D-protein for DNA. Figure 12 illustrates the mode of vitamin D action at the genomic level. To date, the nuclear vitamin D receptor has been found in 34 different cell types and it is quite likely that it is a universal nuclear component. Probably this is because every cell has a need to move calcium into or out of its various compartments as part of its metabolic control systems. Thus, calcium-binding proteins whose synthesis is vitamin D dependent are needed. Among the proteins thus far identified are osteocalcin, vitamin D binding protein, osteopontin, 24-hydroxylase-β3-interferon, calbindin, prepro PTH, calcitonin, Type I collagen, fibronectin, bone matrix GLA protein, interleukin 2 and interleukin γ, transcription factors (GM-CSF, c-myc, c-fos, c-fms), vitamin D receptors, calbindin D_{28x} and $_{9x}$, and prolactin. The transcription of the genes for each of these proteins are affected or regulated by vitamin D.

H. Vitamin D Deficiency

As discussed earlier, bone deformities are the hallmark of the vitamin D-deficient child while porous brittle bones are indications of the deficiency in the adult. In view of the fact that the liver can store large quantities of the previtamin, it is difficult to visualize how the disorder can develop. Rickets was very common in the U.S. prior to the enrichment of milk and other food products. In part, rickets developed because heavy clothing shielded the skin from the ultraviolet rays of the sun. Lacking this exposure, the only other source was food, and because so few foods contain significant quantities of the vitamin, deficiency states developed.

Today, osteomalacia, the adult form of rickets, can be due to inadequate intake or exposure to sunlight and also can be due to disease or damage to either the liver or kidney. As pointed out in Section II.G of this unit, both these organs are essential for the conversion of cholecalciferol to 1,25-dihydroxy-D_3. If either organ is nonfunctional in this respect, the deficient state will develop. On rare occasions, the deficient state will develop not because of any lack of dietary D or sunlight or because of kidney or liver damage, but through a genetic error in which the 1,25-hydroxylase

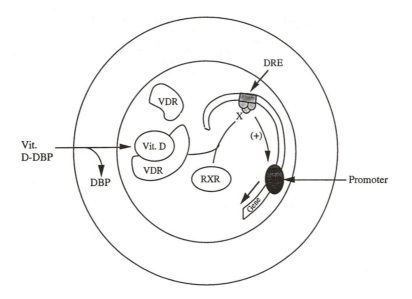

Figure 12   Schematic representation showing vitamin D bound to vitamin D binding protein (DBP) entering the nucleus, binding to receptor (VDR), complexing with retinoid receptor (RXR), and then binding to the vitamin D responsive elements (DRE) as a trans-acting factor enhancing the transcription of a variety of calcium-binding proteins.

enzyme is missing and the 1,25-dihydroxy-D_3 cannot be synthesized. In individuals so afflicted, 1,25-dihydroxy-D_3 must be supplied to prevent the deficiency state from developing.

1,25-Dihydroxy-D_3 must also be provided to the anephritic patient, since these patients cannot synthesize this hormone. Until the realization that the kidney served as the endocrine organ for 1,25-dihydroxy-D_3 synthesis, renal disease was almost always accompanied by a disturbed calcium balance, osteomalacia, and osteoporosis.

I. Hypervitaminosis D

Since previtamin D is fat soluble, like vitamin A, it can be stored. The storage capacity of the liver for the D precursor is much less than its capacity for A and toxic conditions can develop if large amounts of D (in excess of need and storage capacity) are consumed over extended periods of time. Because D's main function is to facilitate calcium uptake from the intestine and tissue calcium deposition, excess D in the toxic range (1,000 to 10,000 IU/day) will result in excess calcification, not only of bone but of soft tissues as well. Renal stones, calcification of the heart, major vessels, muscles, and other tissues have been shown in experimental animals as well as in humans. Seelig has described a series of patients who were unusually sensitive to vitamin D either *in utero* or in infancy. These patients had multiple abnormalities in soft tissues and bones and were mentally retarded. Whether excess D intakes provoke mild, moderate, or severe abnormalities is related not only to the individual's genetic background but also to his/her calcium, magnesium, and phosphorus intake. If any of these are consumed in excess of the others, vitamin D intoxication becomes more apparent.

J. Recommended Dietary Allowances

Because the active D_3 hormone can be synthesized in the body, an absolute requirement is difficult to determine. Few foods naturally contain sufficient preformed vitamin D. In the absence of synthesis *in vivo*, preformed vitamin D must be added to the diet. This is done almost to excess

Table 11   Recommended Dietary Allowances (RDA) for Vitamin D

Group	Age (years)	RDA (μg/day)
Infants	0–6 months	7.5
	7–12 months	10
Children	1–3	10
	4–6	10
	7–10	10
Males	11–14	10
	15–18	10
	19–24	10
	25–50	5
	51+	5
Females	11–14	10
	15–18	10
	19–24	10
	25–50	5
	51+	5
Pregnancy	—	10
Lactation	—	10

in the U.S. Milk is fortified with 10 μg per quart and other food products such as margarine are also fortified with the vitamin. Due to this fortification, infantile rickets is almost unknown today. The level of supplementation for milk was selected based on the concept that the growing child should drink one quart of milk a day in order to optimize growth. Adults usually do not require vitamin supplementation unless they are either pregnant or lactating. Pregnant or lactating females are recommended to consume 10 μg vitamin D per day. Table 11 gives the recommended dietary allowances for vitamin D.

III. VITAMIN E

A. Overview

While much of the excitement of the "vitamin discovery era" was devoted to the work on vitamins A and D, Evans and Bishop in 1922 discovered an unidentified factor in vegetable oil which, if lacking from the diet, resulted in reproductive failure. The term tocopherol was proposed by Emerson for this factor because of its role in reproduction. Rats fed diets lacking this vitamin failed to reproduce. The name tocopherol comes from the Greek work *tokos*, meaning childbirth, *pherein*, meaning to bring forth, and *ol*, the chemical suffix meaning alcohol. Vitamin E, the name suggested by Evans and Bishop, is commonly used for that group of tocol and tocotrienol derivatives having vitamin E activity. The most active of these is α-tocopherol (Figure 13). Much of the earlier work was devoted to tocopherol's role in reproduction such that its function as an antioxidant was ignored. However, in the last 30 years considerable attention has been given to this role in metabolism. It is recognized that vitamin E is an essential nutrient for many animal species. The level of vitamin E in plasma lipoproteins and in the phospholipids of the membrane around and within the cell are dependent on vitamin E intake as well as on the intake of other antioxidant nutrients and on the level of dietary polyunsaturated fatty acids.

B. Structure and Nomenclature

The most active naturally occurring form of vitamin E is D-α-tocopherol. Other tocopherols have been isolated having varying degrees of vitamin activity. Figure 13 shows the molecular

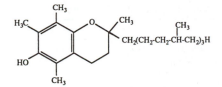

α-Tocopherol (5, 7, 8 Trimethyltocol)

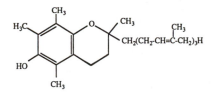

α-Tocotrienol (5, 7, 8 Trimethyltrienol)

Figure 13 Basic structure of vitamin E.

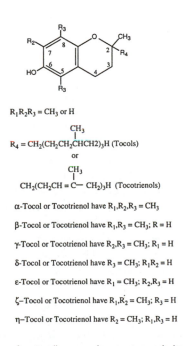

$R_1 R_2 R_3 = CH_3$ or H

$$R_4 = CH_2(CH_2CH_2\overset{\underset{\mid}{CH_3}}{CH}CH2)_3H \text{ (Tocols)}$$

or

$$CH_2(CH_2CH = \overset{\underset{\mid}{CH_3}}{C} - CH_2)_3H \text{ (Tocotrienols)}$$

α-Tocol or Tocotrienol have $R_1,R_2,R_3 = CH_3$

β-Tocol or Tocotrienol have $R_1,R_3 = CH_3$; R = H

γ-Tocol or Tocotrienol have $R_2,R_3 = CH_3$; $R_1 = H$

δ-Tocol or Tocotrienol have $R_3 = CH_3$; $R_1R_2 = H$

ε-Tocol or Tocotrienol have $R_1 = CH_3$; $R_2,R_3 = H$

ζ–Tocol or Tocotrienol have $R_1,\dot{R}_2 = CH_3$; $R_3 = H$

η–Tocol or Tocotrienol have $R_2 = CH_3$; $R_1,R_3 = H$

Figure 14 Structures of naturally occurring compounds having vitamin E activity.

structures of α-tocopherol and α-tocotrienol. Figure 14 shows the other tocopherols and tocotrienols and their relationship to α-tocopherol. To have vitamin activity, the compound must have the double ring structure (chromane nucleus) as shown in Figures 13 and 14 and must also have a side chain attached at carbon 2 and methyl groups attached at carbons 5, 7, or 8. α-Tocopherols have methyl groups attached at all three positions and represent the most active vitamin compounds. β-Tocopherols have methyl groups attached to carbons 5 and 8; γ-tocopherols have methyl groups attached at carbons 7 and 8, and δ-tocopherols have only one methyl group attached at carbon 8. If the side chain attached to carbon 2 is saturated, then the compound is a member of the tocol family of compounds; if unsaturated, it belongs to the tocotrienol family. All forms have a hydroxyl group at carbon 6 and a methyl group at carbon 2. Other forms, ε, ζ, and η, have their methyl groups at carbon 5, or 5 and 7, or 7, respectively. Naturally occurring vitamin E is in the D form

Table 12   Commercially Available Products Having Vitamin E Activity

Form	Units of activity/mg
DL-α-Tocopheryl acetate (all-rac)	1.00
DL-α-Tocopherol (all-rac)	1.10
D-α-Tocopheryl acetate (RRR)	1.36
D-α-Tocopheryl acid succinate (all-rac)	1.49
DL-α-Tocopheryl acid succinate (all-rac)	0.89
D-α-Tocopheryl acid succinate (RRR)	1.21

Note: RRR — only naturally occurring stereoisomers bear this designation.

whereas synthetic vitamin E preparations are mixtures of the D and L forms. Both tocols and trienols occur as a variety of isomers. There are commercially available products usually marketed as acetate or succinate esters. The ester form does not usually occur in nature. Table 12 lists some of these commercially available forms.

C. International Units and Methods of Analysis

The international unit (IU) of vitamin E activity uses the activity of 1 mg of DL-α-tocopherol acetate (all-rac) in the rat fetal absorption assay as its reference standard. Even though D-α-tocopherol is 36% more active than the DL form, the latter was selected as the reference substance because it is more readily available as a standard of comparison. This choice may be a poor one because of the lack of validation of the fetal rat absorption assay as a true test of vitamin E potency. The fetal resorption test uses female vitamin E-depleted virgin rats. These rats are mated to normal males and given the test substance. After 21 days, the number of live fetuses and the number of dead and resorbed ones are counted. The potency of the test material is compared to a known amount of DL-α-tocopherol. Other tests have also been devised and are based on other functions of vitamin E. These tests may yield more reliable comparisons and may result in a redefinition of the IU. Tests of biopotency include the red cell hemolysis test and tests designed to evaluate the potency of the test substance in preventing or curing muscular dystrophy. Using DL-α-tocopherol as the standard with a value of 100, β-tocopherol has a value of 25 to 40 on the fetal resorption test, 15 to 27 on the hemolysis test, and 12 on the preventative muscular dystrophy test using the chicken as the test animal. γ-Tocopherol is even less potent, with values of 1 to 11, 3 to 20, and 5 for the same tests, respectively. The other tocopherols and tocotrienols are even less potent by comparison. Burton and Traber have reviewed the biopotency of vitamin E isomers as antioxidants.

Biochemical methods which utilize changes in enzyme activity rather than functional tests such as the rat fetal resorption test allow for the comparison of the different E vitamin forms. For example, plasma pyruvate kinase, hepatic glutathione peroxidase, and muscle cyclooxygenase activity are reduced in vitamin E-deficient rats. However, a true dose-response curve showing intake vs. changes in enzyme activity patterns, which in turn precede tissue changes, does not clearly provide a basis for biopotency. These enzyme activity studies are not as sensitive with respect to vitamin intake and potency as one would like.

Chemical analyses using thin-layer chromatography, gas-liquid chromatography, and high performance liquid chromatography (HPLC) are now available. These methods are very sensitive and can separate and quantify the various isomers in food, plasma, blood cells, and tissues. The HPLC method is the one of choice because sample preparation is minimal. Amounts of the isomers in the nanogram range can be detected and quantified.

D. Chemical and Physical Properties

The tocopherols are slightly viscous oils that are stable to heat and alkali. They are slowly oxidized by atmospheric oxygen and rapidly oxidized by iron or silver salts. The addition of acetate

Table 13   Characteristics of the Major Tocopherols

Compound	Color	Boiling Point (°C)	Molecular Weight (Da)	Absorption Maxima (nm)	Extraction (Ethanol)
DL-α-Tocopherol	Colorless to pale yellow	200–220	430.69	292–294	71–76
D-α-Tocopherol	Colorless to pale yellow	—	430.69	292–294	72–76
DL-α-Tocopherol acetate	Colorless to pale yellow	224	472.73	285.5	40–44
D-α-Tocopheryl acetate	Colorless to pale yellow	—	472.73	285.5	40–44

Table 14   Vitamin E Content of a Variety of Foods

Food	α-Tocopherol (μg/g)	Food	α-Tocopherol (μg/g)
Corn oil	159	Pork	4–6
Olive oil	100	Chicken	2–4
Peanut oil	189	Almonds	270
Wheat germ oil	1194	Peanuts	72
Palm oil	211	Oatmeal	17
Soft margarine	139	Rice	1–7
Milk	0.2–1.1	Wheat germ	117
Butter	10–33	Apple	3
Lard	2–38	Peach	13
Eggs	8–12	Asparagus	16
Fish	4–33	Spinach	25
Beef	5–8	Carrots	4

or succinate to the molecule adds stability towards oxidation. The tocopherols are insoluble in water but soluble in the usual fat solvents. Ultraviolet light destroys the vitamin activity. Table 13 gives the properties of four of the most potent tocopherols.

E. Sources

The tocopherols have been isolated from a number of foods. Almost all are from the plant kingdom, with wheat germ oil being the richest source. European wheat germ oil contains mostly β-tocopherols while American wheat germ oil contains mostly α-tocopherols. Corn oil contains α-tocopherols and soybean oil δ-tocopherols. Olive and peanut oil are poor sources of the vitamin. Some animal products such as egg yolk, liver, and milk contain tocopherols but, in general, foods of animal origin are relatively poor sources of the vitamin. Table 14 provides values of tocopherols in a variety of foods. Vegetable oils vary from 100 μg/g (olive oil) to nearly 1200 μg/g (wheat germ oil). Some of the animal products shown in this table have a range of values given because of seasonal variations due to differences in intakes of the animal from which these foods come.

F. Metabolism

1. Absorption and Transport

Because of its lipophilicity, vitamin E, like the other fat-soluble vitamins, is absorbed via the formation of chylomicrons and their uptake by the lymphatic system. The tocopherols are transported as part of the lipoprotein complex. Absorption is relatively poor and it is unlikely to involve a protein carrier-mediated process. In humans, studies of labeled tocopherol absorption have shown that less than half of the labeled material appears in the lymph and up to 50% of the ingested vitamin may appear in the feces. Efficiency of absorption is enhanced by the presence of food fat in the intestine. The use of water-miscible preparations enhances absorption efficiency, particularly in those individuals whose fat absorption is impaired, i.e., persons with cystic fibrosis or biliary disease. The commercially prepared tocopherol acetate or palmitate loses the acetate or palmitate through the action of a bile-dependent, mucosal-cell esterase prior to absorption. The pancreatic lipases, bile acids, and mucosal-cell esterases are all-important components of the digestion and absorption of vitamin E from food sources. The same processes required for the digestion and absorption of food fat apply here for the tocopherols. Absorption through penetration of the apical plasma membrane of the enterocytes of the brush border is maximal in the jejunum.

There are some species differences in the process in that mammals absorb the vitamin as part of a lipoprotein complex (chylomicrons) into the lymph whereas birds have the vitamin transported directly into the portal blood. In addition, there are gender differences in absorption efficiency: females are more efficient than males. Unlike the food fats (cholesterol and the acylglycerides), hydrolysis is not followed by reesterification in the absorption process. To date, a specific tocopherol transport protein in the blood has not been identified or described. It appears that the tocopherols are bound to all of the lipid-carrying proteins in the blood and lymph. An excellent antioxidant, vitamin E serves this function very well as it is being transported (from enterocyte to target tissue) with those lipids that could be peroxidized and thus require protection. Some cardiovascular researchers have suggested that one important function of vitamin E is to prevent the peroxidation of lipids in the blood which would, in turn, suppress possible endothelial damage to the vascular tree and thus suppress some of the early events in plaque formation. Whether this hypothesis about the role of vitamin E in preventing such degenerative disease is true remains to be proven.

2. Intracellular Transport and Storage

Although no specific transport protein has been found for the tocopherols in blood and lymph, there appears to be such a protein within the cells. A 30-kDA α-tocopherol-binding protein has been found in the hepatic cytosol and another 14.2-kDa one in heart and liver that specifically binds to α-tocopherol and transfers it from liposomes to mitochondria. No doubt we will also find that either this or another low molecular weight protein transfers the vitamin to the nucleus. Having the vitamin in these two organelles protects them from free radical damage. One of the targets of free radicals is the genetic material, DNA, while another is the membrane phospholipid. In either instance, damage to these vital components could be devastating. The smaller of the two binding proteins is similar in size to the intracellular fatty acid-binding protein, FABP. This protein also binds some of the eicosanoids but not α-tocopherol. The other tocopherols (β, γ, etc.) are not bound to the tocopherol-binding proteins to the same extent as α-tocopherol, nor are these isomers retained as well.

Tocopherols are found in all of the cells in the body, with adrenal cells, pituitary cells, platelets, and testicular cells having the highest concentrations. Adipose tissue, muscle, and liver serve as reservoirs and these tissues will become depleted should intake levels be inadequate to meet the need. The rate of depletion with dietary inadequacy varies considerably. Since its main function is as one of several antioxidants, other nutrients which also serve in this capacity can affect vitamin depletion. The intake of β-carotene and ascorbic acid and the polyunsaturated fatty acids can markedly affect the rate of use of α-tocopherol as an antioxidant. Increased intakes of β-carotene and ascorbic acid protect the α-tocopherol from depletion, whereas increased intakes of polyunsaturated fatty acids drive up the need for antioxidants. A further consideration is the intake of selenium. This mineral is an integral part of the glutathione peroxidase system that suppresses free radical production. In selenium-deficient animals, the need for α-tocopherol is increased, and vice versa. The α-tocopherol-deficient animal has a greater need for selenium. In addition, α-tocopherol protects against iron toxicity in another instance of a mineral-vitamin interaction. In this situation, high levels of iron drive up the potential for free radical formation and this can be overcome with increases in vitamin E intake.

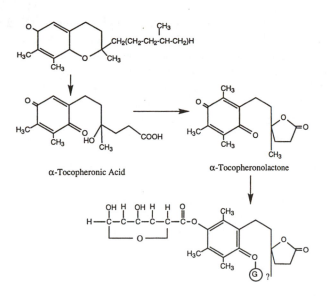

α-Tocopheronic Acid

α-Tocopheronolactone

Figure 15 Excretory pathway for the tocopherols. These compounds are found in the feces.

3. *Catabolism and Excretion*

Upon entry into the cell very little degradation occurs. Usually less than 1% of the ingested vitamin (or its metabolite) appears in the urine. Compounds called Simon's metabolites appear in the urine. These are glucouronates of the parent compound. The degradation and excretion via the intestine is shown in Figure 15.

4. *Function*

As mentioned, the main function of vitamin E is as an antioxidant. This function is shared by β-carotene, ascorbic acid, the selenium-dependent glutathione peroxidase, and the copper-manganese- and magnesium-dependent superoxide dismutases.

Peroxides of fatty acids, amino acids, and proteins are highly reactive materials that can damage cells and tissues. The phospholipids of the membranes within and around the cells are the most vulnerable to this peroxidation because they contain fewer saturated fatty acids than the stored triacylglycerols within the cell. Phospholipids usually contain an unsaturated fatty acid (arachidonate) at carbon 2, a saturated fatty acid at carbon 1, and a phosphate intermediate at carbon 3. In erythrocytes, the selenoenzyme, glutathione peroxidase, protects hemoglobin and the cell membrane from peroxide damage. The enzyme works to maintain glutathione levels, thus regulating the redox state of the cells. In so doing, this enzyme protects hemoglobin and the cell membrane by detoxifying lipid hydroperoxides to less toxic fatty acids, preventing the initial free radical attack on either the hemoglobin protein or the membrane lipids. Vitamin E potentiates glutathione peroxidase action by serving as a free radical scavenger, thus preventing lipid hydroperoxide formation.

Glutathione peroxidase has been found in cells other than red blood cells. It is present in adipose tissue, liver, muscle, and glandular tissue and its activity is complementary to that of catalase, another enzyme which uses peroxide as a substrate. Together, these enzymes and vitamin E protect the integrity of the membranes by preventing the degradation, through oxidation, of the membrane lipids. This function of vitamin E is seen more clearly in animals fed high levels of polyunsaturated fatty acids. As the intake of these acids is increased a larger portion is incorporated into the membrane lipids, which in turn become more vulnerable to oxidation. Unless protected against oxidation, the functionality of the membranes will be impaired and, if uncorrected, the cell will die. Disturbances in the transport of materials across membranes has been shown in liver with respect to cation flux. Liver slices from E-deficient animals lost the ability to regulate sodium/potassium exchange and calcium flux. Investigators have shown a decline in mitochondrial respiration in vitamin E-deficient rats. Such a decline probably represents a decline in the flux of ADP or calcium into the mitochondria to stimulate oxygen uptake by the respiratory chain. Such a decline would permit more oxygen to remain in the cytosol to further stimulate lipid oxidation. In addition to peroxidative damage to the membrane, there is also damage to the DNA, with the possible result of aberrant gene products. Thus, a whole cascade of responses to vitamin E insufficiency can be envisioned. Interestingly, in diseases manifested by an increased hemolysis of the red cells and a decreased ability of the hemoglobin to carry oxygen, red cell vitamin E levels are low. This has been shown in patients with sickle-cell anemia and in patients with cystic fibrosis. In patients with sickle-cell anemia, the low vitamin E level in the erythrocytes is accompanied by an increased level of glutathione peroxidase activity. It has been suggested that the increase in enzyme activity was compensatory to the decrease in vitamin E content.

Vitamin E and zinc have been found to have interacting effects in the protection of skin lipids. In zinc-deficient chicks, supplementation with vitamin E decreased the severity of the zinc deficiency state, suggesting that zinc also may have antioxidant properties or that there may be an interacting effect of zinc with the vitamin.

In addition to the above main function of vitamin E, there are other roles for this substance. One involves eicosanoid synthesis. Thromboxane (TXA_2), a platelet aggregating factor, is synthesized from arachidonic acid (20:4) via a free-radical-mediated reaction. This synthesis is greater in a deficient animal than in an adequately nourished one. Vitamin E enhances prostacyclin formation and inhibits the lipooxygenase and phospholipase reactions. This effect is secondary to the vitamin's role as an antioxidant. As mentioned, phospholipase A_2 is stimulated by lipid peroxides. Other secondary functions also are related to its antioxidant function. Oxidant damage to DNA in bone marrow could explain red blood cell deformation that typifies vitamin E deficiency as well as explain the fragility (due to membrane damage) of these cells. In turn, this would explain why enhanced red cell fragility is a characteristic of the deficient state.

Steroid hormone synthesis as well as spermatogenesis, both processes that are impaired in the deficient animal, could be explained by the damaging effects of free radicals on membranes and/or DNA, which are corrected by the provision of this antioxidant vitamin.

G. Hypervitaminosis E

Even though vitamin E is a fat-soluble vitamin like A and D, there is little evidence that high intakes will result in toxicity in humans. Due to inefficient vitamin uptake by the enterocyte, excess intake is excreted in feces. However, E toxicity has been produced in chickens. It is characterized by growth failure, poor bone calcification, depressed hematocrit, and increased prothrombin times. These symptoms suggest that the excess E interfered with the absorption and/or use of the other fat-soluble vitamins since these symptoms are those of the A, D, and K deficiency states. This suggests that proponents of megadoses of vitamin E as treatment for heart disease, muscular dystrophy, and infertility (amongst other ailments) may unwittingly advocate the development of additional problems associated with an imbalance in fat soluble vitamin intake due to these large E intakes.

H. Deficiency

One of the first deficiency symptoms recorded for the tocopherols was infertility, followed by the discovery that white muscle disease, a peculiar muscle dystrophy, could be reversed if vitamin E

Table 15   Vitamin E Deficiency Disorders

Disorder	Species Affected	Tissue Affected
Reproductive Failure		
Female	Rodents, birds	Embryonic vascular tissue
Male	Rodents, dog, birds, monkey, rabbit	Male gonads
Hepatic necrosis[b]	Rat, pig	Liver
Fibrosis[b]	Chicken, mouse	Pancreas
Hemolysis[a,c]	Rat, chick, premature infant	Erythrocytes
Anemia	Monkey	Bone marrow
Encephalomalacia[a,c]	Chick	Cerebellum
Exudative diathesis[b]	Birds	Vascular system
Kidney degeneration[a,b]	Rodents, monkey, mink	Kidney tabular epithelium
Steatitis[a,c]	Mink, pig, chick	Adipose tissue
Nutritional Myopathies		
Type A muscular dystrophy	Rodents, monkey, duck, mink	Skeletal muscle
Type B white muscle disease[b]	Lamb, calf, kid	Skeletal and heart muscle
Type C myopathy[b]	Turkey	Gizzard, heart
Type D myopathy	Chicken	Skeletal muscle

[a] Increased intake of polyunsaturated acids potentiate deficiency.
[b] Can be reversed by addition of selenium to the diet.
[c] Antioxidants can be substituted for vitamin E to cure condition.

was provided. Later it was recognized that selenium also played a role in the muscle symptom. Listed in Table 15 are the many symptoms attributed to inadequate vitamin E intake. All of these symptoms are related primarily to the level of peroxides in the tissue or to peroxide damage to either the membranes and/or DNA.

I. Recommended Dietary Allowance

Because of the interacting effects of vitamin E with selenium and other antioxidants, the requirement for the vitamin has been difficult to ascertain. It has been estimated that the average adult consumes approximately 15 mg/day but the range of intake is very large. As mentioned earlier, vitamin E requirements are larger when polyunsaturated fat intake is increased. Fortunately, foods containing large supplies of these polyunsaturated fatty acids also contain large quantities of vitamin E. The vitamin E to polyunsaturated fatty acid intake ratio should be 0.6. Table 16 provides the RDA for humans.

IV. VITAMIN K

A. Overview

Even though vitamin K was one of the last fat-soluble vitamins discovered, its existence was suspected as early as 1929. In that year, Henrik Dam was studying cholesterol biosynthesis and observed that chickens fed a semisynthetic sterol-free diet had numerous subcutaneous hemorrhages. Hemorrhages were observed in other tissues as well, and when blood was withdrawn from these birds, it had a prolonged clotting time. At first it was thought that these were symptoms of scurvy in birds, but the addition of vitamin C did not cure the disorder. It was then thought that the hemorrhages characterized the bird's response to a dietary toxin. This hypothesis was also disproved. Finally, it was shown that the inclusion of plant sterols prevented the disease and thus the disease was shown to be a nutrient deficiency.

Table 16   Recommended Dietary Allowances (RDA) for Vitamin E

Group	Age	RDA (mg α-tocopherol equivalents)
Infants	0–6 months	3
	7–12 months	4
Children	1–3	6
	4–6	7
	7–10	7
Males	11–14	10
	15–18	10
	19–24	10
	25–50	10
	51+	10
Females	11–14	8
	15–18	8
	19–24	8
	25–50	8
	51+	8
Pregnancy		10
Lactation	1st 6 months	12
	2nd 6 months	11

Because the condition was characterized by a delayed blood clotting time and because it could be cured or prevented by the inclusion of the nonsaponifiable sterol fraction of a lipid extract of alfalfa, it was named the antihemorrhagic factor. Dam proposed that it be called vitamin K. The letter K was chosen from the German word, koagulation.

B. Structure and Nomenclature

Subsequent to its recognition as an essential micronutrient, vitamin K was isolated from alfalfa and from fish meal. The compounds isolated from these two sources were not identical, so one was named K_1 and the other K_2. Almquist was the first to show that the vitamin could be synthesized by bacteria. He discovered that putrefied fish meal contained more of the vitamin than nonputrefied fish meal. It was also learned that bacteria in the intestine of both the rat and the chicken synthesized the vitamin, thus ensuring a good supply of the vitamin if coprophagy (eating feces) was permitted.

These early studies thus provided the reason to suspect that there was more than one form of the vitamin. A large number of compounds, all related to a 2-methyl-1,4-naphthaquinone possess vitamin K activity (Figure 16). Compounds isolated from plants have a phytyl moiety at position 3 and are members of the K_1 family of compounds. Phylloquinone [2-methyl-3-phytyl-1,4-naph-thaquinone (II)] is the most important member of this family. The K vitamins are identified by their family and by the length of the side chain attached at position 3. The shorthand designation uses the letter K with a subscript to indicate family, and a superscript to indicate the side-chain length. Thus, K_2^{20} indicates a member of the family of compounds isolated from animal sources having a 20-carbon side chain. The character of the side chain determines whether a compound is a member of the K_1 or K_2 family. K_1 compounds have a saturated side chain whereas K_2 compounds have an unsaturated side chain. Chain lengths of the K_1 and K_2 vitamins can vary from 5 to 35 carbons.

A third group of compounds is the K_3 family. These compounds lack the side chain at carbon 3. Menadione is the parent compound name and it is a solid crystalline material menadione sodium bisulfite (a salt), as shown in Figure 16. Other salts are also available. These salts are water soluble and thus have great use in diet formulations or mixed animal feeds. Clinically useful is menadiol sodium diphosphate. The use of this compound must be very carefully monitored as overdoses can

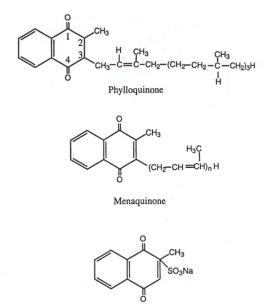

Phylloquinone

Menaquinone

Menadione Sodium Bisulfite

Figure 16 Structures of vitamin K_1 (phylloquinone), K_2 (menaquinone), and K_3 (menadione, a synthetic vitamin precursor that is converted to K_2 by the intestinal flora).

result in hyperbilirubinemia and jaundice. These K_3 compounds can be synthesized in the laboratory. When consumed as a dietary ingredient, the quinone structure is converted by the intestinal flora to a member of the K_2 family.

There are several structural requirements for vitamin activity: there must be a methyl group at carbon 2 and a side chain at carbon 3, and the benzene ring must be unsubstituted. The chain length can vary; however, optimal activity is observed in compounds having a 20-carbon side chain. K_1 and K_2 compounds with similar side chains have similar vitamin activities.

The vitamin can exist in either the cis or trans configuration. All-*trans*-phylloquinone is the naturally occurring form whereas synthetic phylloquinone is a mixture of the cis and trans forms.

C. Biopotency

The various compounds with vitamin activity are not equivalent with respect to potency as a vitamin. The most potent compound of the phylloquinone series is the one with a 20-member side chain. Compounds having fewer or greater numbers of carbons are less active. Table 17 provides this comparison. The most potent compound in the menaquinone series is the one with a 25-member unsaturated side chain.

D. Chemical and Physical Properties

Phylloquinone ($K_1{}^{20}$) is a yellow viscous oil. The physical state of menaquinone ($K_2{}^{20}$) depends on its side-chain length. If the side chain is 5 or 10 carbons long it is an oil, if longer it is a solid. Menadione (K_3) is a solid. All three families of compounds are soluble in fat solvents. Menadione can be made water soluble by converting it to a sodium salt. All the vitamin K compounds are stable to air and moisture but unstable to ultraviolet light. They are also stable in acid solutions but are destroyed by alkali and reducing agents. These compounds possess a distinctive absorption spectra because of the presence of naphthaquinone ring system.

Table 17   Comparative Potency of Various Members of the Phylloquinone and Menaquinone Families of Vitamin K

Side Chain Length (# carbons)	Family	
	Phylloquinone	Menaquinone
10	10	15
15	30	40
20	100	100
25	80	120
30	50	100
35	—	70

Note: Phylloquinone, K_1^{20}, is given a value of 100 and the remaining compounds are compared to this compound with reference to its biological function in promoting clot formation.

E. Chemical Assays

Many different assays have been proposed for vitamin K but they all face the same problem: vitamin K is normally present in very low concentrations and numerous interfering substances such as quinones, chlorophyll, and carotenoid pigments are usually present.

Several colorimetric methods have been developed. One of the first, known as the Dam-Karrer reaction, is the measurement of the reddish-brown color that forms when sodium ethylate reacts with vitamin K. In another method, menadione, as the sodium sulfite, is reduced and then titrated to a green endpoint with ceric sulfate. In yet another, menadione is converted to its 2,4-dinitrophenyl-hydrazone when heated with 2,4-dinitrophenylhydrazine in ethanol. An excess of ammonia causes the solution to become blue-green with an absorption maxima at 635 nm.

As mentioned earlier, the K vitamins have a characteristic ultraviolet absorption spectrum. If the material is sufficiently pure, it can be identified and quantitated. Vitamin K has also been quantitated by a thin-layer and gas chromatographic technique. The menadione content of foodstuffs as been determined with high performance liquid chromatography (HPLC). This technique has been used to determine the blood and tissue levels of the vitamin in humans. As little as 0.5 mmol/l has been detected in the blood of newborns and adults. Regardless of the assay method used, the analytical procedure should include protection of the samples from light. All of the vitamers are sensitive to ultraviolet light and will decompose if exposed. Care also should be exercised with respect to pH. The K vitamers are sensitive to alkali but are relatively stable to oxidants and heat. They can be safely extracted using vacuum distillation.

F. Bioassays

One of the earliest biotechniques for measuring vitamin K content of foods uses the chick. This method is sensitive to 0.1 μg phylloquinone per gram of diet. In this assay, newly hatched chicks are fed a K-free diet for 10 days and thus made deficient. They are then fed a supplement containing the assay food. The prothrombin level of the blood is then compared with a standard curve resulting from the feeding of known amounts of phylloquinone.

Instead of measuring prothrombin concentration, plasma prothrombin times can be measured. Prothrombin time is an indirect and inverse measurement of the amount of prothrombin in the blood: an increase in prothrombin time signifies a decrease in prothrombin concentration. The technique commonly used is a modification of the one-stage method developed by Quick. Blood removed from a patient or animal is immediately oxalated; oxalate binds the calcium and prevents prothrombin from changing into thrombin. Later, an excess of thromboplastic substance (obtained from rabbit or rat brain) and calcium are added to the plasma and the clotting time of the plasma is noted; this time is the prothrombin time. The normal prothrombin time is approximately 12 s; however, the actual time depends to a large extent on the exact procedure employed. To be valid, the "pro time" of a vitamin K-deficient animal must be compared to that of a normal individual.

G. Biosynthesis

Although not too much is known about the biosynthesis of phylloquinone in plants, apparently the synthesis occurs at the same time as that of chlorophyll. The vitamin concentration is richest in that part of the plant that is photosynthetically active: carrot tops are a good source, but not the root; peas sprouted in light contain more than peas sprouted in the dark; and the inner leaves of cabbage have about one-fourth less vitamin than the outer leaves.

Menaquinone is synthesized by intestinal bacteria in the distal small intestine and in the colon. Martius and Esser found that chicks fed a vitamin K-deficient diet and then given menadione (K_3) for long periods of time will synthesize menaquinone (K_2^{20}). Apparently, this synthesis is more complete at small physiological doses than at high doses, such as are used when vitamin K is given as an antidote to dicumarol. Because of intestinal biosynthesis, the experimental animals used in K deficiency studies should be reared in cages that prevent coprophagy.

All of the natural forms of the K vitamins can be stored in the liver. Menadione is not stored as such but is stored as its conversion product, menaquinone. Menadione metabolism by the liver occurs at the expense of the redox state. When menadione is metabolized by Ca^{2+}-loaded mitochondria, there is a rapid oxidation and loss of pyridine nucleotides and a decrease in ATP level. The effects of menadione on Ca^{2+} homeostasis are probably initiated by NAD(P)H: (quinone-acceptor) oxido-reductase. Since it is an oxidant, large amounts of menadione have been shown to alter the surface structure and reduce the thiol content of the liver cell. Because of these changes, menadione is cytotoxic in large quantities. This may explain the induction of jaundice in the newborn of mothers given large doses of menadione just prior to delivery. This once popular obstetric practice has been discontinued.

Using labeled vitamin, it was found that rats stored the vitamin in the liver — 50% of the vitamin was found bound to the endoplasmic reticulum. When cis and trans forms were compared, the biologically active trans isomer was found in the rough membrane fraction (endoplasmic reticulum) whereas the inactive cis isomer was found in the mitochondria.

H. Antagonists, Antivitamins

Blood coagulation can be inhibited by a variety of agents that are clinically useful. Oxalates, heparin, and sodium citrate are but a few of these. These compounds work by binding one or more of the essential ingredients for clot formation. One group of anticoagulants are those which act by antagonizing vitamin K in its role in prothrombin carboxylation. These compounds, shown in Figure 17, are members of a quinone family of compounds. The first of these is 3,3'-methyl-bis-(4-hydroxycoumarin), called dicumarol. It was isolated from spoiled sweet clover and was shown to cause a hemorrhagic disease in cattle. Dicumarol has been found very useful in the clinical setting as an anticoagulant in people at risk for coronary events. It is marketed as Coumarin. Another use is as a rodenticide, marketed as Warfarin®. The structure of Warfarin is also shown in Figure 17. A third group of antivitamin K compounds are the 2-substituted 1,3-indandiones. These are useful as rodenticides but because they can cause liver damage they are not used in the clinical setting.

I. Sources

Phylloquinone serves as the major source of dietary vitamin K in humans. Alfalfa has long been recognized as being most plentifully supplied with vitamin K. In general, studies of the vitamin K content of common foods, as determined by the chick bioassay method, reveal that green

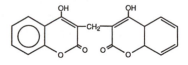

Dicumarol
(Coumarin)

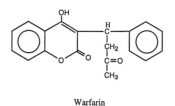

Warfarin

2 phenyl-1,3-indandione

Figure 17 Structures of several compounds that are potent vitamin K antagonists.

leafy vegetables contain large quantities of vitamin K, meats and dairy products intermediate quantities, and fruits and cereals small quantities.

J. Absorption

Under normal physiologic conditions, most nutrients are absorbed before they reach the colon. In large measure, this is true of the K vitamins. However, vitamin K can be absorbed very well by the colon. This is an advantage to the individual since it ensures the uptake of K that is synthesized in the lower intestinal tract by the gut flora. The mechanism by which the K vitamins are absorbed, and the rate at which this occurs, is species dependent. Species such as the chicken, which have a rapid gut passage time, absorb the vitamin more rapidly than do species such as the rat which have a long gut passage time. The absorption of K_1 and K_2 analogs is generally thought to occur via an active, energy-dependent transport process, whereas K_3 (menadione) analogs are absorbed by passive diffusion.

The absorption of K_1 and K_2 requires a protein carrier and, again, species differ in the saturability of the carrier. In rats, the carrier is saturated at far lower vitamin concentrations than occurs in chickens. These differences in carrier saturability led early investigators to suggest that vitamin K absorption was a passive process. Subsequent studies using *in vitro* techniques or using labeled vitamin given *in vivo* showed that absorption was indeed an active process.

In contrast to the absorption of phylloquinone and the menaquinones, menadione appears to be absorbed primarily in the large intestine where the gut bacteria have converted it to a form with a side chain. Without the side chain the absorption of K_3 is a passive process. Biosynthesis by the gut flora is an adequate source of biologically active vitamin K under normal conditions, thus making it difficult to obtain a K deficiency in humans and experimental animals. However, under conditions of stress, such as hypoprothrombinemia induced by coumarin-type anticoagulants, intestinal synthesis does not produce enough of the vitamin to overcome the effects of the drug. Proof of the importance of colonic absorption is seen in the improvement in prothrombin times in chicks and infants when given the vitamin rectally. Excessive intakes of menadione can be harmful due to the quinone structure, which is an oxidant. Quinones can uncouple oxidative phosphorylation.

Absorption of the K vitamins is dependent on the presence of lipid which stimulates the release of bile and pancreatic lipases. As lipids are absorbed into the lymphatic system, so too are the K vitamers. If there is any impairment in the lipid absorption process, less vitamin K will be absorbed. For example, patients with biliary obstruction have been shown to absorb substantially less vitamin K than normal subjects.

Phylloquinone absorption shows a diurnal rhythm. In rats, the highest rate of absorption is at midnight; the lowest is at 6 a.m. This coincides with the rats' eating pattern. The rat is a nocturnal feeder consuming most of its food between 8 p.m. and midnight. Estrogen enhances the absorption of phylloquinone for both intact and castrated males. Castrated rats are more susceptible to uncontrolled hemorrhage due to coumarin than are intact female rats. Female rats also synthesize more prothrombin than do male rats.

K. Metabolism and Function

Historically, vitamin K has been regarded as a vitamin with a single function: the coagulation of blood. While the concept of this function is true, we now know that it serves as an essential cosubstrate in the post-translational oxidative carboxylation of glutamic acid residues in a small group of proteins, most of which are involved in blood coagulation. These proteins are the blood clotting factors II, VII, IX, and X, a calcium-binding bone protein (bone Gla protein), osteocalcin, and plasma proteins C and S.

Blood coagulation is not a single one-step phenomenon. Rather, it involves several phases which must interdigitate if a clot is to be formed. Four phases have been identified: (1) the formation of thromboplastin, (2) the activation of thromboplastin, (3) the formation of thrombin, and (4) the formation of fibrin. Following injury, a blood clot is formed when the blood protein fibrinogen is transformed into an insoluble network of fibers (fibrin) by the reaction cascade illustrated in Figure 18. The change of fibrinogen to fibrin (phase 4) is catalyzed by thrombin which itself must arise from prothrombin. Prior to activation by the protease factor Xa, both the prothrombin and the protease are adsorbed onto the phospholipids of the damaged cells by way of calcium bridges. Without carboxylation, these bridges will not form and the adherence or adsorption of the prothrombin to the phospholipids of the injured cell walls does not take place. The phospholipids are not only important to the binding of prothrombin to the injured cell wall, but are also important determinants of carboxylase activity. Phosphatidyl choline has been found to be an essential component of the carboxylase enzyme system. When depleted of phospholipid the enzyme loses activity; when repleted, its activity is restored. The synthesis of thrombin from prothrombin (phase 3) is catalyzed by prothrombinase, active preaccelerin, and the phospholipid, cephalin. These factors, in turn, are activated by a combination of blood and tissue convertins which represent or reflect the synthesis and activation of the thromboplastin complex (phases 1 and 2). The synthesis and activation of the thromboplastin complex requires several factors which have been named and identified. These factors, studied by different groups, were given different names, and these different names lent considerable confusion to the understanding of the coagulation process. To clarify the literature, it was decided by the International Committee for Standardization of the Nomenclature of Blood Clotting Factors to recommend the use of a numerical system for designating the various factors. This numbering system is given in Table 18 along with some of the other names in use and the function of each in the coagulation process. Note that four of the factors are proteins whose synthesis is dependent on vitamin K. These proteins, prothrombin (factor II), proconvertin (factor VII), the Christmas factor (factor IX), and the Stuart-Prower factor (factor X) are all calcium dependent. That is, calcium ions must be present for their activation and participation in the coagulation cascade (Figure 18). Note, too, that the four proteins which are vitamin K dependent are synthesized in the liver, hence the reason why the liver concentrates and stores this vitamin.

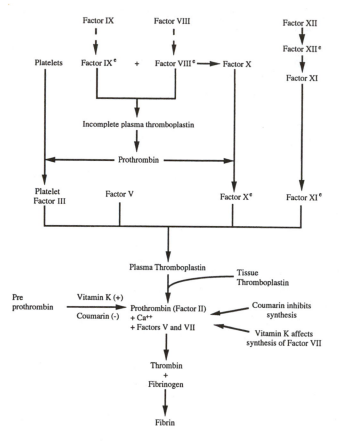

Figure 18   Formation of a clot.

The function of vitamin K is as a cosubstrate in the post-translational oxidative carboxylation of proteins at selected glutamic acid residues. This is a cyclic process (Figure 19). As the vitamin serves as a cosubstrate, it is metabolized by the hepatic microsomes. There are two pathways for vitamin K reduction: (1) the epoxi-quinone cycle, and (2) DT diaphorase and microsomal dehydrogenase. The latter pathway is important for counteracting coumarin toxicity. The metabolism of vitamin K is dependent on adequate intakes of niacin and riboflavin, which are components of the redox systems important in the transfer of reducing equivalents. Vitamin K is reduced to the hydroquinone (vitamin KH_2) with NADH as the coenzyme (NADH is a niacin-containing coenzyme). The K quinone reacts with CO_2 and O_2 in the microsomal carboxylation of glutamyl residues and is then oxidized to form an epoxide. The epoxide is converted back to the quinone form by an epoxide reductase. The reductase is a two-component cytosolic enzyme which catalyzes the reduction of the vitamin K epoxide using a thiol reductant (dithiothreitol *in vitro*) as either a primary or secondary source of reducing equivalents. Warfarin® (coumarin), an antivitamin that binds to the epoxidase and reductase, interferes with both the reduction of vitamin K to the hydroquinone and the conversion of the epoxide back to the original compound.

Vitamin K epoxide can substitute for vitamin K in glutamate carboxylation and prothrombin synthesis. This similarity is probably due to the unhindered conversion of the epoxide to the hydroquinone. The epoxidation reaction is coupled to the carboxylation of the glutamic acid residues protruding from peptides having clusters of this amino acid. Aspartyl residues can also be carboxylated. The epoxidation reaction can be coupled to the oxidation of other peptides as well; however, only those having the clusters of glutamic acid will be oxidatively carboxylated. Unless the proteins

Table 18   Blood Clotting Factors

Factor	Name	Function	Remarks
I	Fibrinogen	Provides the structural network upon which clot is formed.	
II	Prothrombin	Precursor of thrombin, a proteolytic enzyme which causes fibrinogen to lose one or more peptides and polymerize.	Vitamin K dependent, synthesized in liver.
III	Thromboplastin	Serves to stimulate prothrombin conversion to thrombin.	Not a single compound. Includes factors IX, XI, XII, X, V.
IV	Calcium	Combines with prothrombin in presence of agents.	Oxalate acts as an anticoagulant by binding Ca^{++}.
V	Labile factor proaccelerin accelerator (Ac) globule	Has thromboplastic activity. Released by collagen and not ADP; proceeds normally when prostaglandin synthesis is inhibited.	Disappears when plasma is heated or stored with oxalate. In the activated form, may function as the Ka receptor on the platelet membrane.
VII	Proconvertin serum prothrombin conversion accelerator (SPCA), cothromboplastin, autoprothrombin I.	Has thromboplastic activity.	Vitamin K dependent.
VIII	Antihemophilic factor, antihemophilic globulin(AHG)	Activates factor X; associated with platelet membranes. May have a role in the adherence of platelets to subendothelium.	Deficiency of this factor is the cause of the classic form of hemophilia A. The vonWillebrand factor is a carrier of factor VIII.
IX	Plasma thromboplastic component (PTC), Christmas factor	Stimulates conversion of prothrombin to thrombin.	Vitamin K-dependent deficiency results in hemophilia or Christmas disease, named after first patient to have disease.
X	Stuart-Prower factor	Stimulates conversion of prothrombin to thrombin.	Vitamin K-dependent glycoprotein. Gene for human factor X is essentially identical with that for factor IX and Protein C[162a].
XI	Plasma thromboplastin antecedent (PTA)	Has thromboplastic activity.	Patients with PTA are mild hemophiliacs.
XII	Hageman factor	Has thromboplastic activity.	Deficiency does not result in hemophilia.
XIII	Laki-Lorand factor (LLF) Fibrin stabilizing factor	Stabilizes fibrin network; is a proenzyme in the plasma activated by thrombin and which catalyzes the formation of covalent lysyl bonds between the chains of fibrin.	
	Platelet thromboplastic factor	Catalyzes formation of platelet factor.	Appears when platelets disintegrate.

From Walsh, P.N., *Fed. Proc.*, 40:2086, 1981. With permission.

are carboxylated they are unable to bind calcium. For example, the precursor of prothrombin, acarboxyprothrombin has, within the first 33 amino acids at the amino terminal end, 10 tightly clustered glutamic acid residues and binds less than 1 mol of calcium per mole of protein. When carboxylated, the glutamic acid residues are converted to carboxyglutamic acid residues, and now each mole of the prothrombin protein can bind 10 to 12 mol of calcium. Thus, the carboxylated glutamic acid-rich region serves an important function in clot formation.

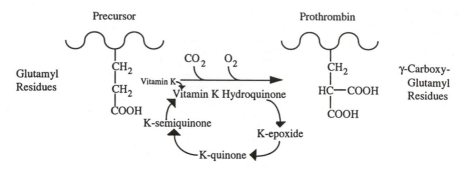

Figure 19 The vitamin K-dependent carboxylation reaction coupled with the epoxi-quinone cycle.

Proteins other than those involved in the coagulation process have also been shown to be vitamin K dependent. Carboxylated proteins have been found in bone matrix. Up to 20% of the noncollagenous proteins (or 1 to 2% of the total bone protein) is a carboxylated protein called osteocalcin. Osteocalcin is synthesized in bone tissue. Bone microsomes are responsible for the post-translational vitamin K-dependent oxidative carboxylation reaction. The synthesis of osteo-calcin is highest during rapid growth periods and coincides with detectable bone mineralization. The osteocalcin appears prior to mineralization and, like the blood coagulation proteins, shows a remarkable avidity for calcium. It will also bind (in order of preference after calcium) magnesium, strontium, barium, and lanthanide. In addition to its ability to bind divalent ions, osteocalcin also binds strongly to hydroxyapatite, the major calcium phosphate salt of the bone. Thus, osteocalcin serves a major role in bone mineralization and this role can not be performed unless its glutamic acid residues have been carboxylated.

Studies of embryonic chicks treated with Warfarin® showed a decrease in both osteocalcin and mineralization. Warfarin-treated animals, in contrast, do not show this same effect; osteocalcin levels are low but bone mineralization is normal. Because the overwhelming effects of vitamin K deficiency induced via Warfarin treatment results in lethal bleeding, the secondary effect on bone mineralization is not observed unless embryonic tissues are used. Evidence of Warfarin injury has been reported in humans. Mothers consuming coumarin during their pregnancy have given birth to infants having defective bone development such as stippled epiphyses, "saddle" nose, punctate calcifications, and frontal bossing.

Another vitamin K-dependent protein involved in the regulation of bone calcium homeostasis is bone Gla protein (BGP). It is a 49-residue protein secreted by osteosarcoma cells having an osteoblastic phenotype and appears in calcifying tissues 1 to 2 weeks after mineral deposition, and at the approximate time that the maturation of bone mineral to hydroxyapatite is thought to occur. The synthesis and secretion of BGP from osteosarcoma cells is regulated by vitamin D. The renal cortex also contains a microsomal vitamin K-dependent oxidative carboxylation system. Its function is to produce a γ-carboxy-glutamic acid-rich protein which serves to bind calcium. It is located in the renal tubule and may function importantly in the conservation of calcium. Unfortunately, these proteins may be entirely too active in calcium uptake and kidney stones may result. Renal stones have been found to contain a unique carboxylated peptide in addition to calcium oxalate. Whether this peptide was responsible for the stone accumulation or was attracted to it because of its high calcium content is not known.

In summary, then, vitamin K functions as a cosubstrate in the production of unique calcium-binding proteins in the blood, bone, and kidney. Further research may reveal the presence of other K-dependent proteins which serve to translocate the calcium ion from one cellular compartment to another. However, evidence of their existence is not now in hand.

In addition to its function as described above, vitamin K serves a role in the inhibition of the carcinogenic properties of benzopyrene. Menadione inhibits aryl hydrocarbon hydroxylase, thus reducing the levels of carcinogenic and mutagenic metabolites in the cell with a resultant reduction in tumor formation. Vitamin K_1 and K_2 have the opposite effect. The different effects probably relate to the previously described effects of these forms on redox state, calcium ion status, and ATP production — all of which are involved in tumorogenesis.

L. Deficiency

Due to the fact that intestinal synthesis of vitamin K usually provides sufficient amounts of the vitamin to the body, primary vitamin K deficiency is rare. However, secondary deficiency states can develop as a result of biliary disease which results in an impaired absorption of the vitamin. Deficiency can also occur as a result of long-term broad-spectrum antibiotic therapy, which may kill the vitamin K-synthesizing intestinal flora, or as a result of anticoagulant therapy using coumarin (Warfarin®) which, as shown in the previous section, interferes with the metabolism and function of the vitamin. The primary characteristic of the deficiency state is a delayed or prolonged clotting time. Deficient individuals may have numerous bruises indicative of subcutaneous hemorrhaging in response to injury. A very sensitive test for deficiency status has been developed. This test uses the measurement of under-γ-carboxylated prothrombin as determined by immunochemical detection and by a decreased urinary excretion of γ-carboxyglutamic acid. This test could be quite useful in assessing not only vitamin K status but also the efficacy of anticoagulant therapy. The objective of such therapy is to slightly impair clotting to prevent vascular occlusions but yet avoid hemorrhages. However, there may be consequences to such therapy.

In women, osteoporosis as well as atherosclerosis are major health concerns. The former has been thought to be related to the loss of estrogen action on bone homeostasis, while the latter involves calcium deposits in the fatty streaks of the vascular system. Although these two conditions may be independent, there is presently some thought that they are not. Indeed, they may be linked via the action or loss of action of vitamin K in the maintenance of calcium homeostasis. Some Dutch workers have shown that markers of bone formation increase whereas bone resorption markers decrease with the administration of pharmacological doses of vitamin K. In addition, these scientists have reported the presence of abdominal aorta atherosclerotic calcifications associated with marginal vitamin K status, as well as reduced bone mass. These observations suggest that there is a relationship between the two processes.

The bone Gla protein is similar to matrix Gla protein (MGP) which inhibits bone mineral resorption as well as inhibits vascular mineralization. Likely, MGP synthesis is vitamin K dependent, and likely its deficiency is the coordinator of the two disorders, osteoporosis and atherosclerosis.

Newborn infants, because they have not yet established their K-synthesizing intestinal flora, have delayed coagulation times. For many years, it was common practice to give the mother an injection of menadione just prior to delivery in order to rectify the newborn's problem. However, it then became apparent that this prophylactic therapy was having no effect on the infant with respect to prothrombin time and, in addition, some infants became jaundiced with this treatment. As a result, vitamin K administration to women just prior to delivery is no longer a routine practice in obstetrics.

M. Recommended Dietary Allowance

Although the gut flora can usually synthesize sufficient vitamin to meet the nutritional need, the Food and Nutrition Board of the National Academy of Science, National Research Council has made recommendations for a daily intake. These are shown in Table 19.

Table 19   Recommended Dietary Allowances (RDA) for Vitamin K

Group	Age	RDA (µg)
Infants	0–6 months	5
	7–12 months	10
Children	1–3	15
	4–6	20
	7–10	30
Males	11–14	45
	15–18	65
	19–24	70
	25–50	80
	51+	80
Females	11–14	45
	15–18	55
	19–24	60
	25–50	65
	51+	65
Pregnancy	—	65
Lactation	—	65

SUPPLEMENTAL READINGS

Vitamin A

Berni, R., Clerici, M., Malpeli, G., Cleris, L., and Formelli, F. 1993. Retinoids: in vitro interaction with retinol-binding protein and influence on plasma retinol, *FASEB J.,* 7:1179-1184.

Chertow, B.S., Blanar, W.S., Rajan, N., Primerano, D.A., Meda, P., Cirulli, V., Krozowski, Z., Smith, R., and Cordle, M.B. 1993. Retinoic acid receptor, cytosolic retinol binding and retinoic acid binding protein mRNA transcripts and proteins in rat insulin-secreting cells, *Diabetes,* 42:1109-14.

Chien, K.R., Zhu, H., Knowlton, K.U., Miller-Hance, W., van Bilsen, M., O'Brien, T.X., and Evans, S.M. 1993. Transcriptional regulation during cardiac growth and development, *Annu. Rev. Physiol.,* 55:77-95.

Chytil, F. and Haq, R. 1990. Vitamin A mediated gene expression, *Crit. Rev. Eukaryotic Gene Expression,* 1:61-73.

DeLuca, U.H. and Sandell, L.J. 1996. Retinoids and their receptors in differentiation, embryogenesis and neoplasia, *FASEB J.,* 5:2924-2933.

Dietz, U.H. and Sandell, L.J. 1996. Cloning of a retinoic acid sensitive mRNA expressed in cartilage and during chondrogenesis, *J. Biol. Chem.,* 271:3311-3316.

Escatante-Alcalde, D., Recillas-Targa, F., Hernandez-Garcia, D., Castro-Obregon, S., Terao, M., Garattini, E., and Covarrubias, L. 1996. Retinoic acid and methylation cis-regulatory elements control the mouse tissue non specific alkaline phosphatase gene expression, *Mech. Dev.,* 57:21-32.

Hathcock, J.N., Hatten, D.G., Jenkins, M.Y., McDonald, J.T., Sundaresan, P.R., and Welkening, V.L. 1990. Evaluation of vitamin A toxicity, *Am. J. Clin. Nutr.,* 52:183-202.

Haq, R., Pfahl, M., and Chytil, F. 1991. Retinoic acid affects the expression of nuclear retinoic acid receptors and tissues of retinol deficient rats, *Proc. Natl. Acad. Sci. U.S.A.,* 88:8272-8276.

Jump, D.B., Lepar, G.J., and MacDougald, O.A. 1993. Retinoic acid regulation of gene expression in adipocytes. In: *Nutrition and Gene Expression,* Berdanier, C.D. and Hargrove, J.L., Eds., CRC Press, Boca Raton, FL, 431-454.

Keller, H., Dreyer, C., Medin, J., Mahfoude, A., Ozato, K., and Wahli, W. 1993. Fatty acids and retinoids control lipid metabolism through activation of peroxisome proliferator activated receptor retinoid X receptor heterodimers, *Proc. Natl. Acad. Sci. U.S.A.,* 90:2160-2164.

Lolly, R.N. and Lee, R.H. 1990. Cyclic GMP and photoreceptor function, *FASEB J.,* 4:3001-3008.

Mano, H., Ozawa, T., Takeyama, K.-I., Yoshizawa, Y., Kojima, R., Kato, S., and Masushige, S. 1993. Thyroid hormone affects the gene expression of retinoid X receptors in the adult rat, *Biochem. Biophys. Res. Commun.*, 191:943-949.

Newcomer, M.E. 1995. Retinoid-binding proteins: structural determinants important for function, *FASEB J.*, 9:229-239.

Olson, J.A. 1991. Vitamin A. In: *Handbook of Vitamins,* Machlin, L.J., Ed., Marcel Dekker, New York, pp. 1-57.

Olson, J.A. 1994. Hypervitaminosis A: contemporary scientific issues, *J. Nutr.*, 124:14615-14665.

Olson, J.A. and Krinsky, N.I. 1995. The colorful fascinating world of the carotenoids: Important physiologic modulators, *FASEB J.*, 9:1547-1550.

Ong, D. 1984. A novel retinol binding protein, *J. Biol. Chem.*, 259:1476-1482.

Rando, R.R. 1991. Membrane phospholipids as an energy source in the operation of the visual cycle, *Biochemisty,* 30:595-602.

Soprano, D.R., Harnish, D.C., Soprano, K.J., Kochhar, D.M., and Jiang, H. 1993. Correlations of RAR isoforms and cellular retinoid-binding proteins mRNA levels with retinoid-induced teratogenesis, *J. Nutr.*, 123:367-371.

Ross, A.C. 1993. Cellular metabolism and activation of retinoids: roles of cellular retinoid binding proteins, *FASEB J.*, 7:317-327.

Suruga, K., Suzuki, R., Goda, T., and Takase, S. 1995. Unsaturated fatty acids regulate gene expression of cellular retinol binding protein type II in rat jejunum, *J. Nutr.*, 125:2039-2044.

Wolf, G. 1991. The intracellular vitamin A binding proteins: an overview of their functions, *Nutr. Rev.*, 49:1-12.

Vitamin D

Beatty, M.M., Lee, E.Y., and Glauert, H.P. 1993. Influence of dietary calcium and vitamin D on colon epithelial cell proliferation and 1,2-dimethylhydrazine-induced colon carcinogenesis in rats fed high fat diets, *J. Nutr.*, 123:144-152.

Bell, N.H. 1995. Editorial: Vitamin D metabolism, aging and bone loss, *J. Clin. Endocrinol. Metab.*, 80:1051.

Brostrom, M.A. and Brostrom, C.O. 1993. Calcium homeostasis, endoplasmic reticular function and the regulation of mRNA translation in mammalian cells. In: *Nutrition and Gene Expression,* Berdanier, C.D. and Hargrove, J.L., Eds., CRC Press, Boca Raton, FL, pp. 117-142.

Bygrave, F.L. and Roberts, H.R. 1995. Regulation of cellular calcium through signaling cross-talk involves an intricate interplay between the actions of receptors, g-proteins and second messengers, *FASEB J.*, 9:1297-1303.

Gill, R.K. and Christakos, S. 1993. Vitamin D dependent calcium binding protein, calbindin-D: regulation of gene expression. In: *Nutrition and Gene Expression* Berdanier, C.D. and Hargrove, J.L., Eds., CRC Press, Boca Raton, FL, pp. 377-390.

Ishimura, E., Shoji, S., Koyama, H., Inaba, M., Nishizawa, Y., and Morii, H. 1994. Presence of gene expression of vitamin D receptor and 24-hydroxylase OK cells, *FEBS Lett.*, 337:48-51.

Jaaskelainen, T., Itkonen, A., and Maenpaa, P.H. 1995. Retinoid X receptor α independent binding of vitamin D receptor to its response element from human osteocalcin gene, *Eur. J. Biochem.*, 228:222-228.

Lian, J.B. and Stein, G.S. 1993. Vitamin D regulation of osteoblast growth and development. In: *Nutrition and Gene Expression,* Berdanier, C.D. and Hargrove, J.L., Eds., CRC Press, Boca Raton, FL, pp. 391-430.

Nishikawa, J.-I., Kitaura, M., Imagawa, M., and Nishihara, T. 1995. Vitamin D receptor contains multiple dimerization interfaces that are functionally different, *Nucleic Acids Res.*, 23:606-611.

Perez, A., Diaz de Barboza, G., Pereira, R., and Tolosa de Talamoni, N. 1995. Vitamin D affects Krebs cycle NAD-linked oxidoreductases from chick intestinal mucosa, *Biochem. Mol. Biol. Int.*, 36:537-544.

Pols, H.A.P., Birkenhager, J.C., and Van Leeiwan, J.P.T.M. 1994. Vitamin D analogues: from molecule to clinical application, *Clin. Endocrinol.*, 40:285-291.

Ray, R. 1996. Molecular recognition in vitamin D-binding protein, *Proc. Soc. Exp. Biol. Med.*, 212:305-312.

Whitfield, G.K., Hsieh, J.-C., Jurutka, P.W., Selznick, S.H., Haussler, C.A., Macdonald, P.N., and Haussler, M.R. 1995. Genomic actions of 1,25 dihydroxyvitamin D_3, *J. Nutr.*, 125:16990S-1694S.

Vitamin E

Buettner, G.R. 1993. The pecking order of free radicals and antioxidants: lipid peroxidation, α-tocopherol and ascorbate, *Arch. Biochem. Biophys.*, 300:535-543.

Burton, G.W. and Traber, M.G. 1990. Vitamin E: antioxidant activity, biokinetics, bioavailability, *Annu. Rev. Nutr.*, 10:357-382.

Chen, H.W., Hendrich, S., and Cook, L.R. 1994. Vitamin E deficiency increases serum thromboxane A$_2$, platelet arachidonate and lipid peroxidation in male Sprague-Dawley rats, *Prostaglandins, Leukotrienes EFA*, 51:11-17.

Dutta-Roy, A.K., Gordon, M.G., Campbell, F.M., Duthrie, G.G., and James, W.P.T. 1994. Vitamin E requirements, transport, and metabolism: role of α-tocopherol-binding proteins, *J. Nutr. Biochem.*, 5:562-570.

Hodis, H.N., Mack, W.J., Labree, L., Cashin-Hemphill, L., Sevanian, A., Johnson, R., and Azen, S.P. 1994. Serial coronary angiographic evidence that antioxidant vitamin intake reduces progression of coronary artery atherosclerosis, *J. Am. Med. Assoc.*, 273:1849-1854.

Jialal, I. and Grundy, S.M. 1992. Effect of dietary supplementation with α-tocopherol on the oxidative modification of low density lipoproteins, *J. Lipid Res.*, 33:899-906.

Meydani, M., Meydani, S.N., and Blumberg, J.B. 1993. Modulation by dietary vitamin E and selenium of clotting whole blood thromboxane A$_2$ and aortic prostacyclin synthesis in rats, *J. Nutr. Biochem.*, 4:322-326.

Morel, D.W., Leera-Moya, M., and Friday, K.E. 1994. Treatment of cholesterol fed rabbits with dietary vitamins E and C inhibits lipoprotein oxidation but not development of atherosclerosis, *J. Nutr.*, 124:2123-2130.

Nair, P.P., Judd, J.T., Berlin, E., Taylor, P.R., Shami, S., Sainz, E., and Bhagavan, H.N. 1993. Dietary fish oil-induced changes in the distribution of α-tocopherol, retinol, and β carotene in plasma, red blood cells and platelets: modulations by vitamin E, *Am. J. Clin. Nutr.*, 58:98-102.

Omara, O.F. and Blakely, B.R. 1993. Vitamin E is protective against iron toxicity and iron-induced hepatic vitamin E depletion in mice, *J. Nutr.*, 123:1649-1655.

Paterson, P.G., Gorecke, D.K.J., and Card, R.T. 1994. Vitamin E deficiency and erythrocyte deformability in the rat, *J. Nutr. Biochem.*, 5:298-302.

Stampfer, M.J., Hinnekins, C.H., Manson, J.E., Colditz, G.A., Rosner, B., and Willett, W.C. 1993. Vitamin E consumption and the risk of coronary disease in women, *N. Engl. J. Med.*, 328:1444-1449; 1450-1456.

Weitzman, S.A., Turk, P.W., Milkowski, D.H., and Kozlowski, K. 1994. Free radical adducts induce alterations in DNA cytosine methylation, *Proc. Natl. Acad. Sci. U.S.A.*, 91:1261-1264.

Vitamin K

Bach, A.U., Anderson, S.A., Foley, A.L., Williams, E.C., and Suttie, J.W. 1996. Assessment of vitamin K status in human subjects administered minidose warfarin, *Am. J. Clin. Nutr.*, 64:894-902.

Chung, A., Suttie, J.W., and Bernatowicz, M. 1990. Vitamin K-dependent carboxylase: structural requirements for propeptide activation, *Biochem. Biophys. Acta.*, 1039:90-93.

Esmon, C.T. 1993. Cell mediated events that control blood coagulation and vascular injury, *Annu. Rev. Cell. Biol.*, 9:1-26.

Gardill, S.L. and Suttie, J.W. 1990. Vitamin K epoxide and quinone reductase activities, *Biol. Pharmacol.*, 40:1055-1061.

Greer, F.R. 1995. The importance of vitamin K as a nutrient during the first year of life, *Nutr. Res.*, 15:289-310.

Jie, K.-S.G., Bots, M.L., Vermeer, C., Witteman, J.C.M., and Grobbee, D.E. 1996. Vitamin K status and bone mass in women with and without aortic atherosclerosis: a population based study, *Calcif. Tissue Int.*, 59:352-356.

Suttie, J.W. 1993. Synthesis of vitamin K dependent proteins, *FASEB J.*, 7:445-452.

Water-Soluble Vitamins

TABLE OF CONTENTS

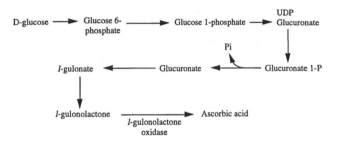

Figure 1 Biosynthesis of ascorbic acid.

I. ASCORBIC ACID

A. Overview

Ascorbic acid, or vitamin C, has been recognized as a needed nutrient for centuries. Although its chemical identity was unknown, foods rich in this micronutrient have long been used as treatment for the symptoms of scurvy. Ancient Egyptians, Greeks, and Romans referred to scurvy as a plague which interfered with victory in military campaigns. Accounts of the scourge of scurvy have appeared in writings of the sixteenth, seventeenth, and eighteenth centuries.

Perhaps the best known treatise on scurvy is that written by a Scottish surgeon, James Lind. Dr. Lind demonstrated that the inclusion of limes, oranges, and lemons in sailors' diets would successfully prevent the development of scurvy. Other reports similar to Lind's were published, but his remains the classic work in this field. Even though the value of citrus fruits was amply demonstrated by Lind, it took 30 years for his recommendations to be adopted. Most nutrition historians credit Captain James Cook, discoverer of the Hawaiian Islands, as the first sea captain to include citrus fruits as part of his ship's stores and part of the sailors' diets. He thus was able to demonstrate that long ocean voyages need not result in scurvy for the crew.

Despite the knowledge that scurvy could be avoided, many sailors and explorers continued to die from scurvy. Even as recently as 1912, Captain Scott and his team died of scurvy as they explored the polar regions of the Southern Hemisphere.

While the knowledge that certain foods prevented or cured scurvy was available in the eighteenth century, the isolation and synthesis of the antisorbutic factor did not occur until early in the twentieth century. The isolation of ascorbic acid was accomplished by two independent groups of chemists in 1928. Szent-Gyorgy isolated a compound which he called hexuronic acid from orange juice, cabbage, and adrenal glands. King likewise isolated the vitamin from lemon juice and showed that it was identical to the compound isolated by Szent-Gyorgy. The structure of the vitamin was accomplished by Haworth and its synthesis by Reichstein. While this exciting chemistry was being pursued an interesting fact became known, and that was that few species required ascorbic acid in their diets. The guinea pig, the primates (including humans), the fruit bat, and some fishes and birds were identified as being unable to synthesize the vitamin *in vivo*. All other species examined were found to be able to synthesize it from glucose (Figure 1). The reason why ascorbic acid-dependent species can not synthesize ascorbic acid is because they lack the enzyme L-gulonolactone oxidase.

B. Structure, Physical and Chemical Properties

Ascorbic acid and dehydroascorbic acid (the oxidized form) are the trivial names for vitamin C. The chemical name is 2,3-didehydro-L-threo-hexano-1,4-lactone. The compound can readily donate

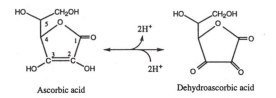

Figure 2   Structures of ascorbic acid and dehydroascorbic acid.

or accept hydrogen ions and thus exists in either state, as shown in Figure 2. In order for the compound to have vitamin activity it must have a 2,3-endiol structure and be a 6-carbon lactone.

L-Ascorbic acid (Figure 2) is a rather simple compound chemically related to the monosaccharide, glucose, with an empiric formula of $C_6H_8O_6$. It is a white crystalline solid with a molecular weight of 176 Da. It is soluble in water, glycerol, and ethanol, but insoluble in fat solvents such as chloroform and ether. It exists in both D and L forms but the L form is the biologically active form. This is in contrast to its related monosaccharide, glucose, which is biologically active as the D form. The vitamin is stable in the dry form but once dissolved in water it is easily oxidized. It is relatively stable in solutions with a pH below 4.0; as the pH rises, the vitamin becomes less stable. Ascorbic acid is easily oxidized by metals such as iron or copper. While ascorbic acid is readily oxidized, it is less perishable in food although it is still oxidized in alkaline environments, especially when heated, exposed to air, or in contact with iron or copper salts. Fortunately, those foods rich in ascorbic acid are relatively acidic and lack iron and copper. If the food is not cooked quickly with a minimum of water, significant losses will occur which will decrease the value of the food as a source of the vitamin.

Ascorbic acid is easily and reversibly oxidized to form dehydroascorbate (Figure 2). The ease with which this interconversion occurs is the basis for its biological function as an acceptor or donor of reducing equivalents. Further oxidation results in the formation of diketogulonic acid, which is biologically inactive. The conversion of ascorbate to dehydroascorbate is aided by sulfhydryl compounds such as glutathione. The strong reducing power of ascorbate can be used to good advantage in its assay. Ascorbate will react with a variety of cyclic compounds to form a color which can be measured spectrophotometrically. Dyes such as dichlorophenolindophenol and 2,4-dinitrophenylhydrazine are the most commonly used compounds in the assay for vitamin C. Chromatographic techniques are also available. An excellent enzymatic assay has been designed using the enzyme ascorbate oxidase. This assay is both sensitive and specific. However, because the need for ascorbic acid and the fact that is prevalent in relatively large amounts in those foods containing the vitamin, the spectrophotometric methods are usually satisfactory. For assays of the vitamin content of tissues such as liver or blood cells, the more sensitive HPLC and thin-layer chromatographic techniques are preferred. In animal and plant tissues vitamin C is present in milligram amounts. Human plasma, for example, contains about 1 mg/dl.

C. Sources

Ascorbic acid is provided mostly by citrus fruits, strawberries, and melons. Some of the vitamin can be found in raw cabbage and related vegetables.

D. Absorption, Metabolism

The metabolic fate of ascorbic acid depends on a number of factors including animal species, route of ingestion, quantity of material, and nutritional status. In species requiring dietary ascorbate, the ascorbate is absorbed in the small intestine, primarily the ileum, by an active transport system which is both sodium dependent and energy dependent. Studies *in vitro* have demonstrated clearly

Table 1 Distribution of Ascorbate in Humans and Rats

Tissue	Human (mg/100 g tissue, wet weight)	Rat (mg/100 g tissue, wet weight)
Adrenals	30–40	280–400
Pituitary	40–50	100–130
Liver	10–16	25–40
Spleen	10–15	40–50
Lungs	7	20–40
Kidneys	5–15	15–20
Testes	3	25–30
Thyroid	2	22
Heart	5–15	5–10
Plasma	0.4–1.0	1.6

that the vitamin moves from the mucosal to the serosal sides of the lumen against a concentration gradient. The influx of the vitamin at the brush border follows saturation kinetics and is specific for the L isomer. Influx can be inhibited by D-isoascorbate, a naturally occurring analog. If sodium is absent, influx does not occur.

Absorption is a sodium-dependent energy-dependent process involving a carrier for ascorbate. The carrier translocates the ascorbate into the enterocyte with sodium, whereupon the sodium must then be pumped out. The sodium dissociates from the carrier mechanism at the inner side of the mucosal membrane and the vitamin moves into the cytosol. The carrier then resumes its original position in the membrane and is available to repeat the process.

Although this process is similar to that envisioned for glucose and alanine, these compounds do not compete with ascorbate for absorption via the above-described carrier. Those species able to synthesize sufficient ascorbic acid do not possess this active transport system and dietary ascorbate is absorbed via passive diffusion. These species differences in transport phenomena lend further evidence of a bifurcation in the evolutionary process which separates guinea pigs, primates, and other ascorbate-requiring species from those species which do not require this vitamin in their diet.

Once absorbed, there appears to be a central pathway for metabolism common to all species. Any excess vitamin consumed beyond need is excreted. There is a very efficient reabsorption mechanism in the kidneys which serves to conserve ascorbic acid in times of need. In the guinea pig, the excess is oxidized to CO_2. In humans very little, if any, oxidation of ascorbate to CO_2 occurs. Ascorbic acid and its metabolites are excreted in the urine. Over 50 metabolites of ascorbate have been detected. Most of these are excreted in minor amounts. The main metabolites in the urine are ascorbate-2-sulfate, oxalic acid, ascorbate, dehydroascorbate, and 2,3-diketogulonic acid. *In vivo*, there is some exchange of ascorbate and ascorbate sulfate in the monkey. The significance of this exchange remains to be elucidated.

E. Distribution

One of the earliest investigations of ascorbic acid function included studies of the distribution of the vitamin throughout the body. Table 1 presents some of these findings in the human and rat. Ascorbic acid is also found uniformly in the brain distributed where it serves as a coenzyme for an enzyme which converts dopamine to norepinephrine.

Ascorbic acid pool sizes and turnover have been estimated using isotopically labeled vitamin. In depleted humans consuming a vitamin C-free diet, about 3% of the total existing pool of ascorbic acid is degraded daily. When the depleted subjects were given doses of vitamin C, this vitamin did not appear in the urine until the body pool approached the size of about 1500 mg. Body pool sizes of more than 1500 mg have not been observed, even when megadoses of the vitamin are consumed.

Table 2 Enzymes Using Ascorbate as a Coenzyme

Cytochrome P_{450} oxidases (several)
Dopamine-β-monooxygenase
Peptidyl glycine α-amidating monooxygenase
Cholesterol 7-α-hydroxylase
4 Hydroxyphenylpyruvate oxidase
Homogentisate 1,2-dioxygenase
Proline hydroxylase
Procollagen-proline 2-oxoglutarate-3-dioxygenase
Lysine hydroxylase
γ-Butyrobetaine, 2-oxoglutarate-4-dioxygenase
Trimethyllysine-2-oxoglutarate dioxygenase

These observations indicate that mega intakes are not useful with respect to the body's vitamin C content. The first signs of scurvy were observed in humans having pool sizes of 300 to 400 mg, and these signs did not disappear until the pool size increased to 1000 mg. Turnover is estimated by measuring the intake rate, the excretion rate, and the total body pool size. This can be accomplished by giving a dose of radioactively labeled vitamin and measuring its distribution and excretion. Vitamin C turnover has been estimated to be 60 mg/day for normally nourished humans. Smokers, incidentally, have higher turnover rates and require more ascorbic acid to maintain their pool sizes.

In contrast to many vitamins, ascorbic acid does not need a carrier for its transport within the body. Like glucose, it is readily carried in the blood in its free form and likewise freely crosses the blood-brain barrier.

F. Function

Although we had an abundance of information about the chemistry of this vitamin, its metabolic function remained elusive for many years. Because it readily converts between the free and dehydro form, it functions in hydrogen ion transfer systems and aids in the regulation of redox states in the cells. Since it is a powerful water-soluble antioxidant it helps to protect other naturally occurring antioxidants which may or may not be water soluble. For example, polyunsaturated fatty acids and vitamin E are protected from peroxidation by ascorbic acid. Ascorbic acid protects certain proteins from oxidative damage and, in addition to its role as an antioxidant, it serves to maintain the unsaturation:saturation ratio of fatty acids. Ascorbic acid aids in the conversion of folic acid to folinic acid and facilitates the absorption of iron by maintaining it in the ferrous state. Ascorbic acid plays a role in the detoxification reactions in the microsomes by virtue of its role as a cofactor in hydroxylation reactions. Table 2 provides a list of those enzymes in which ascorbate is a coenzyme. Many of these are dioxygenases. Again, this is due to the ascorbate-dehydroascorbate interconversion. A number of these enzymes are involved in collagen synthesis. This explains the poor wound healing found in deficient subjects.

The hydroxylation of proline to hydroxyproline, an important amino acid in the synthesis of collagen, is one example of the function of ascorbic acid. The vitamin has been shown to be needed for the incorporation of iron into ferritin. Another function is the role this vitamin plays in maintaining both iron or copper in the reduced state so that the metal can perform as part of an hydroxylation reaction. The hydroxylation of tryptophan to 5-hydroxytryptophan and the conversion of 3,4-dehydroxyphenylethylamine (DOPA) to norepinephrine are further examples. These roles may well explain some of the features of scurvy (Table 3). Poor wound healing is related to the need to form collagen to seal the wound; anemia may be related to the inability of iron and copper to remain in the reduced state in hemoglobin. Ascorbic acid serves as an important cofactor in hydroxylation reactions. Although these reactions will occur in the absence of the vitamin, they occur at a very slow rate.

Table 3   Signs of Ascorbic Acid Deficiency

Hyperkeratosis
Congestion of follicles
Petechial and other skin hemorrhages
Conjunctival lesions
Sublingual hemorrhages
Gum swelling, congestion
Bleeding gums
Papillary swelling
Peripheral neuropathy with hemorrhages into nerve sheaths
Pain, bone endings are tender
Epiphyseal separations occur with subsequent bone (chest) deformities

G. Deficiency

As with other nutrients there are large differences among individuals in their needs for ascorbic acid. As well, there are large differences in the duration of time needed to develop scurvy when consuming a vitamin C-deficient diet. Hodges et al. fed volunteers a diet devoid of vitamin C and described their symptoms as they developed. They noted an increased fatigability, especially in the lower limbs, and a mild general malaise as the symptoms of scurvy became apparent. Mental and emotional changes occurred after 30 days on the diet, with symptoms of depression and suicidal tendencies developing. After 112 days on the ascorbic acid-free diet, some subjects complained of vertigo (feeling of faintness), inappropriate temperature sensing, and profuse sweating. After 26 days of depletion, small petechial hemorrhages were observed on the skin, and after 84 to 91 days small ocular hemorrhages were present. Gingival hemorrhages and swelling in various degrees appeared at different times (42 to 76 days) in the subjects. Hyperkeratosis was observed after two months of depletion. All of these symptoms were reversed when the subjects were repleted.

H. Toxicity

Vitamin C is a water-soluble vitamin and is not usually stored. Thus, there is little evidence of toxicity. As mentioned earlier, oxalate is an end product of ascorbate metabolism and is excreted. Although some investigators have suggested that megadoses of vitamin C may be a risk factor in renal oxalate stores, urinary oxalate levels do not change with increasing intakes of ascorbate. Megadoses of vitamin C have been advocated for the treatment of cancer. However, studies of cancer patients have revealed that such treatment was of little benefit. Massive doses of vitamin C have been shown to reduce serum vitamin B_{12} levels. In part, this may be due to an effect of ascorbic acid on vitamin B_{12} in food. Ascorbic acid destroys B_{12} in food. Ascorbic acid also inhibits the utilization of β-carotene.

I. Recommended Dietary Allowances

Over the years, different countries have had widely different RDAs for ascorbic acid intake. This was due primarily to the differing standards of adequate nutritional status. In Canada, the absence of scorbutic symptoms was used as the indication of adequate nutrient intake. In the U.S., adequate intake has been defined as the saturation of the white blood cell with ascorbic acid. For many years these different definitions have meant that there was a twofold difference in the two countries' recommendations. The U.S. RDA has recently (1989) been revised downward from 75 mg/day for adults to 60 mg/day. Lactating and pregnant women should consume more (+40 and +20 mg, respectively) and children less, depending on age. These recommendations are shown in Table 4.

Table 4 Recommended Dietary Allowances (RDA) for Ascorbic Acid

Group	Age	RDA (mg/day)
Infants	Birth–6 months	30
	7–12 months	35
Children	1–3	40
	4–6	45
	7–10	45
Males	11–14	50
	15–18	60
	19–24	60
	25–50	60
	51+	60
Females	11–14	50
	15–18	60
	19–24	60
	25–50	60
	51+	60
Pregnancy	—	70
Lactation	0–6 months	95
	7–12 months	90

Vitamin C requirements may be higher in stressed or traumatized persons or in persons with diabetes mellitus. In rats, administration of ACTH or cortisone has been shown to lower plasma and hepatic levels of the vitamin. In addition, women taking contraceptive steroids may absorb less of the vitamin or may metabolize it more quickly, and thus may require more than 60 mg/day. Requirements by these groups of people have not been established as yet.

II. THIAMIN

A. Overview

The discovery of the chemical structure and synthesis of thiamin marked the end of a difficult search, spanning continents, to identify the substance in rice polishings responsible for the cure of the disease, beriberi. One of the earliest recorded accounts of the disease was by Jacobus Bonitus, a Dutch physician. He wrote in 1630, "A certain troublesome affliction which attacks men is called by the inhabitants [of Java] beriberi. I believe those whom this disease attacks with their knees shaking and legs raised up, walk like sheep. It is a kind of paralysis or rather tremor: for it penetrates the motion and sensation of the hands and feet, indeed, sometimes the whole body..."

In 1894, Takaki, a surgeon in the Japanese navy, suggested that the disease was diet related. By adding milk and meat to the navy diet, he was able to decrease the incidence of the disease. He thought the problem was a lack of dietary protein. About the same time (1890) a Dutch physician named Eijkman observed a beriberi-like condition (polyneuritis) in chickens fed a polished rice diet. He was able to cure the condition by adding rice polishings. Eijkman suggested that polished rice contained a toxin which was neutralized by the rice polishings.

In 1901, another Dutch physician named Grijens gave the first correct explanation for the cure of beriberi by rice polishings. He theorized that natural foodstuffs contained an unknown factor, absent in polished rice, that prevented the development of the disease.

Jansen and Donath in 1906 and Funk in 1912 reported the isolation of a material from rice polishings which cured beriberi. Funk called the material vita amine or vitamine.

In 1926 Jansen and Donath isolated a crystalline material which cured polyneuritis in birds. Jansen gave the material the trivial name, aneurine. This name was used extensively in the European

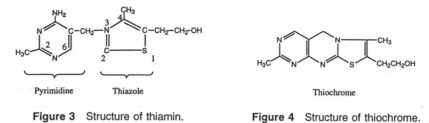

Figure 3 Structure of thiamin.   **Figure 4** Structure of thiochrome.

literature. It is now considered an obsolete term, as are the terms vitamin B_1, oryzamin, torulin, polyneuramin, vitamin F, antineuritic vitamin, and antiberiberi vitamin. All these terms arose as early nutrition scientists identified diseases associated with thiamin deficiency which were reversed when the active principle, now known as thiamin, was provided.

In 1934 Williams et al. isolated enough of the material to make structure elucidation possible. In 1936 thiamin was synthesized by this same group. With synthesis demonstrated, the stage was set for the commercial preparation of thiamin followed by an outburst of publications on its function and metabolism.

B. Structure

Thiamin is a relatively simple compound of a pyrimidine and a thiazole ring (Figure 3). It exists in cells as thiamin pyrophosphate (TPP). TPP used to be called cocarboxylase. The name thiamin comes from the fact that the compound contains both a sulfur group (the thiol group) and nitrogen in its structure. Its biological function depends on the conjoined pyrimidine and thiazole rings, on the presence of an amino group on carbon 4 of the pyrimidine ring and on the presence of a quaternary nitrogen, an open carbon at position 2, and a phosphorylatable alkyl group at carbon 5 of the thiazole ring. In its free form it is unstable. For this reason, it is available commercially as either a hydrochloride or a mononitrate salt. The HCl form is a white crystalline material that is readily soluble (1 g in 1 ml) in water, fairly soluble in ethanol, but relatively insoluble in other solvents. The chemical name for the HCl form is 3-(4'-amino-2'-methyl-pyrimidine-5'-yl)-methyl-5-(2-hydroxyethyl)-4-methylthiazolium chloride hydrochloride. It is stable to acids at up to 120°C but readily decomposes in alkaline solutions, especially when heated. It can be split by nitrite or sulfite at the bridge between the pyrimidine and thiazole rings. The mononitrate form is a white crystalline substance that is more stable to heat than is the hydrochloride form. This form is used more often for food processing than the HCl form. Other forms are also available. These include thiamin allyldisulfide, thiamin propyldisulfide, thiamin tetrahydrofurfuryldisulfide, and o-benzoyl thiamindisulfide. The molecular weight of the disulfide form is 562.7 Da, with a melting point of 177°C. While the hydrochloride form has a molecular weight of 337.3 Da the mononitrate form is 327.4 Da. The latter two are white crystalline powders whereas the disulfide form is a yellow crystal. Thiamin exhibits characteristic absorption maxima at 235 and 267 nm, corresponding to the pyrimidine and thiazole moieties, respectively.

When oxidized, the bridge is attacked and thiamin is converted to thiochrome. Thiochrome is biologically inactive. These structures are shown in Figures 3 and 4.

C. Thiamin Antagonists

Thiamin antagonists include pyrithiamin, a compound with the thiazole ring replaced by a pyridine, and oxythiamin, an analog having the C-4 amino group replaced by a hydroxyl group. It appears that thiamin activity is decreased when the number 2 position of the pyrimidine ring is changed.

Both molecules are potent thiamin antagonists but differ in their mechanisms of action. Oxythiamin is readily converted to the pyrophosphate and competes with thiamin for its place in the

TPP-enzyme systems. Pyrithiamin prevents the conversion of thiamin to TPP by interfering with the activity of thiamin kinase. Oxythiamin depresses appetite, growth, and weight gain and produces bradycardia, heart enlargement, and an increase in blood pyruvate, but it does not produce neurological symptoms. Pyrithiamin results in a loss of thiamin from tissues, bradycardia, and heart enlargement, but does not produce an increase in blood pyruvate.

A type of natural antagonist is a group of enzyme called thiaminases. The first antagonist was discovered by accident when raw fish was incorporated into a commercially available feed for foxes. Foxes fed this diet developed symptoms of thiamin deficiency. When heated, this enzyme is denatured and thus no longer is capable of destroying thiamin. The enzyme has several forms and has been found in fish, shellfish, ferns, betel nuts, and a variety of vegetables. Also found in tea and other plant foods are antithiamin substances that inactivate the vitamin by forming adducts. Tannic acid is one such substance; another is 3,4-dihydroxycinnamic acid (caffeic acid). Some of the flavinoids and some of the dihydroxy derivatives of tyrosine have antithiamin activity.

D. Assays for Thiamin

There are various chemical, microbiological, and animal assays available for thiamin. In animal tissues, thiamin occurs principally as phosphate esters, whereas in plants it appears in the free form. Both forms are protein bound.

The thiochrome method is the most widely used chemical assay for thiamin. It depends upon the alkaline oxidation of thiamin to thiochrome. Thiochrome, in turn, exhibits an intense blue fluorescence which can be measured fluorimetrically. Other chemical tests for thiamin are the formaldehyde-diazotized sulfanilic acid method, the diazotized *p*-aminoacetophenone method, and the bromothymol blue method. All of these assays must be preceded by extraction and removal of protein.

Lactobacillus viridescens is the microorganism most widely used to measure thiamin concentrations. It requires the intact thiamin molecule for growth. Other organisms are available but they are less useful.

Animal assays are used for determining the availability of thiamin in a food source. The rat is the preferred animal to use. The material being tested measures the curative effect of the food source on rats which have been made thiamin deficient and compares it to the curative effect of pure synthetic thiamin hydrochloride. The most sensitive assays are the chromatographic ones. Both HPLC (high performance liquid chromatography) and thin-layer chromatography yield excellent results. They have the advantages of sensitivity and reliability.

E. Sources

Thiamin is widely distributed in the food supply. Pork is the richest source, while highly refined foods have virtually no thiamin. Polished rice, fats, oils, refined sugar, and unenriched flours are in this group. Many products are made with enriched flour and so provide thiamin to the consumer. Enrichment means that the flour (or other food ingredient) has had thiamin added to it to the level that was there prior to processing. Peas and other legumes are good sources; the amount of thiamin increases with the maturity of the seed. Whole-grain cereal products contain nutritionally significant amounts of thiamin. Dried brewer's yeast and wheat germ are both rich in thiamin.

F. Absorption and Metabolism

Thiamin is absorbed by a specific active transport mechanism. In humans and rats, absorption is most rapid in the proximal small intestine. Studies *in vivo* on intact loops of rat small intestine revealed saturation kinetics for thiamin over the concentration range of 0.06 to 1.5 μM. At higher

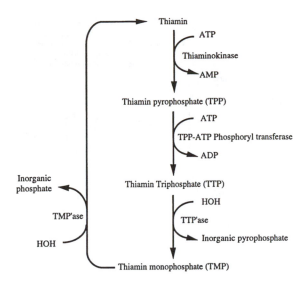

Figure 5 Formation of thiamin pyrophosphate through the phosphorylation of thiamin. About 80% of thiamin exists as TPP, 10% as TTP, and the remainder as TMP or free thiamin.

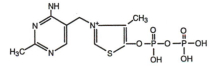

Thiamin pyrophosphate (TPP)

Figure 6 Structure of the coenzyme thiamin phyrophosphate.

concentrations (2 to 560 μM) absorption was linearly related to the luminal thiamin concentration. *In vitro* studies using inverted jejunum sacs indicated an active transport mechanism, which is energy and Na$^+$ dependent and carrier mediated.

Thiamin undergoes phosphorylation either in the intestinal lumen or within the intestinal cells. This phosphorylation is closely related to uptake, indicating that the carrier may be the enzyme thiamin pyrophosphokinase. There is some argument about this, however. Figure 5 illustrates TPP synthesis.

While thiamin can accumulate in all cells of the body, there is no single storage site per se. The body does not store the vitamin and thus a daily supply is needed. Thiamin in excess of need is excreted in the urine. More than 20 metabolites have been identified in urine.

G. Biological Function

Thiamin is a part of the coenzyme thiamin pyrophosphate (TPP) (thiamin with two molecules of phosphate attached to it), also known as cocarboxylase, which is required in the metabolism of carbohydrates. Figure 6 illustrates this structure. The driving force for reactions with thiamin results because of the resonance possible in the thiazolium ring. The thiazolium ion, known as ylid, will form. Because of the formation of the ylid, the thiazole ring of TPP can serve as a transient carrier of a covalently bound "active" aldehyde group. Mg^{2+} is required as a cofactor for these reactions.

The metabolism of carbohydrates involves three stages in which the absence of thiamin as part of a coenzyme (TPP) leads to a slowing or complete blocking of the reactions. There are two

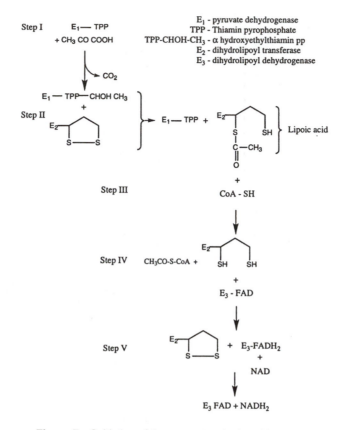

Figure 7   Oxidation of the pyruvate-mitochondria matrix.

oxidative decarboxylation reactions of α-ketoacids: the formation or degradation of α-ketols and the decarboxylation of pyruvic acid to acetyl CoA as it is about to enter the citric acid cycle. This reaction is catalyzed by the pyruvate dehydrogenase complex, an organized assembly of three kinds of enzymes. The mechanism of this action is quite complex. TPP, lipoamide, and FAD serve as catalytic cofactors; NAD and CoA serve as stoichiometric participants in the reaction.

As a consequence of the impairment of this reaction in thiamin deficiency, the level of pyruvate will rise. When thiamin is withheld from the diet, the ability of tissues to utilize pyruvate does not decline uniformly, indicating that there are tissue differences in the retention of TPP. Muscle retains more TPP than does brain. This role of thiamin arose from the discovery that thiamin alone promotes nonenzymatic decarboxylation of pyruvate to yield acetaldehyde and CO_2. Studies of this model revealed that the H at C-2 of the thiazole ring ionizes to yield a carbanion which reacts with the carbonyl atom of pyruvate to yield CO_2 and a hydroxyethyl (HE) derivative of the thiazole. The HE may then undergo hydrolysis to yield acetaldehyde or become oxidized to yield an acyl group. Figures 7 and 8 illustrate pyruvate metabolism and show where thiamin plays a role.

Thiamin is also active in the decarboxylation of α-ketoglutaric acid to succinyl CoA in the citric acid cycle. The mechanism of action is similar to that described above for pyruvate.

Step I.   Similar to nonoxidative decarboxylation of pyruvate in alcohol fermentation.

Step II.   The hydroxyethyl group is dehydrogenated and the resulting acetyl group is transferred to the sulfur atom at C-6 (or C-8) of lipoic acid, which constitutes the covalently bound prosthetic group of the second enzyme of the complex, lipoate acetyl transferase. The transfer of H$^+$ to the disulfide bond of lipoic acid converts the latter to its reduced or dithiol form, dihydrolipoic acid.

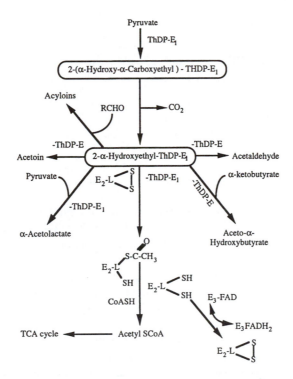

Figure 8 Summary of the metabolic pathways for pyruvate.

Step III. The acetyl group is enzymatically transferred to the thiol group of coenzyme A and a second H⁺ is added to form the dihydrolipoyl transacetylase. The Ac CoA so formed leaves the enzyme complex in free form.

Step IV. The dithiol form of lipoic acid is reoxidized to its disulfide form by transfer of H⁺ and associated electrons to the third enzyme of the complex, dihydrolipoyl (lipoamide) dihydrogenase, whose reducible prosthetic group is FAD. FADH₂, which remains bound to the enzyme, transfers its electron to NAD⁺ to form NADH.

E_1 is regulated by PDH kinase and PDH phosphatase.

The oxidation of αKG to succinyl CoA is energetically irreversible and is carried out by the αKG DH complex:

$$\alpha KG + NAD^+ + CoA \Leftrightarrow succinyl\ CoA + CO_2 + NADH_2$$

$$\Delta G = 8.0\ kcal\ mol^{-1}$$

This reaction is analogous to the oxidation of pyruvate to acetyl-CoA and CO_2 and occurs by the same mechanism with TPP, lipoic acid, CoA, FAD, and NAD participating as coenzymes.

The metabolism of ethanol also requires thiamin. The same pyruvate dehydrogenase complex which converts pyruvate to acetyl-CoA will metabolize acetaldehyde (the first product in the metabolism of ethanol) to acetyl CoA. This system probably accounts for only a small part of ethanol degradation.

TPP participates in the transfer of a glycoaldehyde group from D-xylulose to D-ribose 5P to yield D-sedoheptulose 7P, an intermediate of the pentose phosphate pathway, and glyceraldehyde 3P, an intermediate of glycolysis. Transketolase contains tightly bound thiamin pyrophosphate. In this reaction the glycoaldehyde group (CH_2OH–CO) is first transferred from D-xylulose 5P to

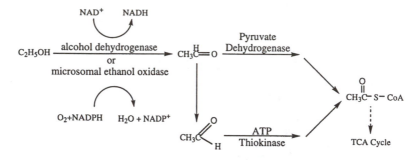

Figure 9   Metabolism of ethanol.

enzyme-bound TPP to form the α,β-dihydroxyethyl derivative of the latter, which is analogous to the α-hydroxyethyl derivative formed during the action of PDH. The TPP acts as an intermediate carrier of this glycoaldehyde group which is transferred to the acceptor molecule D-ribose 5P. This is a reaction in the hexose monophosphate shunt.

From the involvement of vitamin-containing coenzymes in the oxidation of alcohol (see Figure 9), it follows that vitamin deficiency could impair the rate of alcohol oxidation and thus increase the retention of alcohol in the blood of malnourished, chronic alcoholic subjects. Actually, there is little evidence for this assumption in animals or humans. The rate-limiting step appears not to be the level of vitamin concentration, but rather the amount of alcohol dehydrogenase present.

Large dietary intakes of carbohydrates will increase the need for thiamin. Ingestion of lipids, on the other hand, is considered to be thiamin sparing. This is a consequence of the fact that thiamin is required in the metabolism of lipids in fewer places than it is in the metabolism of carbohydrates.

In addition to its role as a coenzyme, it is speculated that thiamin has an independent role in neural tissue since it has been shown that stimulation of nerve fibers results in release of free thiamin and thiamin monophosphate. If a neurophysiologically active form of thiamin exists, it is as thiamin triphosphate. However, thiamin's role in the central nervous system is viewed at present as an intriguing enigma.

H. Deficiency

The major symptoms of thiamin deficiency (beriberi) are loss of appetite (anorexia), weight loss, convulsions, slowing of the heart rate (bradycardia), and lowering of the body temperature. Loss of muscle tone and lesions of the nervous system may also develop. Because the heart muscle can be weakened, there may be a cardiac failure resulting in peripheral edema and ascites in the extremities. The urine of rats with a thiamin deficit contains a higher pyruvate:lactate ratio than that of normal animals. Thiamin-deficient rats also exhibit a reduced erythrocyte transketolase activity. Administration of thiamin to rats brings about a remarkable reversal of deficiency symptoms in less than 24 hr.

Beriberi is classified into several types: acute-mixed, wet, or dry. The acute-mixed type is characterized by neural and cardiac symptoms producing neuritis and heart failure. In wet beriberi, the edema of heart failure is the most striking sign; digestive disorders and emaciation are additional symptoms. In dry beriberi, loss of function of the lower extremities or paralysis predominates; it is often called polyneuritis.

Thiamin deficiency is the most common vitamin deficiency seen in chronic alcoholics in the U.S. Clinical manifestations of the deficiency vary, depending upon the severity of the deprivation. However, all degrees of deficiency involve muscle and/or nerve tissue. The most serious form of thiamin deficiency in alcoholics is Wernicke's syndrome. It is characterized by ophthalmoplegia, 6th nerve palsy, nystagmus, ptosis, ataxia, confusion, and coma which may terminate in death.

Table 5   Clinical Features of Thiamin Deficiency

Wet and dry beriberi	Malaise
	Heaviness and weakness of legs
	Calf muscle tenderness
	"Pins and needles" and numbness in legs
	Anesthesia of skin, particularly at the tibia
	Increased pulse rate and palpitations
Wet beriberi	Edema of legs, face, trunk, and serous cavities
	Tense calf muscles
	Fast pulse
	Distended neck veins
	High blood pressure
	Decreased urine volume
Dry beriberi	Worsening of polyneuritis of early stage
	Difficulty walking
	Wernicke-Korsakoff syndrome; encephalopathy may occur:
	Disorientation
	Loss of immediate memory
	Nystagmus (jerky movements of the eyes)
	Ataxia (staggering gait)

Often the confusional state persists after treatment of the acute thiamin deficiency. This is known as Korsakoff's psychosis.

The next most serious level of thiamin deficiency is sometimes known as alcoholic beriberi. It is seen in those individuals who have had a minimal intake of thiamin. It is characterized by symmetrical foot and wrist drop associated with muscle tenderness. It may also affect cardiac muscle metabolism and may result in congestive heart failure.

The mildest and most common form of thiamin deficiency is the polyneuropathy affecting only the lower extremities of the chronic alcoholic. The signs and symptoms of thiamin deficiency are listed in Table 5. All the signs and symptoms of thiamin deficiency respond to thiamin treatment except the irreversible neurological lesions.

Red cell transketolase activity seems to be a sensitive index of thiamin nutritional status. Brin et al. have suggested an *in vitro* test using transketolase to differentiate between the enzymatic lesions caused by thiamin deficiency and those due to nonspecific causes. This test consists of stimulation of enzyme activity in the presence of saturating amounts of TPP. This so-called TPP effect (TPPE) is claimed to be a true measure of thiamin nutritional status.

In addition to the enzymatic test, a measure of urinary thiamin in relation to dietary intake has been the basis for balance studies to assess the adequacy of intake. When thiamin excretion is low a larger portion of the test dose is retained, indicating a tissue need for thiamin. A high excretion indicates tissue saturation. In the deficient state, excretion drops to zero.

I. Recommended Dietary Allowance

The thiamin needs of an individual are influenced by age, energy intake, carbohydrate intake, and body weight. Table 6 gives the RDAs for humans. The Food and Nutrition Board, on the basis of considerable evidence, recommends 0.5 mg/1000 kcal (4184 kJ). Because there is some evidence that older persons use thiamin less efficiently, it is recommended that they maintain an intake of 1 mg/day even if they consume less than 2000 kcal (8368 kJ) daily.

Since thiamin needs increase during pregnancy and lactation, an additional 0.4 mg/day is recommended during pregnancy and 0.5 mg/day during lactation.

Table 6   Recommended Dietary Allowances for Thiamin

Group	Age	RDA (mg/day)
Infants	Birth–6 months	0.3
	6–12 months	0.4
Children	1–3	0.7
	4–6	0.9
	7–10	1.0
Males	11–14	1.3
	15–18	1.5
	19–24	1.5
	25–50	1.5
	51+	1.2
Females	11–14	1.1
	15–18	1.1
	19–24	1.1
	25–50	1.1
	51+	1.0
Pregnancy	—	1.5
Lactation	—	1.6

Few studies have assessed the thiamin nutritional status of infants and children. The Food and Nutrition Board recommends 0.5 mg/1000 kcal (4184 kJ).

J. Toxicity

Although thiamin produces a variety of pharmacological effects when administered in large doses, the dose required is thousands of times greater than those required for optimal nutrition. Generally, toxic effects are reported with subcutaneous, intramuscular, intraspinal, or intravenous injections, but not with oral administration. In rare cases, thiamin excess has caused reactions in humans resembling anaphylactic shock. These usually develop only in individuals who have been given several large intravenous injections and may be related to the development of hypersensitivity to thiamin.

III. RIBOFLAVIN

A. Overview

While thiamin and niacin were being recognized as the causative factors in beriberi and pellagra, respectively, riboflavin, another B vitamin was ignored. A food fraction isolation by McCollum and Kennedy in 1916 was shown by Emmett and Luros, and later by Goldberger and Lillie, to have several functions: one as beriberi curative, another as a pellagra curative, and a third whose function was not known. These fractions were all water soluble but differed in their stability towards heat and light. In 1932 Warburg and Christian isolated and described a flavoprotein which was recognized by others as having vitamin properties. This became the vitamin, riboflavin. Since it was first isolated with thiamin and niacin it was given a letter designation in England as vitamin B_2 and in the U.S. as vitamin G. As our knowledge of vitamins increased, this nomenclature was dropped in favor of the name riboflavin.

B. Structure, Chemical and Physical Properties

Riboflavin (Figure 10) is a highly colored crystalline substance frequently associated with flavoproteins. As a solid, it is red-orange in color. In solution the color changes to a greenish yellow.

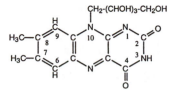

7,8-dimethyl-10-(1' D-ribityl)-isoalloxazine

or

6,7-dimethyl-9-(D-1' ribityl)-isolloxazine
if only the carbons are numbered
as in the older literature.

Figure 10   Structure of riboflavin.

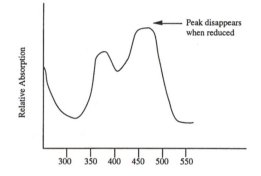

Figure 11   Absorption spectra of riboflavin.

It was first synthesized by Kuhn and also by Karrer et al. in 1935 as needle-like crystals with limited solubility in pure water or in acid solutions. Solubility increases as the pH of the solvent increases; however, as the pH of the solution rises, riboflavin's stability to heat and light decreases. Milk loses 33% of its riboflavin activity in 1 hr of sunlight. In solution, riboflavin is easily destroyed by light and must be protected at all times from exposure. Biochemists working with riboflavin take such precautions as using deep-red glassware and darkened work areas to ensure maximal recovery or assessment of vitamin activity. Because riboflavin has several absorbance maxima and fluoresces due to a shifting of bonds in the isoalloxazine ring, its presence can be quantified by spectrophotometric or photofluorometric techniques. Fluorescence can be measured before and after reduction by such compounds as sodium hydrosulfite. The reduced (hydroquinones) flavins do not fluoresce whereas oxidized flavins do. Fluorescence is pH dependent and is best measured between pH 4 to 8; maximal fluorescence occurs at 556 nm.

The oxidized forms of different flavoenzymes are intensely colored. They are characteristically yellow, red, or green due to strong absorption bands in the visible range. Upon reduction, they undergo bleaching with a characteristic change in the absorption spectrum. Figure 11 shows the change in absorption with changes in wavelength.

In order to have vitamin activity, positions 8 and 7 must be substituted with more than just a hydrogen and the imine group in position 3 must be unsubstituted. There must be a ribityl group on position 10. If the ribityl group is lost then vitamin activity is lost, as depicted in Figure 12 where photodecomposition is shown. There are some antivitamins that interfere with riboflavin's usefulness. These compounds compete for the prosthetic groups or competitively inhibit its phosphorylation and adenylation to form the coenzymes FMN (flavin mononucleotide) or FAD (flavin adenine dinucleotide), respectively. The structures of these coenzymes are shown in Figure 13.

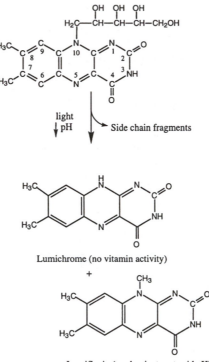

Lumichrome (no vitamin activity)

+

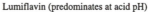

Lumiflavin (predominates at acid pH)

Figure 12   Degradation of riboflavin by light and acid or acidic conditions.

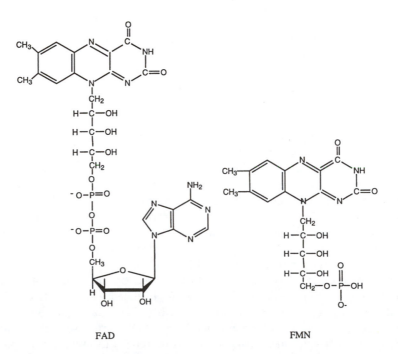

FAD   FMN

Figure 13   Structures of flavin adenine dinucleotide (FAD) and flavin mononucleotide (FMN).

C. Sources

The best sources are foods of animal origin: milk, meat, and eggs. Wheat germ is also a good source.

D. Assay

The most sensitive and selective procedure for the determination of riboflavin is that which uses fluorescence detection coupled with HPLC. The vitamin and coenzymes must be protected from light and acid. The coenzyme forms can be separated from the free form by differential solubility. The free form is soluble in benzyl alcohol while the coenzymes are not.

E. Absorption, Metabolism

Absorption occurs by way of an active carrier and is energy and sodium dependent. Maximum absorption occurs in the proximal segment (the jejunum) of the small intestine, with significant uptake by the duodenum and ileum. After a load dose, peak values in the plasma appear within 2 hr. The phosphorylated forms (coenzyme forms) are dephosphorylated prior to absorption through the action of nonspecific hydrolases from the brush border membrane of the duodenum and jejunum. There is a pyrophosphatase which cleaves FAD and an alkaline phosphatase which liberates the vitamin from FMN. Bile salts appear to facilitate uptake, and a small amount of the vitamin circulates via the enterohepatic system. Prior to entry into the portal blood, some of the vitamin is rephosphorylated to re-form FAD and FMN. After absorption, the vitamin circulates in the blood bound to plasma proteins, notably albumin and certain gamma globulins.

Specific riboflavin-binding proteins have been isolated and identified in several species. These proteins are of hepatic origin. There is facilitated, mediated uptake of the free vitamin by all of the vital organs. For example, isolated liver cells will accumulate up to five times the amount of the vitamin in the fluids which surround them. Although cells will accumulate the vitamin against a concentration gradient, these cells also use the vitamin quite rapidly, so there is little net storage.

The usual blood levels of riboflavin are in the range of 20 to 50 µg/dl while 500 to 900 µg/day are excreted in the urine. Excretion products include 7- and 8-hydroxymethylriboflavin, 8-α-sulfonylriboflavin, riboflavin peptide esters, 10-hydroxyethylflavin, lumiflavin, 10-formylmethyl-flavin, 10-carboxymethylflavin, lumichrome, and free riboflavin. Very small amounts of riboflavin and its metabolites can be found in the feces.

Upon entry into the cell, riboflavin is reconverted to FMN and FAD, as shown in Figure 14. The initial phosphorylation reaction is zinc dependent. FMN and FAD synthesis is responsive to thyroid status. Hyperthyroidism is associated with increased synthesis whereas hypothyroidism is associated with decreased synthesis. FAD is linked to a variety of proteins via hydrogen bonding, and also to the purine portion of FAD, the phenolic ring of tyrosyl residues, and indolic-tryptophanyl residues in flavoproteins. Covalent bonding with certain enzymes also occurs, and involves the riboflavin 8-methyl group which forms a methylene bridge to the peptide histidyl-1 or 3-imidazole functions or to the thioether function of a former cysteinyl residue. When bound to these proteins, these coenzymes are somewhat protected from degradation although the proteins themselves are eventually degraded. However, flavins in excess of that which are protein bound are more rapidly degraded and excreted in the urine.

Degradation involves the oxidation of the ribityl chain and hydroxylation at positions 7 and 8 of the isoalloxazine ring by hepatic microsomal cytochrome P450 enzymes. The methyl groups at these positions are removed and the compound loses its activity as a vitamin. Because degradation and excretion occur at a fairly rapid rate, the rate of riboflavin degradation determines the requirement for the vitamin rather than the need for the vitamin in its function as a coenzyme, that is, the rate of FMN and FAD synthesis.

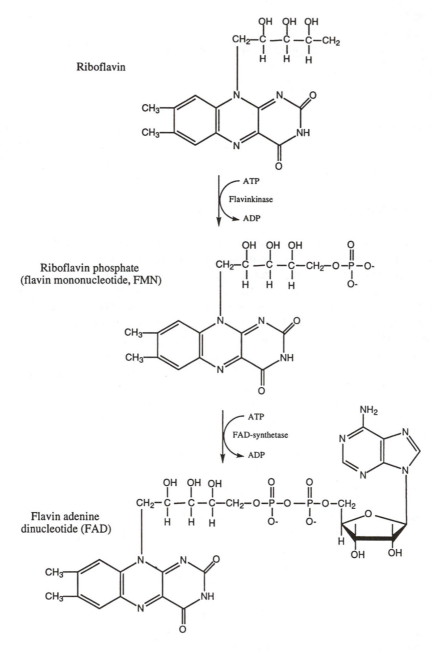

Figure 14   Synthesis of FMN and FAD.

F. Functions

FAD and its precursor FMN are coenzymes for reactions that involve oxidation-reduction. Thus, riboflavin is an important component of intermediary metabolism. The respiratory chain in the mitochondria and reactions in numerous pathways that utilize either FAD or FMN as coenzymes require riboflavin. Shown in Table 7 is a list of some of these enzymes. They include reactions where reducing equivalents are transferred between cellular compartments as part of a shuttle arrangement, as well as reactions that are in a mitochondrial or cytosolic sequence.

Table 7   Reactions Using FAD or FMN

FAD-Linked Enzymes

Ubiquinone reductase	Xanthine oxidase
Monoamine oxidase	Cytochrome reductase
NADH-cytochrome P 450 reductase	Succinate dehydrogenase
D-Amino acid oxidase	α-Glycerophosphate dehydrogenase
Acyl CoA dehydrogenase	Electron transport respiratory chain
Dihydrolipoyl dehydrogenase (component of PDH and α-KGDH)	Glutathione reductase

FMN-Linked Enzymes

NADH dehydrogenase (respiratory chain)	Lactate dehydrogenase
L-Amino acid oxidase	Pyridoxine (pyridoxamine)5'-phosphate oxidase

In most flavoenzymes, the flavin nucleotide is tightly but noncovalently bound to the protein; exceptions given in Table 7 include succinate dehydrogenase and monoamine oxidase, in which the flavin nucleotide, FAD, is covalently bound to a histidine residue of the polypeptide chain in the former case and a cysteinyl residue in the latter. The metalloflavoproteins contain one or more metals as additional cofactors. Flavin nucleotides undergo reversible reduction of the isoalloxazine ring in the catalytic cycle of flavoproteins to yield the reduced nucleotides $FMNH_2$ and $FADH_2$. The enzymes that have a riboflavin-containing coenzyme are of three general types:

1. Enzymes whose substrate is a reduced pyridine nucleotide and the acceptor is either a member of the cytochromes or another acceptor.
2. Enzymes that accept electrons directly from the substrate and can pass them to one of the cytochromes or directly to oxygen.
3. Enzymes that accept electrons from substrate and pass them directly to oxygen (true oxidases).

A simplified mechanism of action is shown in Figure 15.

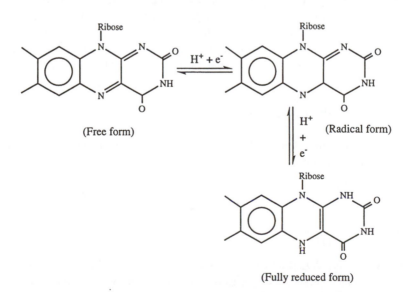

(Free form)

$H^+ + e^-$

(Radical form)

H^+
+
e^-

(Fully reduced form)

Figure 15   Mechanism of action of the riboflavin portion of the coenzyme.

Each of the steps in this sequence is reversible to the extent limited by the flavoprotein's capacity to accept or donate reducing equivalents which, in turn, can be joined to oxygen. Many of the flavoproteins also contain a metal such as iron, molybdenum, or zinc, and the combination of these metals and the flavin structure allows for its easy and rapid transition between single- and double-electron donors.

Note in Table 7 that a number of enzymes are members of the oxidase family of enzymes. The oxidases transfer hydrogen directly to oxygen to form hydrogen peroxide. Xanthine oxidase uses a variety of purines as its substrate, converting hypoxanthine to xanthine which is then converted to uric acid. Xanthine oxidase also catalyzes the conversion of retinal to retinoic acid (see Unit 3).

Among the important enzymes shown in Table 7 are those that are essential to mitochondrial respiration and ATP synthesis as well as to the mitochondrial citric acid cycle. Succinate dehydrogenase is one of these and its activity has been used as a biomarker of riboflavin intake sufficiency. The acyl CoA dehydrogenases catalyze another of the essential pathways, fatty acid oxidation. These are FAD linked. Fatty acid synthesis requires the presence of FMN-linked enzymes. The FMN-dependent pyridoxine (pyridoxamine) 5'-phosphate oxidase is essential for conversion of the two forms of vitamin B_6 to its functional coenzyme, pyridoxal-5'-phosphate. This is another example of vitamin-vitamin interaction. While the list of enzymes shown in Table 7 is by no means complete, it gives evidence of the intimate and essential need for riboflavin in the regulation of metabolism. In its absence, profound impairments can be expected and death should follow in a short time once all of the FAD and FMN are used up. In humans, clinical signs of deficiency appear in less than 6 weeks on intakes of less than 0.6 mg/day.

G. Deficiency

Despite our knowledge about riboflavin's function as a coenzyme, there are few symptoms that are specific to riboflavin deficiency. Poor growth, poor appetite, and certain skin lesions (cracks at the corners of the mouth, dermatitis on the scrotum) have been observed. However, some of these symptoms can occur for reasons apart from inadequate riboflavin intake, as in vitamin B_6 deficiency. As mentioned in the preceding section, the oxidase needed to convert B_6 to its functional form requires riboflavin as FMN. This lack of direct correlation of symptoms to intake is also due to the almost universal need for FAD and FMN as coenzymes in intermediary metabolism. Thus, it is impossible to pinpoint a specific deficiency symptom. Nutrition assessment of adequate riboflavin intake relies upon a few reactions in readily available cells, i.e., blood cells, that can predict intake adequacy. Erythrocyte FAD-linked glutathione reductase is one of these. Low enzyme activity is associated with inadequate intakes. Succinate dehydrogenase is another enzyme frequently used in nutrition assessment.

H. Recommended Dietary Allowance

As mentioned, there is almost no riboflavin reserve. Thus, a daily intake of riboflavin is essential. The RDAs for humans are shown in Table 8.

IV. NIACIN

A. Overview

Few vitamins have as tortuous a history of discovery as niacin, otherwise known as vitamin B_3, or nicotinic acid, or niacinamide. The synthesis of nicotinic acid was accomplished long before it

Table 8   Recommended Dietary Riboflavin Allowances for Humans

	Age	Riboflavin (mg/day)
Infants	Birth to 6 months	0.4
	7 months to 1 year	0.5
Children	1–3	0.8
	4–6	1.1
	7–10	1.2
Males	11–14	1.5
	15–18	1.8
	19–24	1.7
	25–50	1.7
	51+	1.4
Females	11–14	1.3
	15–18	1.3
	19–24	1.3
	25–50	1.3
	51+	1.2
Pregnant	—	+1.6
Lactating	1st 6 months	+1.8
	2nd 6 months	1.7

was discovered to be a vitamin. Some 50 years elapsed before it was connected to the disease pellagra. Pellagra was described in the mid-1800s in Italy and Spain and called "mal de la rosa" in the latter country. Its development was associated with the consumption of low-protein high-corn diets. The disease was more prevalent in very poor populations and associated with the consumption of corn. At one time it was thought to be due to a toxin found in corn; however, as descriptions of pellagra arose in the literature from populations that did not consume corn, this idea was discarded. Some years later, Goldberger demonstrated that pellagra was a nutrient deficiency disease and that the nutrient in question was niacin. The term niacin is a generic term which includes both the acid and amide forms.

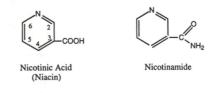

Nicotinic Acid
(Niacin)   Nicotinamide

Figure 16   Structures of nicotinic acid (niacin) and nicotinamide.

B. Structure, Physical and Chemical Properties

Niacin occurs in two forms (as an acid or as an amide) as shown in Figure 16. The vitamin is widely distributed in nature. Nicotinamide is the primary constituent of the coenzymes NAD^+ (nicotinamide adenine dinucleotide) and $NADP^+$ (nicotinamide dinucleotide phosphate). The synthesis of these pyridine nucleotides is shown in Figure 17.

The molecular weight of nicotinic acid is 123.1 Da and that of nicotinamide is 122.1 Da. Nicotinamide is far more soluble in water than is nicotinic acid. Both are white crystals with an absorption maxima of 263 nm. The melting point of the acid form is 237°C while that of the amide is 128 to 131°C. In order to have vitamin activity there must be a pyridine ring substituted with a β-carboxylic acid or corresponding amide and there must be open sites at pyridine carbons 2 through 6.

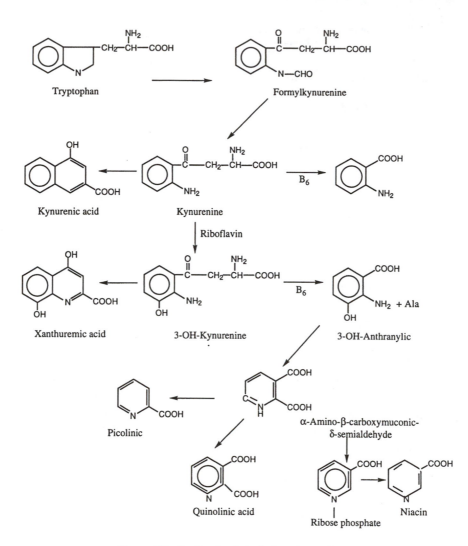

Figure 17 Synthesis of niacin from tryptophan.

Nicotinic acid is amphoteric and forms salts with acids and bases. Its carboxyl group can form esters and anhydrides and can be reduced. Both the acid and amide forms are very stable in the dry form, but when the amide form is in solution it is readily hydrolyzed to the acid form.

Several substituted pyridines can antagonize the biological activity of niacin. These include pyridine-3-sulfonic acid, 3-acetylpyridine, isonicotinic acid hydrazide, and 6-aminonicotinamide. HPLC is the analytical method of choice for this vitamin which does not occur in large amounts as the free form. Most often, it occurs as the coenzyme NAD^+ or $NADP^+$. Chemical analysis using the Koenig reaction, which opens up the pyridine ring with cyanogen bromide, followed by reaction with an aromatic amine to form a colored product, is one technique that is used. The most widely used method employs a chromophore-generating base, p-methylaminophenol sulfate, sulfanilic acid, or barbituric acid. The color intensity so developed is dependent on the concentration of the vitamin.

C. Sources

This vitamin is widely distributed in the human food supply. Especially good sources are whole-grain cereals and breads, milk, eggs, meats, and vegetables that are richly colored.

D. Absorption, Metabolism

Both nicotinic acid and nicotinamide cross the intestinal cell by way of simple diffusion and facilitated diffusion. There are species differences in the mechanism of absorption. In the bullfrog, absorption is via active transport. In the rat there is evidence of a transporter that is saturable and sodium dependent. This suggests facilitated diffusion. After absorption the vitamin circulates in the blood in its free form, as shown. That which is not converted to NAD^+ or $NADP^+$ is metabolized further and excreted in the urine. The excretory metabolites are N'-methylnicotinamide, nicotinuric acid, nicotinamide-N'-oxide, N'-methylnicotinamide-N'-oxide, N'-methylnicotinamide-N'-oxide, N'-methyl-4-pyridone-3-carboxamide, and N'-methyl-2-pyridone-5-carboxamide. Niacin can be synthesized from tryptophan in a ratio of 60 molecules of tryptophan to 1 of nicotinic acid. The pathway for conversion is shown in Figure 17. Note the involvement of thiamin, vitamin B_6, and riboflavin in this conversion.

E. Function

The main function of this vitamin is that of the coenzymes NAD^+ and $NADP^+$. Both function in the maintenance of the redox state of the cell. These coenzymes are bound to the protein (apoenzyme) portions of dehydrogenases relatively loosely during the catalytic cycle and therefore serve more as substrates than as prosthetic groups. They act as hydride ion acceptors during the enzymatic removal of hydrogen atoms from specific substrate molecules. One hydrogen atom of the substrate is transferred as a hydride ion to the nicotinamide portion of the oxidized NAD^+ or $NADP^+$ forms of these coenzymes to yield the reduced forms. The other hydrogen ion exchanges with water. Thus, the reduced coenzyme is represented as $NADH^+H^+$ or $NADPH^+H^+$. Most enzymes are specific for NAD or NADP and these enzymes are members of the oxidoreductase family of enzymes. Some will use either, e.g., glutamate dehydrogenase.

Most of the NAD- or NADP-linked enzymes are involved in catabolic pathways, e.g., glycolysis or the pentose phosphate shunt. NAD turns over quite rapidly in the cell. Its degradation is shown in Figure 18.

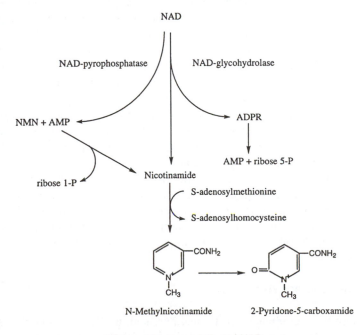

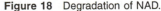

Figure 18 Degradation of NAD.

Beyond its use in biological systems as a precursor of NAD^+ or $NADP^+$, nicotinic acid has a pharmacological use. Nicotinic acid, the drug, is used as a lipid-lowering agent. Large intakes (1 g/day) lower serum cholesterol. However, large doses also result in flushing due to its effect on vascular tone. Nicotinic acid elicits a fibrinolytic activation of very short duration. Both nicotinic acid and nicotinamide can be toxic if administered at levels greater than 10 μmol/kg. Chronic administration of 3 g/day to humans results in a variety of symptoms including headache, heartburn, nausea, hives, fatigue, sore throat, dry hair, inability to focus the eyes, and skin tautness. In experimental animals, nicotinic acid supplements result in a reduction in adipocyte free fatty acid release by streptozotocin-diabetic rats, an inhibition of adipocyte adenylate cyclase activity in normal hamsters, and degenerative changes in the heart muscle of normal rats. All of these responses are those that characterize a defense against a toxic exposure to nicotinic acid rather than a response to a normal intake level.

F. Deficiency

Pellagra has been well described as the niacin deficiency disease. It is characterized by skin lesions that are blackened and rough, especially in areas exposed to sunlight and abraded by clothing. The typical skin lesions of pellagra are accompanied by insomnia, loss of appetite, weight loss, soreness of the mouth and tongue, indigestion, diarrhea, abdominal pain, burning sensations in various parts of the body, vertigo, headache, numbness, nervousness, apprehension, mental confusion, and forgetfulness. Many of these symptoms can be related to niacin deficiency-induced deficits in the metabolism of the central nervous system. This system has glucose as its choice metabolic fuel. Glycolysis, with its attendant need for NAD^+ as a coenzyme, is appreciably less active. As the deficient state progresses, numbness occurs, followed by a paralysis of the extremities. The more advanced cases are characterized by tremor and a spastic or ataxic movement that is associated with peripheral nerve inflammation. Death from pellagra ensues if the patient remains untreated.

More subtle biochemical changes have also been reported in experimental niacin deficiency. It is now well known that NAD^+ is the substrate for poly (ADP-ribose) polymerase, an enzyme associated with DNA repair. In the deficient state this repair does not occur readily, and one of the characteristics of niacin deficiency is an increase in DNA strand breaks. If niacin deficiency accompanies conditions known to increase oxidative damage via free-radical attack on DNA, then the two conditions are additive with respect to cell damage and subsequent tissue pathology. Such has been proposed as a mechanism for the induction of cancer in susceptible cells.

Early indications of niacin deficiency include reductions in the levels of urinary niacin metabolites, especially those that are methylated (N′-methyl-nicotinamide and N′-methyl-2-pyridone-5-carboxamide). Since the discovery of the curative power of nicotinic acid and nicotinamide, pellagra is very rare, except in the alcoholic population. This population frequently substitutes alcoholic beverages for food and thereby is at risk for multiple nutrient deficiencies including pellagra. The metabolism of ethanol is NAD^+ dependent. This dependency drives up the need for niacin in the face of inadequate intake, setting the stage for alcoholic pellagra. In part, the CNS symptoms of alcoholism are those of pellagra as described above.

There is another very small population at risk for developing niacin deficiency. This group carries a mutation in the gene for tryptophan transport. This results in a condition called Hartnup's disease. Its symptoms, apart from tryptophan inadequacy effects on protein synthesis, are very similar to those of niacin deficiency. This is because of the use of tryptophan as a precursor of nicotinic acid. If niacin supplements are given to people with Hartnup's disease, these pellagra-like symptoms disappear.

G. Recommended Dietary Allowance

Because tryptophan can be converted to nicotinic acid, the RDA is stated in terms of niacin equivalents. A niacin equivalent is equal to 1 mg niacin or 60 mg of tryptophan. The need is related to energy intake as well, particularly the carbohydrate intake. However, the RDA takes into account varying diet composition as well as individual differences in nutrient need. Age and gender also influence need and these factors are considered in Table 9.

Table 9 Recommended Dietary Allowances for Niacin Equivalents (NE)

Group	Age	NE (mg/day)
Infants	Birth to 6 months	5
	7–12 months	6
Children	1–3	9
	4–6	12
	7–10	13
Males	11–14	17
	15–18	20
	19–24	19
	25–50	19
	51+	15
Females	11–14	15
	15–18	15
	19–22	15
	23–50	15
	51+	13
Pregnancy	—	17
Lactation	—	20

V. VITAMIN B_6

A. Overview

Of all the B vitamins whose nomenclatures have been changed to trivial names, one vitamin remains known by its letter designation: vitamin B_6. The vitamin was first defined by Gyorgy in 1934 as "that part of the vitamin B complex responsible for the cure of a specific dermatitis developed by rats on a vitamin-free diet supplemented with thiamin and riboflavin." The dermatitis is unlike that seen with other deficiencies of the B complex. There is a characteristic scaliness about the paws and mouth of rats in addition to a loss of hair from the body. The dermatitis is called rat acrodynia.

The vitamin was crystallized in 1938 by three different groups of researchers and was subsequently characterized and synthesized. Even though the vitamin was identified, crystallized, and synthesized in the late 1930s, it was not realized until 1945 that there were three distinct forms of the vitamin. Pyridoxine was isolated primarily from plant sources while pyridoxal and pyridoxamine were isolated from animal tissues. The latter two are more potent growth factors for bacteria and are more potent precursors for the coenzymes pyridoxal phosphate and pyridoxamine phosphate. When commercially prepared (synthesized) the vitamin is commonly available as pyridoxine hydrochloride.

B. Structure, Physical and Chemical Properties

Vitamin B_6 occurs in nature in three different forms which are interconvertible. It can be an aldehyde (pyridoxal), an alcohol (pyridoxine), or an amine (pyridoxamine). These three forms are shown in Figure 19. Vitamin B_6 is the generic descriptor for all 2-methyl-3-hydroxy-5-hydroxymethyl pyridine derivatives. To have vitamin activity it must be a pyridine derivative, be phosphorylatable at the 5-hydroxymethyl group, and the substituent at carbon 4 must be convertible to the aldehyde form.

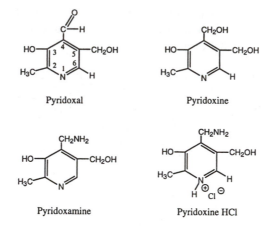

Figure 19   Structures of naturally occurring vitamin B$_6$.

Pyridoxine hydrochloride is the commercially available form of the vitamin and is shown in Figure 19. The molecular weight of pyridoxal is 167.2 Da and pyridoxine HCl has a molecular weight of 205.6 Da. Both occur as white crystals that are readily soluble in water. Pyridoxine is stable to light and heat in acid solutions. In neutral or alkaline solutions it is unstable to light and heat. The aldehyde form (pyridoxal) is much less stable. Its instability to heat is a major concern in food processing since foods that are rich in the vitamin are neutral to slightly alkaline. When heat treated, as is necessary to kill food-borne pathogens and prevent spoilage, vitamin activity may be lost. This is particularly true for foods that are autoclaved (i.e., infant formulas).

Pyridoxine, pyridoxal, and pyridoxamine can be assayed in a variety of techniques. Pyridoxal has an absorption maxima of 293 nm while pyridoxine HCl has absorption maxima of 255 and 326 nm. Microbiological, colorimetric/spectrophotometric, and chromatographic techniques are available. The method of choice is HPLC (high performance liquid chromatography).

C. Sources

Pyridoxine, pyridoxal, and pyridoxamine are widely distributed throughout the food supply. They are present in both plant and animal foods. Meats, cereals, legumes, lentils, nuts, fruits, and vegetables all contain the vitamin. Thus, persons consuming a diet containing a variety of raw and cooked foods likely will not develop a deficiency of the vitamin.

D. Absorption and Metabolism

In vivo and *in vitro* work with the rat and hamster small intestine provided no evidence of an active transport mechanism for the vitamin, however, more recent work suggests that facilitated diffusion may exist. Uptake into everted sacs of rat jejunum over a concentration range of 0.01 to 10 m*M* of pyridoxine was not inhibited by anoxia, DNP, lack of sodium, ouabain, or the presence of a structural analog 4-deoxypyridoxine. Thus, pyridoxine uptake is by passive and facilitated diffusion rather than by active transport (Figure 20). Once absorbed, it is carried by the erythrocytes to all cells in the body. Significant amounts of the vitamin may be found in liver, brain, spleen, kidney, and heart but, like the other water-soluble vitamins, there is no appreciable storage and this vitamin must be present in the daily diet. It is carried in the blood tightly bound to proteins, primarily hemoglobin and albumin. The vitamin binds via the amino group of the N-terminal valine residue of the hemoglobin α chain and this binding has twice the strength of its binding to albumin.

The B$_6$ vitamers are converted via a saturable two-step process to pyridoxal phosphate (PPS). The reactions, shown in Figure 21, are catalyzed by a B$_6$ vitamer kinase — an enzyme present in

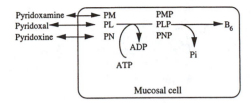

Figure 20 Absorption of the B_6 vitamins.

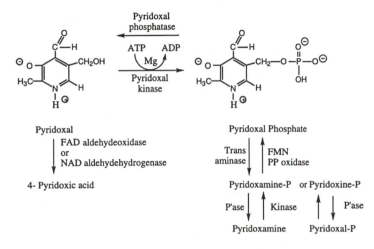

Figure 21 Phosphorylation of pyridoxal.

the cytoplasm of the mucosal cell. When the vitamers are phosphorylated, transmural absorption decreases whereas uptake is unaffected. Phosphorylation thus serves as a means of control of the cellular PMP, PLP, and PNP levels. This is called "metabolic trapping". Pyridoxine phosphate (PNP) and pyridoxamine phosphate (PMP) are oxidized by an FMN-dependent oxidase to form pyridoxal phosphate (PLP). At physiologic pH, zwitterionic structures pyridoxal and pyridoxal phosphate exist. These are shown in Figure 21. Pyridoxal phosphate can be converted (as shown) to either pyridoxine phosphate or pyridoxamine phosphate.

A major metabolite is 4-pyridoxic acid. It accounts for 50% of B_6 excreted in the urine. The reaction sequence is shown in Figure 21. Other metabolites have been found in the urine in addition to the three forms of the vitamin. Amphetamines, chlorpromazine, oral contraceptives, and reserpine all increase B_6 loss. Oral contraceptives had been found to increase tryptophan use and thus increase B_6 use. However, the current use of the minipill with its far smaller dose of hormones may not have this effect. The original observations were made in females using the larger dose of hormones.

E. Function

Pyridoxal phosphate serves as a coenzyme in reactions whose substrates contain nitrogen. Well over 100 reactions are known which involve pyridoxal phosphate. Many of these are transaminase reactions. Reactions such as transamination, racemization, decarboxylation, cleavage, synthesis, dehydration, and desulfhydration have been shown to be dependent on pyridoxal phosphate. In transamination, the α-amino group of amino acids such as alanine, arginine, asparagine, aspartic acid, cysteine, isoleucine, lysine, phenylalanine, tryptophan, tyrosine, and valine is removed and transferred to a carbon chain such as α-ketoglutarate, which in turn can transfer the amino group to the urea cycle for urea synthesis. Pyridoxal phosphate functions in transaminations in a Schiff

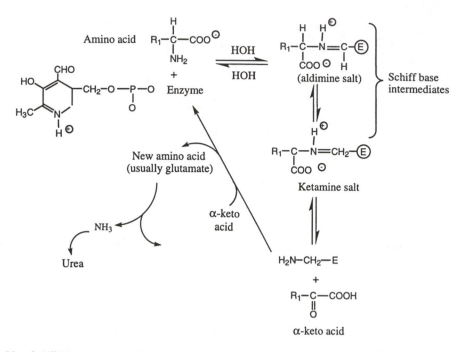

Figure 22   Schiff base mechanism for pyridoxal phosphate. Symbols used are R_1, amino acid; Ⓔ, apoenzyme; +, enzyme.

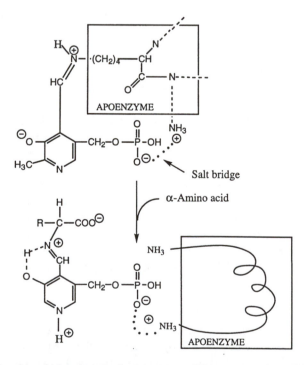

Figure 23   Binding of pyridoxal phosphate to its apoenzyme. When an α-amino acid enters, it displaces the ε-amino group of the lysyl residue of the apoenzyme.

base mechanism as shown in Figure 22. The binding of pyridoxal phosphate to its apoenzyme is shown in Figure 23. The active coenzyme forms of the vitamin B_6 are pyridoxal phosphate and pyridoxamine phosphate.

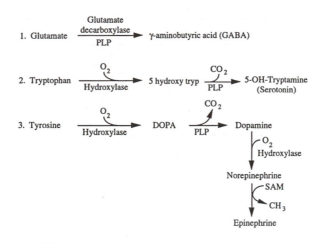

Figure 24 B$_6$ and synthesis of neurotransmitters.

Our present understanding of the role of these coenzymes, in part, is from the early work of Snell et al., who found that pyridoxal will react nonenzymatically at 100°C with glutamic acid to yield pyridoxamine and α-ketoglutarate. This led to the proposal that pyridoxal phosphate functions as a coenzyme by virtue of the ability of its aldehyde group to react with the α-amino group to yield a Schiff's base between the enzyme-bound pyridoxal phosphate and the amino acid, converting it to the α-keto acid. The resulting bound pyridoxamine phosphate enzyme then reacts with another α-keto acid, called an amino acid acceptor, in a reverse reaction to yield a new amino acid and pyridoxal phosphate. The linkage of pyridoxal phosphate to the enzyme is a noncovalent bonding through the charged ring containing the nitrogen atom as well as ionic interaction from the 5′-phosphate moiety to counterionic residues of the transaminase enzyme proteins. In transamination, the unprotonated amino group of the amino donor is covalently bound to the carbon atom of the aldehyde group of enzyme-bound pyridoxal phosphate and, with the elimination of water, forms an aldimine which tautomerizes to the corresponding ketamine. X-ray crystallography has confirmed the covalent aldiminium and ketaminium forms. The step involves the movement of an electron pair from the amino acid to the pyridine ring of the prosthetic group, followed by tautomerization to the ketamine.

Addition of water leads to the formation of a free α-keto acid and Enz-PLP complex. By oscillating between the aldehyde and amino groups, the PLP and PMP act as an amino acid carrier. Thus, the transamination reaction is an example of a double displacement reaction.

Pyridoxal phosphate also acts with cystathionine lyase to catalyze the cleavage of cystathionine and yield free enzyme and free cysteine, with α-ketobutyrate and NH$_3$ as other products. Pyridoxal phosphate is important to the synthesis of the neurotransmitters γ-aminobutyric acid (GABA), serotonin, dopamine, norepinephrine, and epinephrine. These reactions are outlined in Figure 24.

This role of vitamin B$_6$ explains the CNS symptoms associated with the deficient state. Convulsions are a common symptom, together with other derangements in metabolism, as is anemia. The symptom of anemia arises from the role of pyridoxal phosphate in hemoglobin synthesis as is outlined in Figure 25.

More recently, we have come to understand a role of vitamin B$_6$ in steroid hormone-induced protein synthesis. New studies have shown that B$_6$ has an important role as a physiological mediator of steroid hormone function. In this role, B$_6$ binds to a nuclear steroid hormone receptor and, in so doing, inhibits the binding of the steroid hormone-receptor complex to specific DNA sites. In this way, B$_6$ acts as a negative control of steroid hormone action. Progesterone, glucocorticoids, estrogen, and testosterone effects on RNA polymerase II and RNA transcription have been shown to be inhibited by the presence of pyridoxal phosphate. In each of these instances, the pyridoxal phosphate binds to the receptor protein and, in so doing, has a negative effect on hormone-receptor

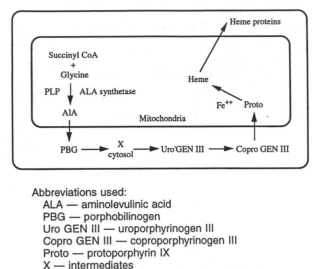

Abbreviations used:
ALA — aminolevulinic acid
PBG — porphobilinogen
Uro GEN III — uroporphyrinogen III
Copro GEN III — coproporphyrinogen III
Proto — protoporphyrin IX
X — intermediates
Enzymes catalyzing heme biosynthesis are omitted,
   except ALA synthetase

Figure 25   Role of pyridoxal-℗ (PLP) in heme biosynthesis.

binding to DNA. This role for B_6 is in addition to its role as a coenzyme in a wide variety of enzymes involved in cell growth and cell division. One of these is ornithine decarboxylase, an enzyme that plays an important role in cell division. In rapidly growing tumor cells, B_6 levels are much lower than in normal cells and some of the major chemotherapies for cancer are based on the need for B_6 by these cells. Antivitamin B_6 compounds are important chemotherapeutic agents in this setting.

F. Deficiency

In laboratory animals, dermatitis (acrodynia) is the chief symptom. Lesions occur on paws, ears, nose, chin, head, and upper thorax. This skin disorder resembles EFA deficiency. A high-fat diet protects somewhat against a B_6 deficiency. Other symptoms include poor growth; muscular weakness; fatty livers; convulsive seizures; anemia; reproductive impairment; edema; nerve degeneration; enlarged adrenal glands; increased excretion of xanthurenic acid, urea, and oxalate; decreased transaminase activity; impaired synthesis of ribosomal RNA, mRNA, and DNA; and impaired immune response. High protein intakes accelerate the development of the deficiency.

In humans, the deficiency syndrome is ill defined. It is characterized by weakness, irritability and nervousness, insomnia, and difficulty in walking. Cheilosis (cracks at the corners of the mouth) appears but is not responsive to biotin or riboflavin. Infants consuming B_6-deficient milk formula have convulsive seizures which can be corrected almost immediately with intravenously administered vitamin. There is a deranged tryptophan metabolism and evidence of increased excretion of xanthurenic acid. In B_6 deficiency, the conversion of tryptophan to niacin is impaired and thus skin lesions develop which resemble those of pellagra and riboflavin deficiency. Behavioral changes have been described and these include depression and irritability.

Hypochromic, sideroblastic anemia is a common finding and is due to the role B_6 plays in hemoglobin synthesis. While B_6 is found in a wide variety of foods, B_6 deficiency can be observed when antivitamin drugs are used. For example, isoniazid, a drug used in the treatment of tuberculosis, results in excessive B_6 loss. Penicillamine, a drug used in the treatment of Wilson's disease, has antivitamin activity. Lastly, higher than normal doses of B_6 have been prescribed for the

Table 10   Recommended Dietary Allowances for B_6

Group	Age	Recommended Daily Allowance (mg/day)
Infants	Birth to 6 months	0.3
	7–12 months	0.6
Children	1–3	1.0
	4–6	1.1
	7–10	1.4
Males	11–14	1.7
	15–18	2.0
	19–22	2.0
	23–50	2.0
	51+	2.0
Females	11–14	1.4
	15–18	1.5
	19–22	1.6
	23–50	1.6
	51+	1.6
Pregnancy	—	2.1
Lactation	—	2.1

treatment of skin disease and for neuromuscular and neurological diseases. Whether this prescription has a positive effect on the pathophysiology of these diseases remains under discussion.

There are several congenital diseases of importance to B_6 status. Homocysteinuria, due to a defect in the enzyme cystathione-β-synthase, is characterized by dislocation of the lenses in the eyes, malformation of skeletal and connective tissue, and mental retardation. Pyridoxal phosphate is a coenzyme for this synthase. Another genetic disease, cystathionuria, due to a defect in cystathione-γ-lyase and characterized by mental retardation, also drives up the need for B_6. A third genetic disorder, GABA deficiency due to mutation in glutamate decarboxylase, is manifested by a variety of neuropathies. Lastly, sideroblastic anemia, due to a mutation in δ-aminolevulinate synthetase, is characterized by anemia, cystathionuria, and xanthurenic aciduria. All of these genetic disorders can be ameliorated somewhat by massive doses of the vitamin. Why this works is not known for all cases, but patients with these disorders do not have any symptoms of B_6 deficiency since the defects are not in the absorption or metabolism of B_6 per se, but in the inadequate function (often due to poor binding of PLP) of specific enzymes involved in amino acid metabolism.

G. Recommended Dietary Allowance

The need for B_6 depends on the composition of the diet and on the age and gender of the individual. The B_6 RDAs are shown in Table 10.

VI. PANTOTHENIC ACID

A. Overview

Pantothenic acid was isolated and synthesized in the late 1940s and recognized as an essential growth factor for yeast. Its essentiality for mammalian species did not become known until it was shown to prevent or cure chick dermatitis. It was subsequently recognized as essential for the rat, mouse, monkey, pig, dog, fox, turkey, fish, hamster and human. Pantothenic acid is synthesized by plant tissues but not by mammalian tissues. It is found in a variety of tissues in the bound form. In 1946, it was discovered to be an essential part of coenzyme A.

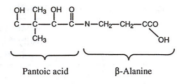

Figure 26   Structure of pantothenic acid.

B. Structure, Chemical and Physical Properties

Pantothenic acid is the trivial name for the compound dihydroxy-β,β-dimethylbutyryl-β-alanine. It has two metabolically active forms: as part of coenzyme A (CoA) and the acyl carrier protein. Pantothenic acid exists as the free acid (molecular weight 219.2 Da) or as a calcium salt (molecular weight 476.5 Da). It is the condensation product of β-alanine and a hydroxyl- and methyl-substituted butyric acid, pantoic acid. Its structure is shown in Figure 26. It is an unstable pale yellow oil, commercially available as a white, stable, crystalline, calcium, or sodium salt. When dry, the salt is stable to air and light but is hygroscopic. The salt is soluble in water and glacial acetic acid. The vitamin is stable in neutral solution but is readily destroyed by heat and either alkaline or acid pH. When heated in aqueous solution, there is hydrolytic cleavage of the molecule yielding β-alanine and 2,4-dihydroxy-3,3-dimethylbutyrate.

Pantothenic acid may be assayed colorimetrically following reaction with 1,2-naphthaquinone-4-sulphonate or ninhydrin. Radioimmunoassay also is used, as are microbiological methods. The method of choice is HPLC (high performance liquid chromatography).

C. Sources

Pantothenic acid is widely distributed in nature. Excellent food sources are organ meats, mushrooms, avocados, broccoli, and whole grains.

D. Absorption and Metabolism

Absorption occurs via facilitated diffusion and travels in the blood within the erythrocytes as well as in the plasma. Large doses of pantothenic acid are rapidly excreted in the urine, indicating no storage (except for that within the red blood cells and the fat cells) and little metabolism/degradation.

E. Function

Pantothenic acid functions in fatty acid metabolism as a component of coenzyme A. Unlike most vitamin coenzymes, pantothenic acid does not comprise the functional unit of CoA; instead, it provides the backbone for its derivative, pantotheine, whose SH group forms the reactive site. The structure of CoA is shown in Figure 27 and its synthesis is shown in Figure 28.

The function of CoA is to serve as a carrier of acyl groups in enzymatic reactions involving fatty acid oxidation, fatty acid synthesis, pyruvate oxidation, and biologic acetylations. It can not cross the cell membrane, and must therefore be synthesized in cells. Acetyl CoA (active acetate) is formed during the oxidation of pyruvate or fatty acids. It may also be generated from free acetate in the presence of the enzyme acetyl CoA synthetase. Acetyl CoA may then react with an acyl group acceptor such as choline to yield acetylcholine or oxaloacetate for citrate (Figure 29).

The sulfhydryl group of the β-mercaptoethylamine is the site at which acyl groups are linked for transport by the coenzyme. The ability of the CoASH to form thioesters with carboxylic acids is responsible for the vital role of the coenzyme in numerous metabolic processes.

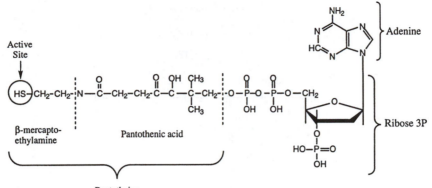

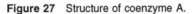

Figure 27 Structure of coenzyme A.

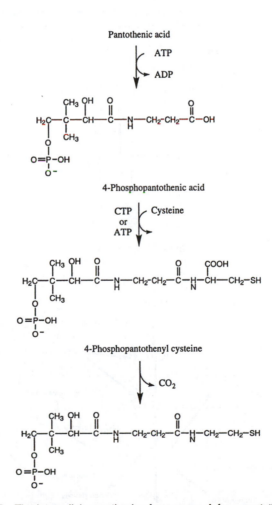

Figure 28 The intracellular synthesis of coenzyme A from pantothenic acid.

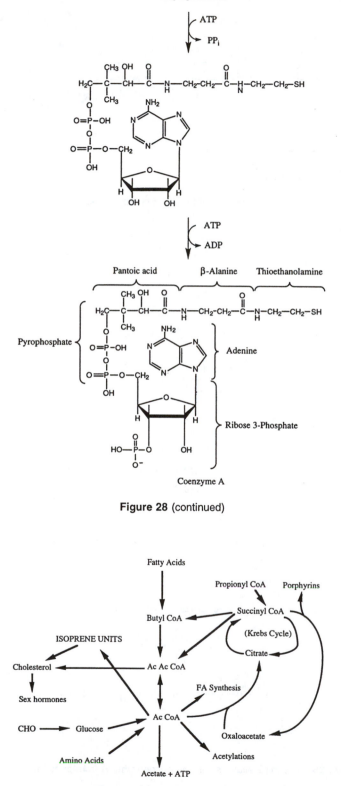

4-Phosphopantetheine

Pantoic acid   β-Alanine   Thioethanolamine

Pyrophosphate

Adenine

Ribose 3-Phosphate

Coenzyme A

Figure 28 (continued)

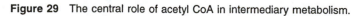

Fatty Acids

Propionyl CoA   Porphyrins

Butyl CoA   Succinyl CoA

(Krebs Cycle)

ISOPRENE UNITS   Citrate

Cholesterol ← Ac Ac CoA

FA Synthesis

Sex hormones

Ac CoA

CHO → Glucose   Oxaloacetate

Amino Acids   Acetylations

Acetate + ATP

Figure 29   The central role of acetyl CoA in intermediary metabolism.

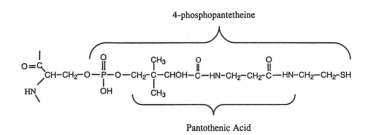

Figure 30 Structure of acyl carrier protein.

All known acyl derivatives of CoA are thiol esters. These acyl derivatives of CoA may participate in a number of metabolic reactions: condensation, addition, acyl group interchanges, and nucleophilic attack.

These reactions fall into three general categories:

1. Acetylation of choline and certain aromatic amines such as sulfonamides.
2. Oxidation of fatty acids, pyruvate, α-ketoglutarate, and acetaldehyde.
3. Synthesis of fatty acids, cholesterol, sphingosine, citrate, acetoacetate, porphyrin, and sterols.

Thus, CoA serves not only as an acetyl donor/acceptor but also as an acyl donor/acceptor and thus CoA serves as a central integrator of intermediary metabolism.

Fatty acid synthesis in the cytoplasm involves an additional role of pantothenic acid in the form of a cofactor, 4′-phosphopantetheine. This factor is bound to a protein commonly called acyl carrier protein (ACP). ACP plus 4′-phosphopantetheine appears to be involved in all fatty acid syntheses. Its structure attached to a seryl residue is shown in Figure 30. The acyl intermediates formed during fatty acid synthesis are esterified to the SH group. Phosphopantetheine is a cofactor bound to the GTP-dependent acyl CoA synthetase. Thus, 4′-phosphopantotheine serves in a capacity analogous to CoA during fatty acid oxidation.

Carnitine reacts with fatty acyl CoA esters to form carnitine esters capable of crossing the mitochondrial membrane. CoA does not travel across membranes and thus must be synthesized within each cell as the need for it arises.

F. Deficiency Symptoms

Deficiency symptoms are species specific (see Table 11). Pantothenic acid deficiency has not been described in humans as a single entity. If it occurs, it is accompanied by other deficiency disorders as well. The exception to this is in patients treated with the pantothenic acid antagonist, ω-methylpantothenic acid. In these patients, neurological symptoms (paresthesia of toes and feet), depression, fatigue, insomnia, vomiting, and muscle weakness have been reported. Changes in glucose tolerance, increased sensitivity to insulin, and decreased antibody production have also been noted.

G. Recommended Dietary Allowance

An RDA for pantothenic acid has not been determined, however, a provisional range for intake of 4 to 7 mg/day was suggested in 1980.

VII. BIOTIN

A. Overview

At the end of the nineteenth century, it was discovered that yeast needed a factor for growth that was not any of the already discovered essential nutrients. This factor was called "bios". Later,

**Table 11   Pantothenic Acid
Deficiency Symptoms
in Rats, Dogs, and Pigs**

Rat
  Dermatitis
  Achromotrichia (graying)
  Adrenal necrosis
  Hemorrhage
  Spectacle eye
  Spastic gait
  Anemia
  Leukopenia
  Impaired antibody formation
  Gonadal atrophy
  Infertility
Dog
  Appetite
  Hair loss
  Runny nose
  Fatty liver
  Irritability
  Hypoglycemia
Pig
  Spastic gait
  Hair loss
  As above

scientists realized that bios was a mixture of inositol and biotin and that bios could overcome "egg white injury". At this point it was named vitamin H or factor H and was found to be needed for cellular respiration. Because of its essentiality for respiration, it was named coenzyme R. In the late 1930s Gyorgy finally integrated all these bits and pieces, and together with Kögl, du Vigneaud, and Harris realized the essential nature of a material they had isolated and synthesized. Biotin was chosen as its name.

B. Structure, Physical and Chemical Properties

Biotin is the trivial name for the compound *cis*-hexahydro-2-oxo-1H-thieno-(3,4-d) imidazole-4-pentanoic acid. Its structure is shown in Figure 31. In order to have vitamin activity the structure must contain a conjoined ureido and tetrahydrothiophene ring with the ureido 3′N sterically hindered, preventing substitution. The ureido 1′N is a poor nucleophile.

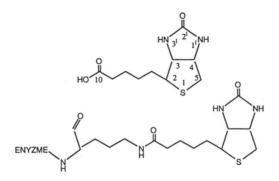

Figure 31   Structure of biotin and enzyme-bound biotin.

Biotin occurs in eight isomeric forms but only D-biotin has vitamin activity. Several biotin analogs have been synthesized or isolated from natural sources. Among these are oxybiotin or biotinol, biocytin, dithiobiotin, and biotin sulfoxide. The latter two are inactive as vitamins whereas the first two have some vitamin activity, albeit less than that of D-biotin.

Biotin is a white crystalline substance that, in its dry form, is stable to air, heat, and light. Its molecular weight is 244.3 Da and melting point is 167°C. It decomposes at 230 to 232°C. It has a limited solubility in water (22 mg/ml HOH) and is more soluble in ethanol. When in solution it is unstable to oxygen and strong acid or alkaline conditions and will be gradually destroyed by ultraviolet light. The analytical method of choice is HPLC; however, microbiological methods are also available. These methods use *Lactobacillus casei*, *Lactobacillus plantarum*, *Neurospora crassa*, *Ochromonas danica,* or *Saccharomyces cerevisiae*. These microorganisms require biotin for growth and are sensitive to varying quantities of biotin in the growth media. Using avidin, a protein found in egg white which binds biotin at the ureido group, an isotope dilution assay has been developed and is sensitive in the range of 4 to 41 pmol. Colorimetric assays based on the reaction of biotin with *p*-(dimethylamino)-cinnamaldehyde or on the absorbance of iodine formed during the oxidation of biotin to its sulfone with potassium iodide have been developed. The colorimetric assays are not as sensitive as HPLC or the avidin binding assays.

C. Sources

There are numerous food sources for biotin. Biotin is found in every living cell in minute amounts where it exists either in its enzyme-bound form or as a biotin ester or amide. Rich sources include organ meats, egg yolk, brewer's yeast, and royal jelly. Soy flour or soybean, rice polishings, various ocean fish, and whole grains are good sources of the vitamin.

D. Absorption, Metabolism

Biotin in food exists in the free and enzyme-bound form. The protein-bound form can be digested, which in turn yields biocytin, a combination of biotin and lysine. Biocytin is hydrolyzed via the action of biotinidase to its component parts. The resultant biotin is then available for absorption. Biotin is absorbed via facilitated diffusion. The jejunum is the major site for this absorption. Once absorbed, it circulates as free biotin. There may be some species differences in absorptive mechanisms. In addition, there is synthesis of the biotin by the gut flora.

Biotinidase is present in plasma as well, where it has a similar function. This enzyme plays a major role in biotin recycling. It acts as a hydrolase by cleaving biocytin and biotinyl peptides, thereby liberating biotin for reuse. Biotinidase, if mutated, results in an autosomal recessive disorder that causes a secondary biotin deficiency that can be overcome with biotin supplements. The clinical symptoms of this genetic disorder are the same as those of the biotin-deficient state and relate to the function of biotin as a coenzyme in intermediary metabolism, especially the carboxylase reactions.

Biotinidase has been cloned and sequenced and its distribution throughout the body has been determined. Although active in the intestinal tract, its activity is not sufficient to catalyze all of the bound biotin found in food. It has been estimated that less than 50% of the bound biotin found in foods of plant origin is hydrolyzed to provide the free form. The availability of biotin in food depends on the percent that is bound. In general, bound biotin found in foods of animal origin is more available than that of foods from plant origin. Biotin can be rendered unavailable by avidin, a protein found in raw egg white. Once the egg is cooked, the avidin is denatured and no longer binds the biotin. This binding is the explanation of the disorder "egg white injury". Other proteins, particularly membrane and transport proteins, bind biotin and are responsible for its entry into all cells that use the vitamin.

E. Function

Biotin serves as a mobile carboxyl carrier as it is attached to enzymes that catalyze carboxy group transfer. The formation of this biotin-enzyme complex is shown in Figure 32. A number of enzymes require biotin as a coenzyme for their function. These are listed in Table 12.

F. Deficiency

In humans the symptoms of severe deficiency include dermatitis, skin rash, hair loss (alopecia), developmental delay, seizures, conjunctivitis, visual and auditory loss, metabolic ketolactic acidosis, hyperammonemia, and organic acidemia. These symptoms have been reported in persons lacking normal biotinidase activity through a genetic error. In a genetically normal human population, a true biotin deficiency in the absence of other nutrient deficiencies is extremely rare. Only a few instances have been reported. In one instance, the deficient state was caused by the chronic consumption of 30 raw eggs per day for several months. In this individual, the symptoms were primarily related to the skin. Biotin deficiency may, however, be a secondary consequence of severe protein-energy malnutrition. Studies of severely malnourished children have shown improvement in biotin status with biotin supplements.

G. Recommended Dietary Intake

At present there is no RDA for biotin. Because the vitamin is present in a wide variety of foods, and because it can be synthesized by the intestinal flora, a fixed intake figure has been difficult to determine. However, the National Academy of Sciences Food and Nutrition Board has published a safe and adequate dietary intake for this vitamin. These suggested intakes are shown in Table 13.

VIII. FOLIC ACID

A. Overview

More than 50 years ago, folate was discovered to be a necessary constituent of every living cell of every organism, whether plant or animal. It took years of meticulous work to separate its function from that of vitamin B_{12}, for both are involved in the one-carbon transfers so important in the synthesis of the purines and pyrimidines that are constituents of DNA and RNA. Actually, until the genetic material and its function in the cell was worked out, there was no progress in understanding the role of the folates in nucleic acid synthesis. With the advent of our knowledge of how genes are made and how they work, we finally have come to understand the importance of folic acid in cellular function.

B. Structure, Chemical and Physical Properties

Folic acid, folate, or folacin are the generic terms for pteroylmonoglutamic acid and its related biologically active compounds. A number of derivatives (Table 14) have vitamin activity. The basic structure of pteroylglutamic acid is shown in Figure 33. The derivatives include the addition of hydrogen at N-5 and N-8 and to C-6 and C-7, with only one glutamate attached to p-aminobenzoic acid. This derivative is called tetrahydrofolic acid (THF). Other derivatives can have a methenyl group attached at N-5, a methenyl bridge between N-5 and N-10 or a methylene bridge at this position, or an aldehyde group at either N-5 or N-10, or an imino group at N-5. All of these derivatives have vitamin activity because vitamin activity is dependent on the presence of a pterin structure with variable hydrogenation or a methyl addition at N-5 or N-10 and the presence of at

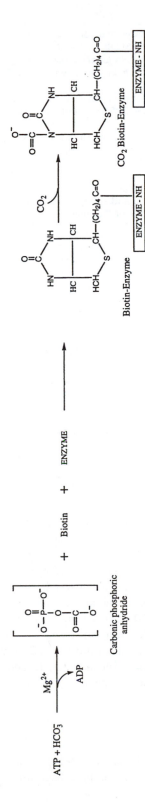

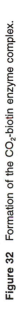

Figure 32 Formation of the CO_2-biotin enzyme complex.

Table 12   Biotin-Dependent Enzymes in Animals

Enzyme	Role	Location
Pyruvate carboxylase	First reaction in pathway that converts 3-carbon precursors to glucose (gluconeogenesis). Replenishes oxaloacetate for citric acid cycle.	Mitochondria (rate-limiting step in gluconeogenesis).
Acetyl-CoA carboxylase	Commits acetate units to fatty acid synthesis by forming malonyl-CoA.	Cytosol (rate-limiting step in fatty acid synthesis).
Propionyl-CoA carboxylase	Converts propionate to methylmalonyl-CoA which can be converted to succinyl CoA, an intermediate of the citric acid cycle.	Mitochondria
β-Methylcrotonyl-CoA carboxylase	Catabolism of leucine and certain isoprenoid compounds.	Mitochondria

Table 13   Safe and Adequate Dietary Intake of Biotin (μg/day)

Infants	0–6 months	35
	7–12 months	50
Children	1–3 years	65
	4–6 years	85
	7–10 years	120
Adolescents, Adults		100–200

Table 14   Derivatives of Folic Acid

Derivatives	N-5	N-10
Tetrahydrofolic acid	–H	–H
5-Methylfolic acid	–CH$_3$	–H
5,10-Methanylfolic acid	–CH=	–CH=
5,10-Methylenefolic acid	–CH$_2$–	–CH$_2$=
5-Formylfolic acid	–HCO	H
10-Formylfolic acid	–H	–HCO
5-Formiminfolic acid	–HCNH	H

least one glutamyl residue linked via peptide bonds to p-aminobenzoic acid. Methotrexate (4-amino-N^{10}-methyl folic acid, an antineoplastic agent) and aminopterin (4-amino folic acid, a rodenticide) are folate antagonists and as such are useful pharmaceutical agents against cell growth. Other drugs, sulfasalazine and diphenylhydantoin, for example, interfere with folacin uptake and use.

The pteroylmonoglutamate form has a molecular weight of 441.4 Da and is moderately soluble in water (0.0016 mg/ml water). It has absorption maxima at 256, 283, and 368 nm. It is an orange-yellow crystal with a melting point of 250°C. It is unstable to ultraviolet light, heat, oxygen, acidic conditions, and divalent metal ions such as iron and copper. As mentioned, it is present in all living cells in small amounts, so until the advent of sensitive HPLC techniques its determination in food and animal tissues relied on microbiological techniques. In addition to the HPLC methodology there is also a radioimmunological technique which involves the competitive binding of the vitamin to a protein, followed by quantification.

C. Sources

Folate is found in a wide variety of foods of both animal and plant origin. However, because it is so unstable, reliable food composition data have been difficult to obtain and it is altogether

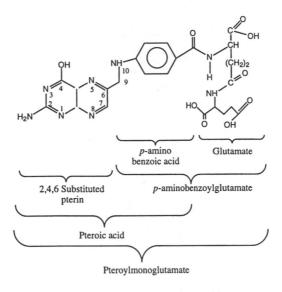

Figure 33   Structure of folic acid.

possible that food sources may be insufficient to meet dietary need. Good sources include meats, fruits, vegetables (especially asparagus), dry beans, peas and nuts, and whole-grain cereal products.

D. Absorption, Metabolism

Folate transport in the intestine is a carrier-mediated, pH-dependent process with maximum transport occurring after deconjugation to the monoglutamate form in the jejunum. There are specific folate-binding proteins that function in the absorption process. One is a low-affinity folate-binding protein found in the brush border membrane of the absorptive cell. There is another high-affinity folate-binding protein that is localized to the jejunal brush border cells. Affinity is optimized at pH 5.5 to 6.0. The high-affinity binding protein is similar to one found in the kidney.

A number of drugs inhibit or compete with folate for transport. These include ethacrynic acid, sulfinpyrazone, phenylbutazone, sulfasalazine, and furosemide. All of these are amphipathic substances. That is, they are compounds with a polar-apolar character. Absorption is also inhibited by cyanide and 2,4-dinitrophenol — drugs that poison oxidative phosphorylation and thus reduce the ATP supply. ATP is necessary for the active transport process to work. Absorption can also occur by passive diffusion but this is a secondary means for folate uptake. Very little folate appears in the feces.

After folate is absorbed it circulates in the plasma as pteroylmonoglutamate. That which is not used by the cells is excreted in the urine as pteroylglutamic acid, 5-methyl-pteroylglutamic acid, 10-formyltetrahydrofolate, or acetamidobenzoylglutamate. Uptake by cells is mediated by a highly specific folate binding protein. This protein has been isolated from the membranes of a variety of cells and a cDNA probe has been prepared. Folate appears to stimulate the transcription of the mRNA for this protein. In this role folate binds to a specific DNA binding protein (a folate receptor) which, in turn, serves as a transcription factor enhancing the transcription of the mRNA for the highly specific folate-binding protein.

Some of the food folate exists as 5,10-methylenetetrahydrofolate, which must be converted to 5-methyltetrahydrofolate, the circulatory folate form. This conversion requires the enzyme methylenetetrahydrofolate reductase. The gene for this enzyme has been mapped in the mouse to chromosome 4, and a common mutation that results in a substitution of valine for alanine at position 299

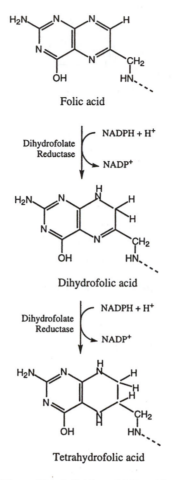

Figure 34 Activation of folic acid.

has been linked to neural tube defects. This mutation requires low folate status in the plasma for the development of mild hyperhomocysteinemia which in turn has been linked to neural tube defects.

E. Function

Folate's main function is as a coenzyme in one-carbon transfer. However, before it can do this it must be activated. Activation consists of the reduction of folic acid to dihydrofolic acid and thence to tetrahydrofolic acid as shown in Figure 34.

A number of folate derivatives have vitamin activity and these derivatives are interconvertible, as shown in Figure 35. Methyl-group transfer also involves vitamin B_{12}, as illustrated in Figure 36.

The regulation of methyl-group transfer is complex and involves a number of enzymes and substrates. Enzymes requiring folate as a coenzyme are listed in Table 15. While serine is a good source for the methyl group, methyl groups arise from other substrates as well. The major source of single methyl groups involves a cycle of reactions catalyzed by serine hydroxymethyltransferase, 5,10-methylene-FH_4 reductase, and methionine synthetase. The last of these reactions is rate limiting for the cycle, whereas the second is inhibited by a S-adenosylmethionine (SAM) as well as 5-methyl-FH_4. As described in Section IX on vitamin B_{12}, methionine synthesis depends on the transfer of labile methyl groups from 5-methyl-folate to B_{12} which, as methyl-B_{12}, donates this methyl group to homocysteine, making methionine.

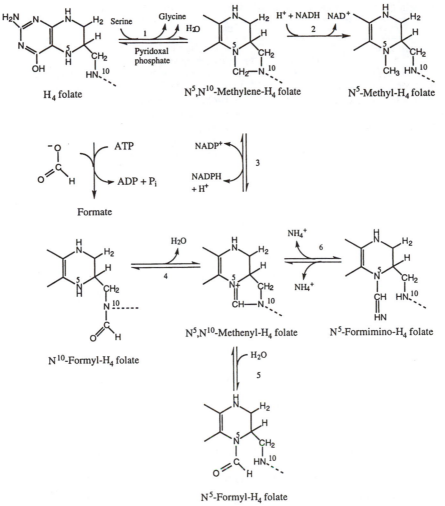

Figure 35 The interconversions of one-carbon moieties attached to tetrahydrofolate.

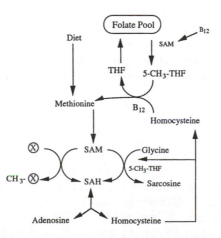

Figure 36 Involvement of B_{12} in methyl group transfer via S-adenosylation (SAM).

Table 15   Metabolic Reactions in Which Folate Plays a Role as a Coenzyme

Enzyme	Role
Thymidylate synthetase	Transfers formaldehyde to C-5 of dUMP to form a dTMP in pyrimidine synthesis (see Figure 5).
Glycinamide ribonucleotide transformylase	Donates formate in purine synthesis (see Unit 2).
5-Amino-4-imidazolecarboxamide transformylase	Donates formate in purine synthesis (see Unit 2).
Serine hydroxymethyl transferase	Accepts formaldehyde in serine catabolism.
10-Formyl-FH$_4$ synthetase	Accepts formaldehyde from tryptophan catabolism.
10-Formyl-FH$_4$ dehydrogenase	Transfers formate for oxidation to CO_2 in histidine catabolism.
Methionine synthase	Donates methyl group to homocysteine to form methionine.
Formiminotransferase	Accepts formimino group from histidine.

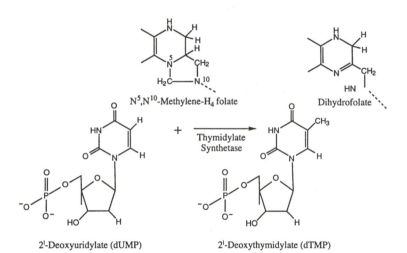

Figure 37   Addition of methyl groups to deoxyuridylate using the methyl-group transfer function of folate.

One-carbon transfer is particularly important in purine and pyrimidine synthesis. The mechanism of this transfer that involves folate (and also B_{12}) is illustrated in Figure 37. The whole reaction sequence for purine and pyrimidine synthesis is presented in Unit 2. In this sequence, methyl transfer via thymidylate synthetase converts 2′-deoxyuridylate to 2′-deoxythymidylate.

From this reaction (Figure 37) it is immediately apparent why folate and vitamin B_{12} are so important to gene expression. While nuclear DNA, once made, merely reproduces itself within the cell cycle, new messenger RNA is made every minute as new proteins are needed by the cell. While some of the purine and pyrimidine bases can be salvaged and reused, this recycling is not 100% efficient. Messenger RNA has a *very* short half-life (seconds to hours) compared to the other nucleic acid species in the cell. Thus, newly synthesized purines and pyrimidines must be available. If not available, mRNA synthesis, *de novo* protein synthesis, and, of course, cell renewal will be adversely affected.

F. Deficiency

While anemia, dermatitis, and impaired growth are the chief symptoms of folate deficiency in the human, scientists are now beginning to recognize the importance of adequate folate intake in early embryonic development. Inadequate intake by the mother prior to and/or during the early stages of development can have teratogenic effects on the embryo. Embryonic development, particularly closure of the neural tube, is impaired in folate deficiency. As a result, infants are born with spina bifida and other neural tube defects. It is estimated that about 2500 infants per year are

Table 16   1989 Recommended Dietary Allowances (RDA) for Folate

Group	Age	RDA (μg/day)
Infants	0–6 months	25
	7–12 months	35
Children	1–3	50
	4–6	75
	7–10	100
Males	11–14	150
	15–18	200
	19–24	200
	25–50	200
	51+	200
Females	11–14	150
	15–18	180
	19–24	180
	25–20	180
	51+	180
Pregnancy		400
Lactation		280

born with these defects, but not all of these infant defects are attributable to inadequate folate nutrients. Available evidence indicates that women contemplating pregnancy should consume 400 μg/day as a prophylactic measure. Low folate intake has been suggested as a factor in the development of colon cancer as well as in the bronchial squamous metaplasia (premalignant lesions) of smokers, and cervical dysplasia (another premalignant lesion) in women. Folate deficiency in rats has been shown to induce DNA strand breaks and hypomethylation within the p53 tumor suppressor gene. Whether this occurs in humans and can explain the link between folate status and cancer development remains to be explored. Other symptoms of deficiency are leukopenia (low white-cell count), general weakness, depression, and polyneuropathy. The latter sign is probably related to the folate-B_{12} interaction.

G. Recommended Dietary Allowance

Because of the concern over the folate deficiency effect on embryonic development, the RDA for folacin is under revision. The 1989 RDAs are given in Table 16. However, as mentioned in the preceding section, women contemplating pregnancy should at least double their intake (from an RDA of 180 to 400 μg/day). Since folate is not toxic this is probably a good idea, with the caveat that B_{12} status is normal. If this is not the case, excess folate could mask a B_{12} deficiency somewhat until the irreversible neurologic features of B_{12} deficiency appear. To avoid this consequence of masking, an evaluation of B_{12} status should be conducted. Alternatively, supplementation of B_{12} and folacin could be considered assuming that there is no deficit in intrinsic factor (see Section IX).

IX. VITAMIN B_{12}

A. Overview

Vitamin B_{12} is one of the most recently discovered micronutrients and is the most potent. Very little of the vitamin is required to prevent the symptoms of pernicious anemia and subsequent neurological change. It was isolated in 1948 and shortly thereafter was shown to be the required substance needed to prevent pernicious anemia.

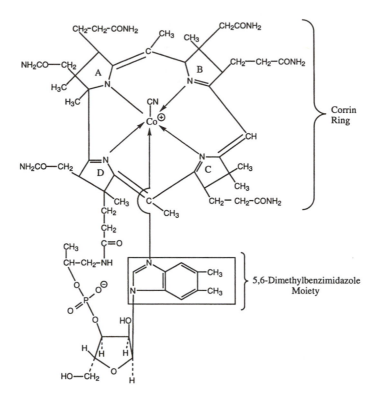

Figure 38   Cyanocobalamin; vitamin B_{12} ($C_{63}H_{88}N_{14}PCo$).

B. Structure, Chemical and Physical Properties

Vitamin B_{12} is a very complex structure as shown in Figure 38. The term B_{12} is the generic descriptor for all corrinoids — those compounds having a corrin ring. Cyanocobalamin is the trivial designation for this compound. In order to have vitamin activity it must contain a cobalt-centered corrin ring. Below the ring it may have a heterocyclic nitrogen side chain or may have nothing attached here. Above the ring it may have a hydroxo, aquo, methyl, 5-deoxyadenosyl, CN, Cl⁻, Br⁻, nitro, sulfito, or sulfato group. There are a number of structural analogs that have vitamin activity. Regardless of the substituents present above or below the cobalt-centered corrin ring, unless the ring is present there will be no vitamin function. The ring consists of four reduced pyrrole rings linked by three methylene bridges and one direct bond. The cobalt atom is in the 3+ state and can form up to 6 coordinate bonds. It is tightly bound to the four pyrrole N atoms and can also bond a nucleotide and a small ligand below and above the ring, respectively. Commercially viable synthesis of this compound is very difficult although one such process has been developed using 2 mol of 5-aminolevulinate to form porphobilinogen, a pyrrole ring with an aminomethyl group on C-2, an acetate group on C-3, and a proprionate on C-4. Four of these are linked together and cyclized to form hydroxymethylcobalamin to which cobalt is attached. Vitamin B_{12} has a molecular weight of 1355.4 Da and is moderately soluble in water (12.5 mg/ml). It is insoluble in fat solvents. Its absorption maxima occur at 278, 361, and 550 nm. It is a heat-stable red crystal but will decompose at temperatures above 210°C. The crystal will melt at temperatures above 300°C. It is unstable to ultraviolet light, acid conditions, and the presence of metals such as iron and copper. Vitamin B_{12} is very difficult to assay. It is primarily the product of microbial synthesis and thus is not usually present in large amounts in most foods. Organ meats are good sources of B_{12}. It is synthesized in the gastrointestinal system by the resident flora. One assay system uses B_{12}-dependent microorganisms. The most responsive and specific of these is *Ochromonas malhamensis*. Although sensitive to small amounts of the vitamin, these procedures are tedious. Spectrophotometric assays that can detect as little as 25 μg/ml are also available but not practical because the sensitivity is so limited. HPLC is the best system for detection and quantitation.

C. Absorption, Metabolism

Most mammals depend on a very complex system to extract vitamin B_{12} and absorb it. The process of absorption begins in the stomach, where preformed B_{12} is bound to a carrier protein called intrinsic factor. As B_{12} is made by the gut flora, it, too, is bound to a carrier protein. Whether this carrier is identical to that available in the stomach is not known. It probably is. Likely, future research will show that the synthesis of this carrier is directed by the vitamin in a manner analogous to that of retinol and the retinol receptor protein (see Unit 3).

Actually, there are four structurally distinct B_{12} carrier proteins. Intrinsic factor (IF) is one of these, and another, called R binder, is found in the proximal part of the alimentary tract. R binder is degraded by the pancreatic peptidases and proteases, while the intrinsic factor-B_{12} complex proceeds intact to the distal portion of the ileum where, in the presence of calcium and neutral pH, the complex binds to IF on the surface of the luminal epithelial cell. Subsequent to binding to IF, the vitamin appears in the portal blood bound to another protein called transcobalamin II or TCII. The blood contains an additional R-type protein called transcobalamin I (TCI) which assists in the transport of the vitamin to its target cells.

Although absorption occurs mainly in the distal ileum, it also occurs in the large intestine. This takes advantage of the fact that B_{12} is synthesized by the flora in this part of the intestinal tract. The mechanism of absorption by the ileum is mediated by a carrier, the intrinsic factor; however, the details of this mechanism are unknown except for the need for the carrier as described above. Passive diffusion also occurs when large B_{12} doses are given. Once absorbed, the transport of B_{12} within the enteral cell also involves a carrier and divalent ions. Calcium, in particular, is needed for the attachment of the intrinsic factor-B_{12} complex to its cognate receptor on the enteral cell plasma membrane. Likely, other factors are also involved; persons with a variety of diseases such as pancreatitis, tropical sprue, fluoroacetate poisoning, and pancreatic insufficiency do not absorb B_{12} efficiently and often show signs of pernicious anemia until provided with oral B_{12} supplements or injected with B_{12}. Absorption by the large intestine likely occurs via passive diffusion.

Once absorbed, B_{12} is transported in the blood bound to one of three transport proteins: transcobalamin I, II, or III. Small amounts are stored (as methylcobalamin) in the liver, kidney, heart, spleen, and brain. Thus, if an individual lacks intrinsic factor due perhaps to a genetic disease or surgical loss of the stomach (gastrectomy) or, as described above, has one or more diseases that affect B_{12} absorption, an injection of B_{12} can be given once a month (rather than daily) and this will correct the problem of inadequate supply.

D. Function

Vitamin B_{12} functions in one of two ways: (1) it participates as a coenzyme in reactions that utilize 5′-deoxyadenosine linked covalently to the cobalt atom (adenosylcobalamin), and (2) it participates as a substrate in reactions that utilize the attachment of a methyl group to the central cobalt atom (methylcobalamin). The conversion of cobalamin to methylcobalamin is catalyzed by the enzyme, B_{12} coenzyme synthetase. It catalyzes the reduction of the molecule then catalyzes the reaction with deoxyadenosyl derived from ATP. In addition to ATP, this reaction needs a diol or a dithiol group, a reduced flavin, or a reduced ferredoxin as the biological alkylating agent. The enzymes requiring B_{12} as a coenzyme are listed in Table 17. The first of these is required for L-methionine synthesis. This reaction removes a methyl group from methyl folate via methyl-B_{12} and delivers it to homocysteine. This allows recycling of the folate coenzymes required for purine

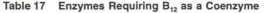

Table 17   Enzymes Requiring B$_{12}$ as a Coenzyme

N^5-Methyltetrahydrofolate homocysteine methyltransferase
Acetate synthetase
Glutamate mutase
Methylmalonyl-CoA mutase
α-Methyleneglutarate mutase
Dioldehydrase a
Dioldehydrase b
Glyceroldehydrase
Ethanolamine ammonia-lyase
L-β-Lysine mutase
D-α-Lysine mutase
Ornithine mutase
L-β-Leucine aminomutase

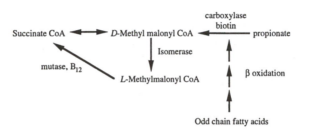

Figure 39   Overall reaction in the conversion of proprionate to succinate using biotin and vitamin B$_{12}$ as coenzymes.

and pyrimidine biosynthesis. Thus, in B$_{12}$ deficiency nucleic acid synthesis is arrested because it is indirectly dependent on adequate B$_{12}$ intake. This process is directly dependent on folacin. B$_{12}$-deficient animals show decreased methylation of tetrahydrofolate and decreased cellular folate levels despite dietary folate sufficiency. One of the characteristics of the B$_{12}$ deficient state is an anemia characterized by few mature red cells. Immature nucleated cells (megaloblasts) can be found, but not mature ones. Among the other enzymes listed in Table 17 is methylmalonyl CoA mutase, which participates in propionate metabolism. The overall reaction using B$_{12}$ as a coenzyme in proprionate metabolism is shown in Figure 39.

Propionate metabolism, although a minor pathway in monogastric animals, is of some importance in neural tissue. Loss of this metabolic activity may explain the peripheral neural loss that characterizes long-term B$_{12}$ deficiency.

Methylmalonic aciduria characterizes the B$_{12}$-deficient individual. Studies with rats made B$_{12}$ deficient show an increase in odd-numbered fatty acids in the serum and in the neural and hepatic lipids and low hepatic methylmalonyl-CoA mutase activity. Replacement of B$_{12}$ in the diet corrects both these responses. The effect of B$_{12}$ on mutase activity is such that it is likely that the vitamin serves not only as the coenzyme in the reaction but also serves a role in the synthesis of that enzyme. Several reports of B$_{12}$ activity vis à vis protein synthesis have appeared in the literature in addition to the one concerning the synthesis of the mutase. Whether this relates to the indirect role of B$_{12}$ in DNA and RNA synthesis, i.e., the synthesis of pyrimidines and purines, or whether a B$_{12}$-protein complex acts as a *cis*- or *trans*-acting factor in the pathway for the expression of the specific genes for these enzymes is unknown.

E. Deficiency

As described in the preceding section, the deficiency state has as its main characteristic, megalobastic anemia. While inadequate B$_{12}$ intake can result in this anemia, this is a rather unusual nutritional state because most foods of animal origin contain B_{12} and so little is needed. More common as a cause of vitamin B_{12} deficiency is a genetically determined deficiency in the synthesis of intrinsic factor. This trait is inherited as an autosomal dominant trait and occurs in about 1 person in 1000. It can be treated with monthly B_{12} injections (~60 to 100 μg per dose). In the absence of this trait, the people most at risk for B_{12} deficiency are those who abstain from eating foods of animal origin. In addition to these are those who have had one of the illnesses described earlier that impair absorption. Humans that have had a gastrectomy or some disease of the gastric mucosa or some disease resulting in malabsorption are in this category.

Following the development of megaloblastic anemia, which is reversible, is the irreversible loss of peripheral sensation. This is due to the degenerative changes in the peripheral nerve tracts that include demyelination or loss of the lipid protective coat that surrounds the nerve tracts. Once the myelin is lost the nerve dies. Neural loss begins in the feet and hands and progresses upward to the major nerve trunks such that a progressive neuropathy can be followed. Sometimes this pattern of loss is not followed; instead the patient may have problems with balance or coordination of limb motions as in walking or picking up objects. Because both folate and B_{12} are interactively involved in DNA and RNA synthesis it used to be difficult to segregate one deficiency anemia from the other. Folacin supplements might mask the symptoms of B_{12} deficiency. However, measuring the presence of methylmalonic acid in urine and blood will allow for the differential analysis in the cause of the anemia. In addition to folacin and B_{12}, deficient intakes of ascorbic acid, vitamin B_6, niacin, iron, copper, and zinc can also explain anemia (see Units 1 and 6) and deficiencies of these nutrients must be ruled out.

F. Recommended Dietary Allowance

The daily dietary requirements for B_{12} are very small. The normal turnover rate is about 2.5 μg/day thus the recommendation for adults is close to this turnover rate or 2 μg/day. Table 18 gives the RDA for humans of different ages. The need for B_{12} is also related to the intake of ascorbic acid, thiamin, carnitine, and fermentable fiber. Each of these nutrients affects the production of propionate, and in their absence or relative deficiency, propionate production is increased and this, in turn, drives up the need for B_{12}. As already mentioned, the needs for B_{12} and folate are related.

Table 18 Recommended Dietary Allowances for Vitamin B_{12}

Group	Age	RDA (μg/day)
Infants	Birth to 6 months	0.3
	7–12 months	0.5
Children	1–3	0.7
	4–6	1.0
	7–10	1.4
Males	11–14	2.0
	15–18	2.0
	19–24	2.0
	25–50	2.0
	50 +	2.0
Females	11–14	2.0
	15–18	2.0
	19–24	2.0
	25–50	2.0
	51 +	2.2
	Pregnant —	2.6
	Lactation —	2.6

SUPPLEMENTAL READINGS

Ascorbic Acid

Barja, G., Lopez-Torres, M., Perez-Campo, R., Rojas, C., Cadenas, S., Prat, J., and Pamplona, R. 1994. Dietary vitamin C decreases endogenous protein oxidative damage, malonaldehyde, and lipid peroxidation and maintains fatty acid unsaturation in guinea pig liver, *Free Rad. Biol. Med.*, 17:105-115.

Bieri, J.G. 1973. Effects of excessive vitamins C and E on vitamin A status, *Am. J. Clin. Nutr.*, 26:382.

Bowers-Komro, D.M. and McCormick, D.B. 1991. Characterization of ascorbic acid uptake by isolated rat kidney cells, *J. Nutr.*, 121:57-64.

Creagen, E.T., Moertel, C.G., O'Fallon, J.R., Schutt, A.J., O'Connell, M.J., Rubin, J., and Frytak, S. 1979. Failure of high dose vitamin C therapy to benefit patients with advanced cancer, *N. Engl. J. Med.*, 301:687.

Harris, A.B., Hartley, J., and Moor, R. 1973. Reduced ascorbic acid excretion and oral contraceptives, *Lancet*, 2:201.

Herbert, V. and Jacob, E. 1974. Destruction of vitamin B_{12} by ascorbic acid, *J. Am. Med. Assoc.*, 230:241.

Hodges, R.E., Baker, E.M., Hood, J., and Sauberlich, H.E. 1969. Experimental scurvy in man, *Am. J. Clin. Nutr.*, 22:535.

Kallner, A., Hartmann, D., and Hornig, D. 1979. Steady state turnover and body pool of ascorbic acid in man, *Am. J. Clin. Nutr.*, 32:530.

Kallner, A.B., Hartmann, D., and Hornig, D.H. 1981. On the requirements of ascorbic acid in man: steady state turnover and body pool in smokers, *Am. J. Clin. Nutr.*, 34:1347.

Mayfield, H.L. and Roehm, R.R. 1956. The influence of ascorbic acid and the source of B vitamins on the utilization of carotene, *J. Nutr.*, 58:203.

McLeroy, V.J. and Schendel, H.E. 1973. Influence of oral contraceptives on ascorbic acid concentrations in healthy, sexually mature women, *Am. J. Clin. Nutr.*, 26:191.

Padh, H. 1991. Vitamin C: newer insights into its biochemical functions, *Nutr. Rev.*, 49:65-70.

Rivers, J. and Devine, M.M. 1970. Plasma ascorbic acid concentrations and oral contraceptives, *Fed. Proc.*, 29:295.

Will, J.C. and Byers, T. 1996. Does diabetes mellitus increase the requirement for vitamin C?, *Nutr. Rev.*, 54:193-202.

Thiamin

Brin, M. 1980. Red cell transketolase as an indicator of nutritional deficiency, *Am. J. Clin. Nutr.*, 33:169-171.

Caster, W.O. and Meadows, J.S. 1980. The three thiamin requirements of the rat, *Int. J. Vitam. Nutr. Res.*, 50:125-130.

Lonsdale, D. and Shamberger, R.J. 1980. Red cell transketolase as an indicator of nutritional deficiency, *Am. J. Clin. Nutr.*, 33:205-211.

Massey, V. 1994. Activation of molecular oxygen by flavins and flavoproteins, *J. Biol. Chem.*, 269:22459-22462.

McCormick, D.B. 1991. Coenzymes, Biochemistry. In: *Encyclopedia of Human Biology*, Vol. 2, Academic Press, Orlando, FL, pp. 1009-1028.

Molina, P.E., Yousef, K.A., Smith, R.M., Tepper, P.G., Lang, C.H., and Abumrad, N.N. 1994. Thiamin deficiency impairs endotoxin-induced increases in hepatic glucose output, *Am. J. Clin. Nutr.*, 59:1045-1049.

Sklan, D. and Trostler, N. 1977. Site and extent of thiamin absorption in the rat, *J. Nutr.*, 107:353-356.

Riboflavin

Addison, R. and McCormick, D.B. 1978. Biogenesis of flavoprotein and cytochrome components in hepatic mitochondria from riboflavin deficient rats, *Biochem. Biophys. Res. Commun.*, 81:133-138.

Aw, T.Y., Jones, D.P., and McCormick, D.B. 1983. Uptake of riboflavin by isolated liver cells, *J. Nutr.*, 113:1249-1254.

Casirola, D., Gastaldi, G., Ferrari, G., Kasai, S., and Rindi, G. 1993. Riboflavin uptake by rat small intestinal brush border membrane vesicles. A dual mechanism involving specific membrane binding, *J. Membr. Biol.*, 135:217-223.

Hoppel, C., DiMarco, J.P., and Tandler, B. 1979. Riboflavin and rat hepatic cell structure and function, *J. Biol. Chem.*, 254:4164-4170.

Joseph, T. and McCormick, D.B. 1995. Uptake and metabolism of riboflavin 5-a-D glucoside by rat and isolated liver cells, *J. Nutr.,* 125:2194-2198.

Massey, V. 1994. Activation of molecular oxygen by flavins and flavoproteins, *J. Biol. Chem.,* 269:22459-22463.

McCormick, D.B. and Zhang, Z. 1993. Cellular assimilation of water soluble vitamins in the mammal: riboflavin B_6, biotin, and C, *Proc. Soc. Exp. Biol. Med.,* 202:265-270.

McCormick, D.B. 1989. Two interconnected B vitamins, *Physiol. Rev.,* 69:1170-1198.

Muller, E.M. and Bates, C.J. 1977. Effect of riboflavin deficiency on white cell glutathione reductase in rats, *Int. J. Vitam. Nutr. Res.,* 47:46-51.

Ross, N.S. and Hansen, T.P.B. 1992. Riboflavin deficiency is associated with selective preservation of critical flavoenzyme-dependent metabolic pathways, *Biofactors,* 3:185-190.

Zaman, Z. and Verwilghen, R.L. 1975. Effects of riboflavin deficiency on oxidative phosphorylation, flavin enzymes and coenzymes in rat liver, *Biochem. Biophys. Res. Commun.,* 67:1192-1198.

Niacin

Aktories, K., Jakobs, K.H., and Shultz, G. 1980. Nicotinic acid inhibits adipocyte adenylate cyclase in a hormone like manner, *FEBS Lett.,* 115:11-14.

Horwitt, M.K., Harper, A.E., and Henderson, L.M. 1981. Niacin-tryptophan relationships for evaluating niacin equivalents, *Am. J. Clin. Nutr.,* 34:423-427.

Jacob, R.A., Sweinseid, M.E., McKee, R.W., Fu, C.S., and Clemens, R.A. 1989. Biochemical markers for assessment of niacin status in young men: urinary and blood levels of niacin metabolites, *J. Nutr.,* 119:591-598.

McCormick, D.B. 1991. Coenzymes, Biochemistry. In: *Encyclopedia of Human Biology,* Vol. 2, Academic Press, Orlando, FL, pp. 1009-1038.

Melax, H., Singh, D.N.P., Cookson, F.B., and Jeria, M.J. 1981. Degenerations of the myocardium in rats fed nicotinic acid diet, *IRCS Med. Sci.,* 9:293-294.

Rose, R.C. 1990. Water soluble vitamin absorption in intestine, *Annu. Rev. Physiol.,* 42:157-171.

Van Eys, J. 1991. Nicotinic acid. In: *Handbook of Vitamins,* Machlin, L.J., Ed., Marcel Dekker, New York, pp. 311-340.

Zhang, J.Z., Henning, S.M., and Swenseid, M.E. 1993. Poly (ADP-ribose) polymerase activity and DNA strand breaks are affected in tissues of niacin-deficient rats, *J. Nutr.,* 123:1349-1355.

Pyridoxine

Allgood, V.E., Powell-Oliver, F.E., and Cidlowski, J.A. 1990. Vitamin B_6 influences glucocorticoid receptor-dependent gene expression, *J. Biol. Chem.,* 265:12424-12433.

Heiskanen, K., Salmenpera, L., Perheentupa, J., and Sümes, M.A. 1994. Infant vitamin B_6 status changes with age and with formula feeding, *Am. J. Clin. Nutr.,* 60:907-910.

Leklem, J.E. 1991. Vitamin B_6. In: *Handbook of Vitamins,* Machlin, L., Ed., Marcel Dekker, New York. pp. 341-392.

Miller, J.W., Nadeau, M.R., Smith, D., and Selhub, J. 1994. Vitamin B_6 deficiency vs. folate deficiency: comparison of responses to methionine loading in rats, *Am. J. Clin. Nutr.,* 59:1033-1039.

Rebaya-Mercado, J.D., Russell, R.M., Sahyoun, N., Morrow, F.D., and Gershoff, S.N. 1991. Vitamin B_6 requirements of elderly men and women, *J. Nutr.,* 121:1062-1074.

Rogers, K.S. and Mohan, C. 1994. Vitamin B_6 metabolism and diabetes, *Biochem. Med. Metab. Biol.,* 52:10-17.

Schaumburg, H., Kaplan, J., Windebank, A., Vick, N., Rasmus, S., Pleasure, D., and Brown, M.J. 1983. Sensory neuropathy from pyridoxine abuse, *N. Engl. J. Med.,* 309:445-448.

Thanassi, J.W., Nutter, L.M., Meisler, N.T., Commers, P., and Chiu, J.-F. 1980. Vitamin B_6 metabolism in Morris hepatomas, *J. Biol. Chem.,* 256:3370-3375.

Tully, D.B., Allgood, V.E., and Cidlowski, J.A. 1993. Vitamin B_6 modulation of steroid-induced gene expression. In: *Nutrition and Gene Expression,* Berdanier, C.D. and Hargrove, J.L., Eds., CRC Press, Boca Raton, FL, pp 547-567.

Zhang, Z., Gregory, J.F., and McCormick, D.B. 1993. Pyridoxone-5'-b-D-glucoside competitively inhibits uptake of vitamin B_6 into isolated liver cells, *J. Nutr.,* 123:85-89.

Pantothenic Acid

Eissenstat, B.R., Wyse, B.W., and Hansen, R.G. 1986. Pantothenic acid status of adolescents, *Am. J. Clin. Nutr.,* 44:931-937.

Fenstermacher, D.K. and Rose, R.C. 1986. Absorption of pantothenic acid in rat and chick intestine, *Am. J. Physiol.,* 250:G155-G160.

Fox, H.M. 1991. Pantothenic acid. In: *Handbook of Vitamins,* Machlin, L.J., Ed., Marcel Dekker, New York, pp. 429-451.

Sugarman, B. and Munro, H.N. 1980. ^{14}C Pantothenate accumulation by isolated adipocytes from adult rats of different ages, *J. Nutr.,* 110:2297-2301.

Biotin

Cole, H., Reynolds, T.R., Lockyer, J.M., Bucks, G.A., Denson, T., Spence, J.E., Hymes, J., and Wolf, B. 1994. Human serum biotinase. cDNA cloning sequence and characterization, *J. Biol. Chem.,* 269:6566-6570.

Hynes, J. and Wolf, B. 1996. Biotinidase and its roles in biotin metabolism, *Clin. Chim. Acta,* 255:1-11.

Li, S.-J. and Cronan, J.E. 1992. The gene encoding the biotin carboxylase subunit of *E. coli* acetyl CoA carboxylase, *J. Biol. Chem.,* 267:855-863.

Mock, D.M., Johnson, S.B., and Holman, R.T. 1988. Effects of biotin deficiency on serum fatty acid composition: evidence for abnormalities in humans, *J. Nutr.,* 118:342-348.

Mock, D.M., Mock, N.I., and Dankle, J.A. 1992. Secretory patterns of biotin in human milk, *J. Nutr.,* 122:546-552.

Mock, D.M., Mock, N.I., and Langbehn, S.E. 1992. Biotin in human milk: methods, location, and chemical form, *J. Nutr.,* 122:535-545.

Utter, M.F. and Sheu, K.-F.R. 1980. Biochemical mechanisms of biotin and thiamin action and relationships to genetic diseases, *Birth Defects,* 16:289-304.

Valazquez, A., Teran, M., Baez, A., Gutierrez, J., and Rodriquez, R. 1995. Biotin supplementation affects lymphoctye carboxylase and plasma biotin in severe protein-energy malnutrition, *Am. J. Clin. Nutr.,* 61:385-391.

Vesely, D.L., Kemp, S.F., and Eldres, M.J. 1987. Isolation of a biotin receptor from hepatic plasma membranes, *Biochem. Biophys. Res. Commun.,* 143:913-916.

Watanabe, T. 1993. Dietary biotin deficiency affects reproductive function and prenatal development in hamsters, *J. Nutr.,* 123:2101-2108.

Weiner, D. and Wolf, B. 1991. Biotin uptake, utilization and efflux in normal and biotin deficient rat hepatocytes, *Biochem. Med. Metab. Biol.,* 46:344-363.

Xia, W.-L., Zhang, J., and Ahmad, F. 1994. Biotin holocarboxylase synthetase: purification from rat liver cytosol and some properties, *Biochem. Mol. Biol. Int.,* 34:225-232.

Folic Acid

Anon. 1992. Morbidity and Mortality Weekly Report. Recommendations for the use of folic acid to reduce the number of cases of spina bifida and other neural tube defects. U.S. Department of Health and Human Services, Centers for Disease Control, Atlanta, GA, Vol. 41:1-7 (9/11/92).

Antony, A. 1996. Folate receptors. In: *Annual Review of Nutrition,* McCormick, D., Bier, D., and Goodridge, A., Eds., Annual Reviews, Palo Alto, CA, pp. 501-521.

Appling, D.R. 1991. Compartmentation of folate-mediated one-carbon metabolism in eukaryotes, *FASEB J.,* 5:2645-2651.

Bailey, L.B. 1992. Evaluation of a new RDA for folate, *J. Am. Diet. Assoc.,* 92:463-468.

Balaghi, M., Horne, D.W., and Wagner, C. 1993. Hepatic one-carbon metabolism in early folate deficiency in rats, *Biochem J.,* 291:145-149.

Branda, R.F. and Nelson, N.L. 1981. Inhibition of 5-Methyltetrahydrofolic acid transport by amphipathic drugs, *Drug Nutr. Interact.,* 1:45-53.

Chu, E., Takimoto, C.H., Voeller, D., Grem, J.L., and Allegra, C.J. 1993. Specific binding of human dihydrofolate reductase protein to dihydrofolate reductase messenger RNA *in vitro, Biochemistry,* 32:4756-4760.

Halsted, C.H. 1979. Intestinal absorption of folates, *Am. J. Clin. Nutr.,* 32:846-855.

Iwakura, M. and Tanaka, T. 1992. Dihydrofolate reductase gene as a versatile expression marker, *J. Biochem.*, 111:31-36.

Kim, Y.-I., Pogribny, I.P., Basnakian, A.G., Miller, J.W., Selhub, J., James, S.J., and Mason, J.B. 1997. Folate deficiency in rats induces DNA strand breaks and hypomethylation within the p53 tumor suppressor gene, *Am. J. Clin. Nutr.*, 65:46-52.

Libbus, B.L., Borman, L.S., Ventrone, C.H., and Branda, R.F. 1990. Nutritional folate deficiency in Chinese hamster ovary cells, *Cancer Genet. Cytogenet.*, 46:231-242.

Mason, J.B. 1994. Folate and colonic carcinogenesis: searching for a mechanistic understanding, *J. Nutr. Biochem.*, 5:170-175.

Rose, R.C., Koch, M.J., and Nahrwold, D.L. 1978. Folic acid transport by mammalian small intestine, *Am. J. Physiol.*, 235(6):E678-E685.

Sadasivan, E. and Rothenberg, S.P. 1988. Molecular cloning of the complementary DNA for a human folate binding protein, *Proc. Soc. Exp. Biol. Med.*, 189:240-244.

Shane, B. 1982. High performance liquid chromatography of folates. Identification of poly-g-glutamate chain lengths of labeled and unlabeled folates, *Am. J. Clin. Nutr.*, 35:598-599.

Shoda, R., Mason, J.B., Selhub, J., and Rosenberg, I.H. 1990. Folate binding in intestinal brush border membranes. Evidence for the presence of two binding activities, *J. Nutr. Biochem.*, 1:257-261.

Steinberg, S.E. 1984. Mechanisms of folate homeostasis, *Am. J. Physiol.*, 246:G319-G324.

Vitamin B_{12}

Brass, E.P. and Ruff, L.J. 1989. Effect of carnitine on proprionate metabolism in the vitamin B_{12}-deficient rat, *J. Nutr.*, 119:1196-1201.

Cullen, R.W. and Oace, S.M. 1989. Fermentable dietary fibers elevate urinary methylmalonate and decrease propionate oxidation in rats deprived of vitamin B_{12}, *J. Nutr.*, 119:1115-1120.

Ellenbogen, L. 1991. Vitamin B_{12}. In: *Handbook of Vitamins*, Machlin, L.J., Ed., Marcel Dekker, New York, pp. 491-536.

Marcoullis, G., Rothenberg, S.P., and Labombardi, V.J. 1980. Preparation and characterization of proteins in the alimentary tract of the dog which bind cobalamin and intrinsic factor, *J. Biol. Chem.*, 255:1824-1829.

Merzbach, D. and Grossowicz, N. 1987. Absorption of vitamin B_{12} from the large intestine of rats, *J. Nutr.*, 87:41-51.

O'Sullivan, D. 1991. New studies pinpoint pathway of B_{12} biosynthesis, *C & E News*, Feb. 4, pp. 30-31.

Peifer, J.J. and Cleland, G. 1987. Metabolic demands for coenzyme B_{12}-dependent mutase increased by thiamin deficiency, *Nutr. Res.*, 7:1197-1201.

Peifer, J.J. and Lewis, R.D. 1981. Odd numbered fatty acids in phosphatidyl choline versus phosphatidyl ethanolamine of vitamin B_{12}-deprived rats, *Proc. Soc. Exp. Biol. Med.*, 167:212-217.

Sennett, C. and Rosenberg, L.E. 1981. Transmembrane transport of cobalamin in prokaryotic and eukaryotic cells, *Annu. Rev. Biochem.*, 50:1053-1086.

Thenen, S.W. 1989. Megadose effects of vitamin C on vitamin B_{12} status in the rat, *J. Nutr.*, 119:1107-1114.

Watanabe, F., Saido, H., Toyoshima, S., Tamura, Y., and Nekano, Y. 1994. Feeding vitamin B_{12} rapidly increases the specific activity of hepatic methylmalonyl CoA mutase in vitamin B_{12} deficient rats, *Biosci. Biotech. Biochem.*, 58:556-557.

Other Organic Nutrients

TABLE OF CONTENTS

I. CHOLINE

A. Overview

While many nutrition scientists consider that the list of required vitamins is complete, others would argue that there are certain circumstances where a dietary supply of a compound is essential for the support of normal metabolism. Choline is one of these compounds. In rats given a choline-deficient diet, one can observe a fatty liver as well as certain central nervous system deficits. Human cells grown in culture also have an absolute requirement for choline, and humans sustained by choline-free parenteral solutions develop symptoms similar to those of the deficient rat. It is on this basis that the inclusion of choline in a list of "conditionally" essential nutrients is argued.

B. Structure, Chemical and Physical Properties

Choline is the trivial name for 2-hydroxy-N,N,N-trimethyl-ethanaminium. The structure for this compound is shown in Figure 1. Choline is freely soluble in water and ethanol but insoluble in organic solvents such as ether or chloroform. It is extremely hygroscopic. It is a strong base and readily decomposes in alkaline solutions, resulting in the production of trimethylamine. Because of its unique structure, choline serves as a donor of methyl groups. It has a molecular weight of 121.2 Da and belongs to a class of compounds that function either as methyl donors or as membrane constituents. Related compounds are listed in Table 1. Because of its instability, the determination of choline in food and biological tissues is fraught with difficulty. Commonly used is the reineckate method which involve the precipitation of choline as a reineckate salt and the development of a characteristic color. Unfortunately this method lacks the sensitivity and specificity provided by newer chromatographic and isotopic methods that are combined with rapid inactivation, via microwave, of choline degradative enzymes. Work is ongoing for the development of sensitive and specific methods for choline assay.

C. Sources

Choline is widely distributed in foods and is consumed mainly in the form of lecithin (phosphatidylcholine). Lecithin is not only a naturally occurring common food ingredient but is also a

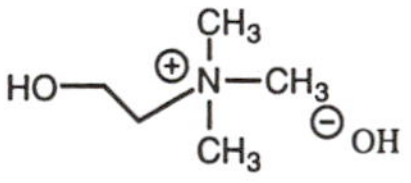

$$HO-\!\!\!\diagdown\!\!\!\!\diagup\!\!\!\!\overset{\displaystyle CH_3}{\underset{\displaystyle CH_3}{\overset{\oplus}{N}}}\!\!-CH_3 \quad \overset{\ominus}{}OH$$

Figure 1 Structure of choline.

Table 1   Choline and Related Metabolites

As methyl donor:
   Choline
   S-Adenosyl-L-methionine
   Methyltetrahydrofolate
   Betaine
As choline metabolite:
   Choline, acetylcholine
   Phosphorylcholine
   Betaine
   Phosphatidylcholine (lecithin)
   Lysophosphatidylcholine (lysolecithin)
   Sphingomyelin

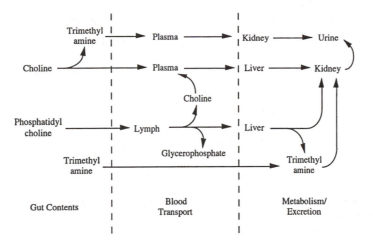

Figure 2 Absorption and metabolism of choline.

common additive to processed foods. It serves as a good food stabilizer and emulsifying agent. Choline chloride and choline bitartrate are added to infant formulas to assure equivalency to breast milk, which contains 7 mg/100 kcal (7 mg/420 kJ): 7 mg is about 0.05 mmol or 50 µmol. Recent assessments of commercial infant formulas, however, showed less choline in the preparation than shown on the label. The choline content of the infant formulas in this report ranged from 100 to 647 µmol. In part, this discrepancy may be due to the lability of choline once in a solution (the infant formula) that is mildly alkaline, and in part due to the relative difficulty in assessing the choline content accurately. If the energy requirement of the infant is 650 kcal (2720 kJ), this infant would need 45.5 mg or 375 µmol of choline a day. Depending on which of the infant formulas is used, the infant could be at risk of insufficient intake.

D. Absorption, Metabolism

There is a good bit of difficulty in assessing choline absorption. Currently it is believed to be absorbed via a sodium-dependent carrier-mediated mechanism. If large amounts of choline are consumed, uptake of the excess is by passive diffusion. One study using labeled choline showed that about 65% of the dose was found in the urine as trimethylamine within 12 hr of ingestion. When labeled choline was incorporated into lecithin and ingested, significantly less of the label was recovered in the urine as trimethylamine. About 50% of the ingested labeled lecithin entered the thoracic duct intact. The use of antibiotics to reduce the population of gut flora reduced the loss of trimethylamine in the urine. This showed that one of the major degradative steps in the loss of choline is through the action of the gut flora. The route of choline and lecithin metabolism and degradation is shown in Figure 2. In addition to the action of the gut flora, phosphatidylcholine is subject to enzymatic degradation. Phospholipase A_1, A_2, and B catalyze the cleavage of the ester bonds that link the fatty acids from the glycerol backbone, resulting in free fatty acids and glycerophosphocholine. Most of the lecithin that is ingested has only one of its fatty acids removed prior to absorption. Sphingomyelin, a related complex lipid containing choline, is not degraded at all in the intestinal lumen. All of the phospholipids are transported into the lymphatic circulation from the gut and appear in the plasma lipoproteins. All classes (high-density lipoproteins, low-density lipoproteins, very-low-density lipoproteins, and chylomicrons) contain phosphatidylcholine. The chylomicrons are the major carriers from the gut, but once into the blood the phosphatidylcholine is redistributed among the lipoprotein classes. From the blood it is then taken up by all cell types.

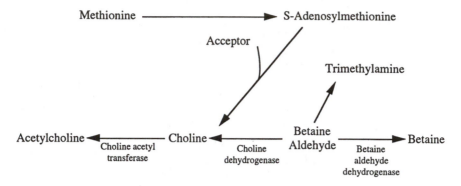

Figure 3 Use of methionine in the synthesis of choline and subsequent use of choline in betaine and acetyl-choline synthesis.

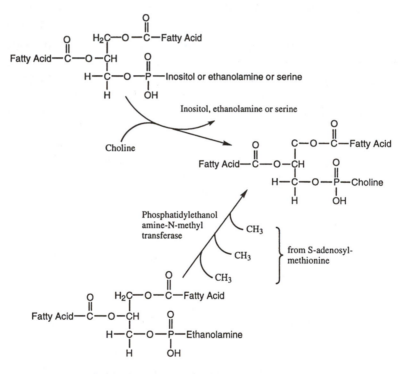

Figure 4 Biosynthesis of phosphatidylcholine.

Most species including humans can synthesize choline using methionine as the methyl donor. This synthesis is shown in Figure 3. Methionine is converted to S-adenosylmethionine (SAM). The methyl groups are then successively transferred to ethanolamine and its monomethyl and dimethyl derivatives to form choline. Aside from its use in the synthesis of acetylcholine, choline's other essential function is as part of the phospholipid, phosphatidylcholine. The synthesis of this lipid occurs via an exchange reaction using phosphatidylethanolamine, another phospholipid, as the starting material. This synthesis is outlined in Figure 4. Also shown in Figure 4 is the interconversion of other phospholipids, through base exchange, to phosphatidylcholine.

E. Function

Choline serves as a precursor for the neurotransmitter, acetylcholine. The intake of choline can affect brain levels of acetylcholine and this may be a benefit to patients showing acetylcholine deficits as in tardive dyskinesia. Some benefit is also claimed to be achieved with people having short-term memory loss as in Alzheimer's disease.

As important as the synthesis of acetylcholine, is the synthesis of the membrane phospholipid, phosphatidylcholine. This phospholipid is an important structural element of the membrane and, depending on the chain length and saturation of the fatty acids attached to carbons 1 and 2, contributes to the degree of fluidity of that membrane. The consideration of fluidity is important to the function of the membrane-embedded proteins. Many of these proteins change shape as part of their action, and the fluidity of the surrounding lipid determines the ease with which they can do this.

Phosphatidylcholine functions in the transport of lipids not only as part of the lipoproteins but also in the transmembrane lipid transport system. In this role, phosphatidylcholine serves as a lipotrope.

Lastly, because choline is a precursor of betaine, it serves as a methyl donor in the one-carbon metabolic pathways. These pathways include the formation of methionine from homocysteine and the formation of creatine from guanidoacetic acid.

F. Deficiency

Because choline can be synthesized in the body and because it is universally present in our food supply, a true deficiency in normal humans is rare indeed. Choline deficiency can occur in poultry fed a low-choline diet or one deficient in methionine and/or methyl donors. Depressed growth, fatty liver, and hemorrhagic renal disease have been reported to occur in deficient animals of a number of species. Of interest is an early report of an effect of choline deficiency on body carnitine pools. A 50% reduction has been reported and, due to the importance of carnitine in fatty acid oxidation, this relationship may explain the fatty liver of deficient animals.

G. Requirement

There are no stated requirements for choline. Zeisel has recently pleaded the case for developing intake guidelines. His arguments have merit and probably will be explored in the coming years.

II. CARNITINE

A. Overview

As is the case with choline and inositol, carnitine can be synthesized in the body in amounts usually sufficient to meet needs. Thus, carnitine is not considered an essential nutrient at all stages of life. However, just as there may be instances where choline or inositol must be provided from external sources, this is also true for carnitine. Interest in the conditional essentiality of carnitine was stimulated by Broquist and colleagues, who showed that carnitine was synthesized from lysine, an amino acid frequently in short supply in Third World malnourished patients. Follow-up work by Borum showed that the premature infant cannot synthesize sufficient carnitine to meet the needs for growth and normal metabolism. These reports thus stimulated the consideration of carnitine as a nutrient that becomes required under some circumstances.

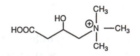

Figure 5   Structure of carnitine.

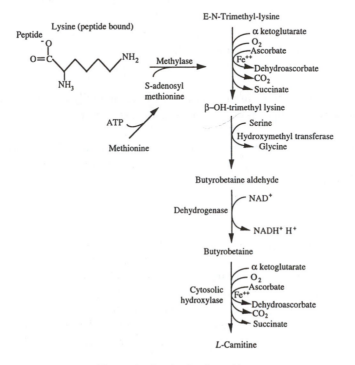

Figure 6   Synthesis of carnitine.

B. Structure, Physical and Chemical Properties

Carnitine is a quaternary amine, β-hydroxy-γ-N-trimethyl aminobutyric acid. Its structure is shown in Figure 5. It is very hygroscopic with a molecular weight of 161.2 Da. As mentioned, it is synthesized in the body (primarily the liver) from lysine. This pathway is shown in Figure 6. There are a number of essential nutrients involved: niacin as part of NAD, iron in the ferrous state, ascorbate to keep iron in its ferrous state and, of course, lysine together with methionine as a methyl donor. As long as the diet provides these nutrients, carnitine will be synthesized to meet the needs of the normal individual. There are instances, however, where despite the provision of these essential nutrients, carnitine synthesis does not take place to the extent that is needed. In this instance, carnitine becomes an essential nutrient. This occurs in the premature infant. Due to its prematurity, its biochemical pathways, especially that for carnitine synthesis, are not well developed. The severely traumatized individual also has a need for carnitine that exceeds endogenous synthesis. The whole-body response to trauma involves a catecholamine-glucocorticoid response that greatly increases lipolysis and fatty acid oxidation. This drives up the need for carnitine, and in this situation endogenous synthesis is inadequate.

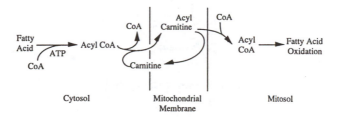

Figure 7   Carnitine acyltransferase system.

C. Sources

The techniques for carnitine analysis of foods are not well developed. However, despite the inadequacies of the methodology, it is safe to indicate that good sources of carnitine include red meats and some organ meats. Milk, whole grains, and some vegetables (i.e., spinach, cauliflower, avocado, and peanuts) contain modest amounts.

D. Absorption, Metabolism

Carnitine is absorbed via an active process involving sodium and a carrier. Carnitine in large amounts is also absorbed by passive diffusion. Concurrent with its absorption is its acetylation. It is transported in both the free and acetylated form to the muscles, where 90% of the total body carnitine may be found. The turnover of carnitine is quite slow. Although needed for fatty acid oxidation, particularly by the working muscle, it is continuously recycled rather than degraded and excreted. The kidney plays an important role in carnitine conservation in that 90% of the carnitine that arrives at the kidney is reabsorbed by the glomerulus and returned to the circulation. In instances of kidney failure this conservation is lost and again we have a situation where exogenous carnitine must be supplied. A small amount of acylcarnitine ester may be found in the urine of normal subjects. This probably represents less than 1% of the total body carnitine pool.

E. Function

Carnitine serves as part of the carnitine acyltransferase system located in the mitochondrial membrane. This system is shown in Figure 7. There are two transferases involved: carnitine acyltransferase I located on the outer side of the inner mitochondrial membrane, and carnitine acyltransferase II located on the matrix side of the membrane. These enzymes catalyze the synthesis and hydrolysis of the fatty acylcarnitine esters as well as work with the transporter protein (acyltranslocase) that catalyzes the movement of the fatty acids into the mitochondrial matrix. There is no other known function for carnitine.

F. Deficiency

Low levels of carnitine in tissues and blood typify the carnitine-deficient individual in addition to hyperlipidemia, cardiomyopathy, and muscle spasm.

G. Requirement

Because carnitine can be synthesized in the body no recommended intake levels have been set for normal children and adults. Work continues on developing intake recommendations for preterm infants and others with special needs.

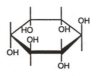

Figure 8 Myoinositol structure.

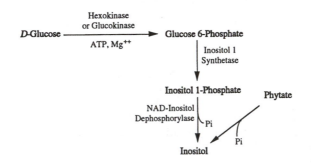

Figure 9 *De novo* synthesis of free inositol from either glucose or phytate. The conversion of glucose to inositol is an insulin-dependent pathway, whereas the dephosphorylation of phytate (phytic acid) is not.

III. INOSITOL

A. Overview

Until fairly recently, little attention has been paid to the role of inositol in the diet. This has occurred despite the recognition that dietary inositol has been shown to prevent the development of a fatty liver in rats and to cure alopecia in rats and mice, and despite a report published over a 100 years ago that diabetic humans excreted large quantities of this substance in the urine. Inositol is an essential part of every cell. It is a key ingredient for one of the membrane lipids, phosphatidylinositol. It is not considered an essential nutrient for humans.

B. Structure, Physical and Chemical Properties

Inositol is a six carbon sugar that is configuratively related to D-glucose. Its structure is shown in Figure 8. It occurs in nature in nine possible isomeric forms. However, only one, myoinositol, is biologically important as a nutrient. Myoinositol is a water-soluble, cyclic, six-carbon compound (*cis*-1,2,3,5 *trans*-4,6-cyclohexane-hexanol). It is widely distributed in foods of both plant and animal origin. In plants and animals it exists as part of the phosphatidylinositol (PI) of the cell membranes or as free inositol. Phytic acid, a component of many grain products, can be converted to myoinositol with the removal of the phosphate groups (see Figure 9). Phytate or phytic acid can bind calcium, magnesium, and other divalent ions within the intestinal compartment, making them unavailable for absorption by mucosal cells. Once the phytate is dephosphorylated through the action of phytase, the inositol residue remains. The divalent ions are released and the free inositol is absorbed. Both free inositol and cell membrane phosphatidylinositol are found in foods of animal origin.

C. Absorption, Metabolism

Dietary phosphatidylinositol is acted on by the luminal enzyme, phospholipase, and converted to lysophosphatidylinositol. This compound can then be further hydrolyzed to produce glycerophosphorylinositol and then free inositol, or acted upon by an acyltransferase in the intestinal cell

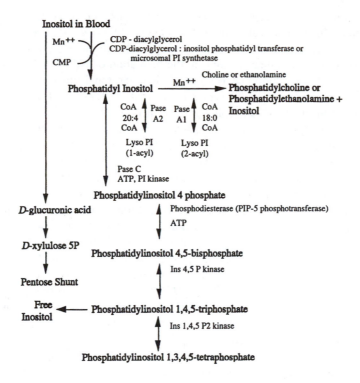

Figure 10 Inositol metabolism and the PI cycle.

which converts it back to phosphatidylinositol. This is then transported out of the gut absorptive cell as a component of the lipoproteins.

Free inositol in the lumen is transported into the luminal cells via an active, energy-dependent, sodium-dependent transport process quite similar to that which transports glucose. Although similar, it is not identical to it. Free inositol is then transported in the blood at a concentration of about 30 µm/l.

As mentioned, inositol can be synthesized from glucose by a variety of mammalian cells. Synthesis in the testes, brain, kidney, and liver has been reported. Humans can synthesize up to 4 g/day in the kidneys alone. Synthesis from glucose proceeds from glucose to glucose-6-phosphate to inositol-1-phosphate to inositol. The enzymes are glucokinase or hexokinase, followed by inositol-1-synthetase and then NAD-inositol-dephosphorylase. Figure 9 illustrates the pathway for the production of inositol from glucose and also from phytate.

D. Function

Inositol functions as a constituent of the membrane phospholipid, phosphatidylinositol. Free inositol is added to diacylglycerol via a CDP reaction producing phosphatidylinositol and CMP. The enzyme catalyzing this reaction is CDP diacylglycerol:inositol phosphatidyltransferase, sometimes called phosphatidylinositol synthetase. This synthesis takes place in the microsomes and the enzyme has a Km of 4.6 mM for inositol. This reaction is illustrated in Figure 10. Phosphatidylinositol can also be synthesized via an exchange reaction where free inositol can exchange for either choline or ethanolamine in either phosphatidylcholine or phosphatidylethanolamine. The Km for the Mn^{2+}-dependent reaction is 0.024 mM. Once formed, the phosphatidylinositol migrates from the microsomes where it is formed to any one of the membranes within and around the cell. It comprises approximately 10% of the phospholipids in the cellular membranes. Recently, its function as a part of a unique cellular second messenger system (different from the cyclic AMP system) has been explored. This system, called the PIP system or PIP cycle, has been reported to function in insulin release by the pancreatic insulin-producing β cells, in the regulation of protein kinase C, in the mobilization of intracellular calcium, in the regulation of Na⁺K⁺ ATPase activity, and may have a role in blood clotting, blood pressure regulation, and renal function.

Once formed, phosphatidylinositol serves as a substrate for one of several enzymes. These reactions are shown in Figure 10. Phospholipase A1 acts on phosphatidylinositol to produce lyso PI (2-acyl PI). Phospholipase A2 acts to produce a 1-acyl PI. Both A1 and A2 act to remove one of the fatty acids from the phospholipids; A1 removes the fatty acid (usually stearic acid, 18:0) from the glycerol carbon 1, while A2 removes the fatty acid (usually arachidonic acid, 20:4) from the glycerol carbon 2. When phospholipase A2 is activated, arachidonic acid is released and this fatty acid serves as the substrate for prostaglandin synthesis. Prostaglandins are another group of hormone-like substances that are important in the regulation of blood pressure and blood clotting.

A third enzyme also has phosphatidylinositol as its substrate. This enzyme is ATP PI kinase (Phospholipase C) and initiates the PIP cycle also illustrated in Figure 10. Phospholipase C action is mediated by the guanine nucleotide-binding protein called the G protein. Phospholipase C cleaves the phosphorylated inositol from the glycerol backbone, producing diacylglycerol (DAG) and phosphatidylinositol-4,5-bisphosphate (PIP_2). DAG serves to activate protein kinase C, an important regulatory enzyme discovered in 1979. Neutral DAG remains within the membrane while the liberated inositol-4,5-bisphosphate migrates into the cytoplasm and, in the process, is again phosphorylated to form inositol-1,4,5-triphosphate (PIP_3). This compound causes a release of calcium ion from nonmitochondrial vesicular intracellular stores. The triphosphate inositol binds to a receptor protein associated with these stores to effect this release. Ca^{2+} release from the endoplasmic reticulum is elicited via an opening of a gated channel. Cyclic AMP dependent-phosphorylation of the receptor protein seems to be involved. The magnesium ion is also involved. Inositol-1,4,5-triphosphate can then either be dephosphorylated to release free inositol or be phosphorylated once again to form inositol-1,3,4,5-tetraphosphate (PIP_4) via the enzyme D-myoinositol-1,4,5-triphosphate-3-kinase. This kinase is stimulated by a Ca^{2+} in the presence of calmodulin and protein kinase C and thus the level of the inositol-1,4,5-triphosphate is carefully regulated. Inositol 1,3,4,5-tetraphosphate also is an active metabolic regulator in that it modulates calcium ion through either the re-uptake of Ca^{2+} into the intracellular stores or through control of the Ca^{2+} transfer process between inositol-1,4,5-phosphate sensitive and insensitive pools. The kinase enzyme might be the target for the enzyme protein tyrosine kinase.

All of the above phosphorylations of inositol are reversible and the amounts of each of the phosphorylated intermediates depend on the hormonal status of the individual as well as on the availability of inositol for phosphatidylinositol synthesis. Insulin, various growth factors, and PGF2α (one of the prostaglandins) have all been shown to stimulate the phosphatidylinositol cycle. Of particular interest are the reports that inositol turnover is increased in acute diabetes. Other observations on the relationship of diabetes to inositol status include the following: anti-insulin antiserum treatment of the diabetic neutralizes the effect of the exogenous insulin on inositol turnover; insulin treatment of acute insulin deficiency reverses the effect of diabetes on inositol turnover; and insulin increases the synthesis of phosphatidylinositol, DAG, and protein kinase C activity in a variety of cells from normal animals. All of these findings suggest that there may be circumstances where the synthesis of inositol by the body might be inadequate to meet the body's need and that this substance must be provided in the diet. Under these circumstances inositol becomes an essential nutrient. One of these circumstances is the disease, diabetes mellitus.

Diabetes, regardless of whether it is insulin dependent or non insulin dependent, is characterized by a failure to appropriately regulate blood glucose levels. With high blood levels of glucose the sorbitol pathway is stimulated. If this pathway is stimulated, endogenous synthesis of myoinositol is reduced. Further, cellular uptake of glucose is impaired in the diabetic state. If cellular glucose uptake is impaired, less inositol is synthesized from that glucose and thus less is available for phosphatidylinositol synthesis. Hence, the diabetic excretes more inositol in the urine while having an intracellular deficiency because of inadequate endogenous synthesis. In turn, this means that more preformed inositol should be provided to the body via the diet. Thus, the diabetic may have a significantly greater requirement for inositol than the nondiabetic. Indeed, there may be as broad a range in inositol requirements as there is in the range of severity of diabetes.

Recently, there have been reports in the medical literature that have suggested that the secondary complications of diabetes, i.e., renal disease, could be ameliorated by dietary inositol supplementation. Some investigators have shown a reversal of the diabetes-induced increased glomerular filtration rate with a seven- to tenfold increase in dietary levels of myoinositol. At any rate, it would appear that diabetics have a larger than normal need for dietary inositol because (1) they excrete more than do normal people; (2) when hyperglycemic they synthesize less from glucose because less glucose is available inside the cell and because the first two steps in glucose metabolism are insulin dependent; (3) they absorb less from the diet; and (4) when hyperglycemic they have greater sorbitol production which, in turn, inhibits the pathway for inositol synthesis.

E. Deficiency

In normal humans, inositol needs are presumed to be met by endogenous synthesis, so detailed studies have not been performed using healthy volunteers. Indirect evidence of need has been reported sparsely in the medical literature but detailed, controlled feeding studies have not been conducted. Such studies have been performed in laboratory rats and mice. In these animals the most striking feature of the deficient state was the development of a fatty liver. This was reversed with dietary inositol supplementation. Hair loss and poor growth were also reported for deficient animals. At the time these animal studies were conducted (1979–1980) the PIP cycle was not known. Researchers knew about the presence of phosphatidylinositol in the cell membrane but they did not recognize its importance in the lipid signal transduction process. Studies on the PIP cycle in rats made inositol deficient have yet to be conducted.

F. Requirement

Inositol is a conditionally essential nutrient because the body can synthesize it from glucose, but there may be circumstances where this synthesis is inadequate and exogenous inositol might become essential. At this time this information is only suggestive.

IV. OTHER COMPOUNDS WITH BIOLOGIC ACTIVITY

A. Overview

The bulk of the work identifying and describing compounds we now know as vitamins occurred in the first part of the twentieth century. Recent work has suggested other compounds that may also be essential to the maintenance of normal metabolism of some organisms, but for which there is no direct proof for mammals including humans. In this list are pyrroloquinoline quinone, ubiquinone, orotic acid, para-aminobenzoic acid, lipoic acid, and the bioflavinoids. Brief descriptions of these substances follow.

B. Pyrroloquinoline Quinone

Pyrroloquinoline quinone, sometimes called methoxatin, serves as a cofactor for certain methane-forming bacteria. The structure of pyrroloquinoline quinone is shown in Figure 11. It is a tricarboxylic acid with a fused heterocylic (*o*-quinone) ring system. Its C-5 carbonyl group is very reactive towards nucleophiles and it is this action that allows this substance to function in metabolic reactions. At present, information is scarce with respect to its food sources and essentiality. Likely, it can be endogenously synthesized in organisms that can use it, but whether this compound meets the definition of a vitamin has yet to be established for any species.

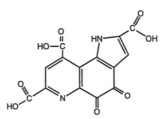

Figure 11   Structure of pyrroloquinoline quinone.

C. Ubiquinone

Ubiquinone is an essential component of the mitochondrial respiratory chain and it has been shown to be synthesized endogenously. Actually, ubiquinone is one of a group of related substances. They are a group of tetra-substituted 1,4-benzoquinone derivatives with isoprenoid side chains of various lengths. The biochemists have termed these substances as coenzyme Q. They function as reversible donors/acceptors of reducing equivalents from NAD, passing electrons from flavoproteins to the cytochromes via cytochrome b_5. Because the ubiquinones can be synthesized endogenously in large amounts even when diets lacking the ubiquinones are offered, these substances fail to meet the definition of the word vitamin.

D. Orotic Acid

Orotic acid is an important metabolic intermediate in the synthesis of pyrimidines. Its structure is shown in Figure 12. It is synthesized endogenously from N-carbamyl phosphate by dehydration and oxidation. It is another of those substances that fails to meet the definition of a vitamin. When used as a dietary supplement (0.1% of diet) orotic acid had deleterious effects. It resulted in a fatty, enlarged liver and increased the levels of hepatic uracil, presumably due to an influence on pyrimidine synthesis. Orotic acid-induced fatty liver is accompanied by falling plasma cholesterol levels and falling activity of HMG CoA reductase. This hepatic enzyme is greatly influenced by its product (cholesterol) and so if the liver does not export it, it feeds back to inhibit synthesis.

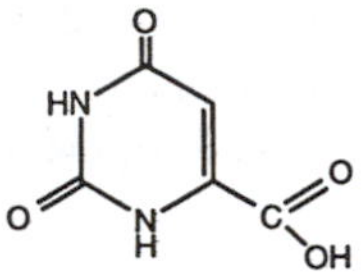

Figure 12   Structure of orotic acid.

E. Para-Aminobenzoic Acid (PABA)

p-Aminobenzoic acid is an essential growth factor for a number of bacteria which use it as a precursor of folacin. Animals, however, cannot synthesize folacin so *p*-aminobenzoic acid does not meet the definition of a vitamin. Its involvement in folacin use is discussed in Unit 4, Section VIII.

F. Lipoic Acid

Lipoic acid is essential to oxidative decarboxylation of α-keto acids. It participates in the pyruvate dehydrogenase complex (see Figures 7 and 8 in Unit 4 on pages 84 and 85). This is a multienzyme complex where lipoic acid is linked to the ε-amino group of a lysine residue from the enzyme dihydrolipoyl transacetylase. As the lipoamide undergoes reversible acylation/deacylation it transfers acyl groups to coenzyme A and results in reversible ring opening/closing in the oxidation of the α-keto acid. Lipoic acid can be synthesized endogenously in amounts sufficient to meet the need. Therefore, it does not meet the definition of the word vitamin.

G. Bioflavinoids

Bioflavinoids are a group of compounds that are presumed by some to augment the action of ascorbic acid in the prevention of scurvy . They are mixtures of phenolic derivatives of 2-phenyl-1,4-benzopyrone. The bioflavinoids are present in a large variety of foods and were first isolated by Szent-Gyorgy from lemon juice and red peppers. More than 800 different flavinoids have been found. They occur naturally as glycosides which are hydrolyzed by the gut flora prior to absorption. No single unique deficiency syndrome has been found or reported in animals fed a bioflavinoid-free diet. Furthermore, there has not been a unique response to the addition of bioflavinoids to the diet. On this basis, despite their activity as potentiators of ascorbic acid, bioflavinoids can not be considered vitamins.

H. Pseudovitamins

The term vitamin was coined many years ago to designate those organic dietary compounds that cannot be made endogenously but are needed in small amounts to sustain normal growth and metabolism throughout life. This term, developed by nutritional biochemists and physiologists, has been used commercially as well as scientifically. Unfortunately, there have been (and continue to be) commercial uses of the term that are inappropriate. Hence we have compounds such as laetrile (an extract from fruit pits), pangamic acid or vitamin B_{15}, and methylsulfonium salts of methionine called vitamin U, and gerovital. Gerovital, also called vitamin H_3 or CH_3, is a buffered solution of procaine hydrochloride (Novocaine™), a local anesthetic. To be effective as an anesthetic it must be injected. Gerovital is advertised as an antiaging substance but claims of its effects have not been substantiated. The advertised use of methylsulfonic salts of methionine to prevent peptic ulcers likewise has not been substantiated. Pangamic acid, another of these pseudovitamins, is not a chemically defined substance. Rather it is a mixture of compounds. Of the materials labeled pangamic acid, one of the compounds is N,N-diisopropylamine dichloroacetate. This is a drug, and when administered to normal rats it caused death preceded by respiratory failure, extreme hypotension, and hypothermia. There is no evidence of essentiality for pangamic acid.

Lastly, laetrile is included in this list of pseudovitamins. This compound has been the focus of a number of litigations due to the claim by its suppliers that it can serve as an anticancer drug. This claim was investigated and found wanting by the U.S. Food and Drug Administration (FDA). The term laetrile has several synonyms: amygdalin and vitamin B_{17}. Amygdalin is a β-cyanogenic glucoside and is a major constituent in preparations named laetrile. Amygdalin is a substance found in peach pits, apricot pits, and the kernels and seeds of many fruits. Neither the U.S. FDA or the Canadian equivalent of this regulatory agency recognize laetrile as a vitamin.

SUPPLEMENTAL READINGS

Choline

Chan, M.M. 1991. Choline. In: *Handbook of Vitamins,* Machlin, L.J., Ed., Marcel Dekker, New York, pp. 537-556.
Mehlman, M.A., Therriault, D.G., and Tobin, R.B. 1971. Carnitine-^{14}C metabolism in choline-deficient, alloxan diabetic choline deficient and insulin treated rats, *Metabolism,* 20:100-107.
Zeisel, S.H. 1990. Choline deficiency, *J. Nutr. Biochem.,* 1:332-349.

Carnitine

Borum, P. 1991. Carnitine. In: *Handbook of Vitamins,* Machlin, L.J., Ed., Marcel Dekker, New York, pp. 557-563.

Inositol

Best, L. and Malaise, W.J. 1983. Phospholipids and islet function, *Diabetologia,* 25:299-305.
Farese, R.V. 1990. Lipid derived mediators in insulin action, *Proc. Soc. Exp. Biol. Med.,* 312:324.
Flier, J.S. and Underhill, L.H. 1990. Sorbitol, phosphoinositides, and sodium-potassium-ATPase in the pathogenesis of diabetic complications, *N. Engl. J. Med.,* 316:599-606.
Han, O., Failla, M., Hill, A.D., Morris, E.R., and Smith, J.C. 1994. Inositol phosphates inhibit uptake and transport of iron and zinc by a human intestinal cell line, *J. Nutr.,* 124:580-587.
Holub, B.J. 1986. Metabolism and function of myoinositol and inositol phospholipids, *Annu. Rev. Nutr.,* 6:563-597.
Martin, T.F.J. 1991. Receptor regulation of phosphoinositidase C, *Pharmacol. Ther.,* 49:329-345.
Olgemoller, B., Schwaabe, S., Schleicher, E.D., and Gerbitz, K.D. 1993. Upregulation of myoinositol transport compensates for competitive inhibition by glucose, *Diabetes,* 42:1119-1125.
Saltiel, A.R. 1990. Signal transduction in insulin action, *J. Nutr. Biochem.,* 1:180-188.

Minerals and Living Systems

TABLE OF CONTENTS

I. OVERVIEW

Minerals are found in every cell, tissue, and organ. They are important constituents of essential molecules such as thyroxine, hemoglobin, and vitamin B_{12}. They serve as critical cofactors in numerous enzymatic reactions, and form the hard mineral complexes that comprise bone. Minerals serve in the maintenance of pH, osmotic pressure, nerve conductance, muscle contraction, energy production, and in almost every aspect of life. While minerals are essential to normal health and development, they can also be toxic. The body defends itself against such toxicity through a variety of mechanisms. For the microminerals, the protective mechanisms center primarily around the regulation of uptake by the mucosal cells of the intestine. Many of the minerals are poorly absorbed and this, in itself, can be viewed as a protection against lethality. This protection is absolutely essential because in many of these same instances the means for excretion is very inefficient, if it exists at all.

Optimal intake is a balance between an intake that is too little and one that is toxic. With some minerals, the range of intake for optimal benefit is very large; for others it is quite small. This is illustrated in Figure 1 that arbitrarily plots a generic function against an intake of a mineral upon which that function depends. This plot has a typical bell-shaped curve with an optimal range in the middle. Almost any mineral function can be plotted in this way. In hemoglobin synthesis, too much iron results in a condition known as hemosiderosis; too little iron results in anemia. Other mineral-related functions likewise can be demonstrated, with the caveat that the body protects itself from excess intake through a reduction in mineral absorption, through deposition in the mineral apatite of bone and through a variety of excretions such as bile, urine, sweat, expired air, hair, and desquamated epithelial cells. Some of these excrements are not usually considered important pathways of excretion, but under toxic conditions they become avenues of loss of the excess mineral.

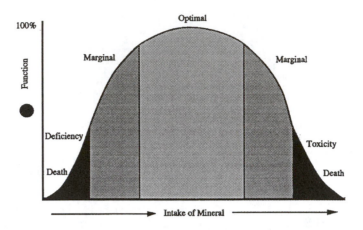

Figure 1   Dependence of biological function on intake of a mineral.

The illustration in Figure 1 is indeed quite simplistic of the need for a given mineral. Just as was discussed in the vitamin units, there are numerous interactions that affect mineral uptake and use. The ratio of calcium to phosphorus, the ratio of iron to copper and to zinc, the ratio of calcium to magnesium, and other factors both mineral and nonmineral affect the mineral status. Some of these interactions are mutually beneficial while others are antagonistic. Most of these interactions occur at the level of the gut in that most are concerned with mineral absorption. For example, zinc absorption is impaired by high iron intakes; high zinc intake impairs copper absorption. Molybdenum and sulfur antagonize copper, tungsten interferes with molybdenum, and so forth. These interactions are itemized in the individual mineral sections. These antagonisms contribute to the relative inefficiency of absorption of minerals that are poorly absorbed and just as poorly lost once absorbed.

II. BIOAVAILABILITY

One concept that nutritionists have developed relates not only to absorption efficiency but also to mineral interactions at the site for absorption and the site of use. This concept is that of bioavailability. Bioavailability is defined as the percent of the consumed mineral that enters via the intestinal absorptive cell, the enterocyte, and is used for its intended purpose. Thus, bioavailability includes not only how much of a consumed mineral enters the body, but also how much is retained and available for use. An example might be the comparison of iron from red meat to the same amount of iron in spinach. Iron from red meat has a greater bioavailability than iron from spinach because it is an integral component of the protein heme. It is this form (heme iron) that is efficiently absorbed and used. The iron in the spinach is bound to an oxalate, and, even though some of this iron can be released from the oxalate, it is in the ferric state and poorly absorbed.

III. APPARENT ABSORPTION

There is another term referring to absorption that is frequently used. That is the term "apparent absorption". This term refers to the difference between the amount of mineral consumed and that which appears in the feces. Some minerals are recirculated via the bile while others are not. This recirculation, especially in a poorly absorbed mineral, can contribute to the mineral content of the feces, but there is no correction for the biliary contribution to the fecal mineral content. The term "apparent absorption" refers *only* to the difference between intake and fecal excretion.

Table 1   Periodic Table of the Elements

Group	I	II										III	IV	V	VI	VII	0
Period																	
1	H																He
	1																2
2	Li	Be										B	C	N	O	F	Ne
	3	4										5	6	7	8	9	10
3	Na	Mg				Transition elements						Al	Si	P	S	Cl	Ar
	11	12										13	14	15	16	17	18
4	K	Ca	Sc	Ti	V	Cr	Mn	Fe	Co	Ni	Cu	Zn	Ga	Ge	As	Se	Br	Kr
	19	20	21	22	23	24	25	26	27	28	29	30	31	32	33	34	35	36
5	Rb	Sr	Y	Zr	Nb	Mo	Tc	Ru	Rh	Pd	Ag	Cd	In	Sn	Sb	Te	I	Xe
	37	38	39	40	41	42	43	44	45	46	47	48	49	50	51	52	53	54
6	Cs	Ba	*	Hf	Ta	W	Re	Os	Ir	Pt	Au	Hg	Ti	Pb	Bi	Po	At	Rn
	55	56	57–71	72	73	74	75	76	77	78	79	80	81	82	83	84	85	86
7	Fr	Ra	**															
	87	88	89–102															

*Lanthanide series	La	Ce	Pr	Nd	Pm	Sm	Eu	Gd	Tb	Dy	Ho	Er	Tm	Yb	Lu
	57	58	59	60	61	62	63	64	65	66	67	68	69	70	71
**Actinide series	Ac	Th	Pm	U	Np	Pu	Am	Cm	Bk	Cf	Es	Fm	Md		
	89	90	91	92	93	94	95	96	97	98	99	100	101		

IV. THE PERIODIC TABLE AND MINERAL FUNCTION

Of the 109 known elements in the periodic table (Table 1) 30 are essential to life — 19 of these are trace elements and, of these, 12 are transition elements. Transition elements are those which have more than one charged state. For example, iron can exist as the ferrous ion (Fe^{++}) and the ferric ion (Fe^{+++}), while chromium has several oxidation states, as does copper. However, biological systems usually use only one of these states. The multivalent characteristic of iron is unique in that it allows it to serve as an oxygen carrier in hemoglobin or as an hydrogen carrier in enzymatic reactions using an iron-sulfur center within a large structure. Most transition elements are not this variable.

Because of their ionic nature, minerals can form electrovalent bonds with a variety of substances. Although ingested as salts, minerals ionize to their component parts and it is the resultant ions that are absorbed, used, stored, or excreted. For some ions there are very efficient retainment cycles. Sodium, potassium, chloride, calcium, and phosphorus fall into this category. For sodium, potassium, and chloride, conservation is energy driven via the sodium-potassium ATPase. There are several ATPases that serve in this role. The $Ca^{2+}Mg^{2+}$ATPase of the mitochondrial membrane works to optimize the ion content of this organelle. These ATPases are proteins and illustrate a further mechanism of mineral metabolism. As ions, minerals react with charged amino acid residues of intact proteins and peptides. Table 2 provides a list of minerals and the amino acids with which they react. Depending on their valence state these electrovalent bonds can form very strong, moderate, or very weak associations. The marginally charged ion (either an electron acceptor or an electron donor) will be less strongly attracted to its opposite number than will an ion with a strong charge.

Table 2   Mineral-Amino Acid Interactions

Minerals	Amino Acid
Calcium	Serine, carboxylated glutamic acid (GLA)
Magnesium	Tyrosine, sulfur-containing amino acids
Copper	Histidine
Selenium	Methionine, cysteine
Zinc	Cysteine, histidine

Table 3   Hard and Soft Acids and Bases: Some *Properties* that Can Be Used as Guidelines for Classifying Species

ACID (Electron acceptor)			BASE (Electron donor)		
Hart	**Property**	**Soft**	**Hard**	**Property**	**Soft**
Low	Polarizability	High	Low	Polarizability	High
High	Electropositivity	Low	High	Electronegativity	Low
Large	Positive charge or oxidation state	Small	Large	Negative charge	Small
Small	Size	Large	Small	Size	Large
Ionic, electrostatic	Types of bond usually associated with the acid	Covalent, π	Ionic, electrostatic	Types of bond usually associated with the base	Covalent, π
Few and not easily excited	Outer electrons on donor atoms	Several, easily excited	High energy and inaccessible	Available empty orbitals or donor atom	Low lying and accessible

Note: The entire column need not be true before a species is called hard or soft. The more factors that are true, the greater the degree of hardness or softness.

A. Lewis Acids and Bases

In biological systems, the princples of Lewis acids and bases apply. According to this concept, a Lewis base is an ion which has at least one pair of valence electrons available for sharing (an electron donor). A Lewis acid is an ion that can accept or share at least one pair of valence electrons (an electron acceptor). Thus, an acid-base reaction which produces a product is represented as A+:B → A:B. The product of this reaction can be called a coordination complex, an adduct, or an acid-base complex. Examples of this type of reaction have already been shown in Units 3 and 4. In particular, the reader should reexamine the structure of vitamin B_{12} where cobalt is held in a coordinate structure involving pterin rings.

Within the Lewis system there is a subdivision of hard and soft acids and bases. The hydrochloric acid released by the gastric parietal cells is an example of a hard acid. It meets the definition because the constituent ions, H^+ and Cl^-, readily polarize, have high electropositivity, have a large positive and negative charge, are small in size, are almost exclusively ionic in their bonding, and have few outer electrons to be donated or accepted. The constituent ions of hydrochloric acid are single-valence ions. In contrast, consider a number of compounds that are soft Lewis acids. These have properties that are the opposite of those listed above. In many instances the electron donor is one of the multivalent ions, i.e., copper or iron, and the electron acceptor is an amino acid or an organic ring structure. Some organic substances can be both an acid and a base. Consider ethyl acetate — it çan be a Lewis base when it forms complexes through one of its oxygen atoms to a proton or other Lewis acid. It acts as a Lewis acid when it adds bases such as the hydroxide ion. Tables 3 to 5 provide further information about Lewis acids and bases. These reactions are important mechanisms for the hydrolysis of an ester bond (as in triacylglyceride metabolism) or in understanding the basis for ligand (mineral-protein) formation. Throughout the individual units dealing with the minerals the reader will encounter instances of ligand binding. Many minerals are carried in the blood by specific transport proteins. This is an example of a Lewis acid-base reaction.

The specificity of the transport protein has yet to be unraveled. There are preferred ligand bonding groups, as shown in Table 6, but why these are the preferred groups is not known. There are instances where a transport protein will carry more than one ion. An example is metallothionein, which will carry both zinc and copper. It will also carry some of the heavy metals, but its affinity is greater for zinc and copper. Many of the ions can be chelated by organic materials. Ethylenedi-aminetetraacetic acid (EDTA) is a potent chelator and is used to remove lead or other heavy metals from the body. It will also chelate calcium and magnesium, so the clinician using EDTA to treat

Table 4   Hard and Soft Acids and Bases: The HSAB Classification of Acids

Hard	Soft
H^+, Li^+, Na^+, K^+	Cu^+, Ag^+, Au^+, Tl^+, Hg^+
Be^{2+}, Mg^{2+}, Ca^{2+}, Sr^{2+}, Mn^{2+},	Pd^{2+}, Cd^{2+}, Pt^{2+}, Hg^{2+}, CH_3Hg^+, $Co(CN)_5^{2-}$, Pt^{4+}, Te^{4+}
Al^{3+}, Sc^{3+}, Ga^{3+}, In^{3+}, La^{3+}	Tl^{3+}, $Tl(CH_3)_3$, BH_3, $Ga(CH_3)_3$
N^{3+}, Cl^{3+}, Gd^{3+}, Lu^{3+}	$GaCl_3$, GaI_3, $InCl_3$
Cr^{3+}, Co^{3+}, Fe^{3+}, As^{3+}, CH_3Sn^{3+}	RS^+, Rse^+, Rte^+
Si^{4+}, Ti^{4+}, Zr^{4+}, Th^{4+}, U^{4+}	I^+, Br^+, HO^+, RO^+
Pu^{4+}, Cc^{3+}, Hf^{4+}, WO^{4+}, Sn^{4+}	
UO_2^{2+}, $(CH_3)_2Sn^{2+}$, VO^{2+}, MoO^{3+}	I_2, Br_2, ICN, etc.
$BeMc_2$, BF_3, $B(OR)_3$	Trinitrobenzene, etc.
$Al(CH_3)_3$, $AlCl_3$, AlH_3	Chloranil, quinones, etc.
RPO_2^+, $ROPO_2^+$	Tetracyanoethylene, etc.
RSO_2^+, $ROSO_2^+$, SO_3	O, Cl, Br, I, N, Ro^*, RO^*2
I^{7+}, I^{5+}, Cl^{7+}, Cr^{6+}	$M°$ (metal atoms)
RCO^+, CO_2, NC^+	Bulk metals
HX (hydrogen bonding molecules)	CH_2, carbenes

Borderline

Fe^{2+}, Co^{2+}, Ni^{2+}, Cu^{2+}, Zn^{2+}, Pb^{2+}, Sn^{2+}, Sb^{2+}, Bi^{2+}, Rh^{2+}, Ir^{2+}, $B(CH_3)_3$, SO_2, $NO+$, Ru^{2+}, Os^{2+}, $R3C^+$, $C_6H_5^+$, GaH_3

From Pearson, R.G., *J. Chem. Educ.*, 45, 581, 1968. With permission.

Table 5   HSAB Classification of Bases

Hard	Soft
H_2O, OH^-, F^-	R_2S, RSH, RS^-
$CH_3CO_2^-$, PO_4^{3-}, SO_4^{2-}	I^-, SCN^-, $S_2O_3^{2-}$
Cl^-, CO_3^{2-}, ClO_4^-, NO_3^-	R_3P, R_3As, $(RO)_3P$
ROH, RO^-, R_2O	CN^-, RNC, CO
NH_3, RNH_2, N_2H_4	C_2H_4, C_6H_6
	H^-, R^-

Borderline

$C_6H_5NH_2$, C_5H_5N, N_3^-, Br^-, NO_2^-, SO_3^{2-}, N_2

Note: The symbol R stands for an alkyl
group such as CH_3 or C_2H_5.

From Pearson, R.G., *J. Chem. Educ.*, 45, 581,
1968. With permission.

lead overload will have to be aware of this feature as well. Penicillamine is another chelator of importance. It is used to remove excess copper in patients with the genetically inherited disease called Wilson's disease. 2,3-D-Dimercaptopropanol-1 is a chelator of lead, mercury, arsenic, copper, cadmium, tin, and other toxic metals. It solubilizes these metals and chelates them, allowing for their excretion in the urine. The mechanism of action is that of a Lewis base. Other chelates in metabolism are well known: heme, shown in Figure 2, chelates iron, and thus we have heme acting as a Lewis base and iron as a Lewis acid.

The formation of mineral-organic compound bonds is also seen when one examines the roles of minerals in gene expression. Almost every mineral is involved in one or more ways. Mineral response elements (MREs) can be found in the promoter regions of almost all genes encoding products of interest to nutritionists and biochemists. These MREs can be located very near the start site of the structural gene and thus serve as cis-acting transcription factors. Alternatively, they can be located fairly far away from the start site and, indeed, some may be located at sites some distance

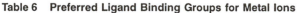

Table 6   Preferred Ligand Binding Groups for Metal Ions

Metal	Ligand Groups
K^+	Singly charged oxygen donors or neutral oxygen ligands
Mg^{2+}	Carboxylase, phosphate, nitrogen donors
Ca^{2+}	$=Mg^{2+}$, but less affinity for nitrogen donors, phosphate, and other multidentate anions
Mn^{2+}	Similar to Mg^{2+}
Fe^{2+}	$-SH$, NH_2 > carboxylates
Fe^{3+}	Carboxylate, tyrosine, $-NH_2$, porphyrin (four 'hard' nitrogen donors)
Co^{3+}	Similar to Fe^{3+}
Cu^+	$-SH$ (cysteine)
Cu^{2+}	Amines >> carboxylates
Zn^{2+}	Imidazole, cysteine
Mo^{2+}	$-SH$
Cd^{2+}	$-SH$

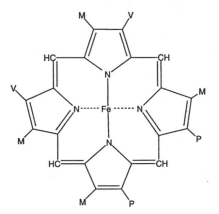

Figure 2   Heme as a chelator of iron. Abbreviations used: A, acetate (CH_2-COO_3H); M, methyl ($-CH_3$); P, proprionate ($-CH_2$-CH_2-COOH); V, vinyl ($-R$-CH=CH_2).

away such that there may be intervening noncoding sequences which separate the MRE from the promoter region. In this instance the MRE serves as the bending site for a mineral containing a trans-acting transcription factor. Table 7 provides some examples of minerals and the gene products that require these minerals. Zinc bonds with certain base sequences to form the zinc fingers so necessary for transcription. In fact, a large number of genes are turned on (or off) by these fingers. For example, the vitamin A receptor (RAR, RXR) protein contains several zinc fingers (see Unit 3) without which retinoic acid could not function as a transcription factor. The details of these zinc fingers are provided in the last unit (Unit 8). Minerals can bond either by themselves or in complexes with proteins to inhibit or enhance translation and, lastly, minerals by themselves or in a complex can influence post-translation protein modification. The details, where known, will be provided in the individual mineral sections.

V. MINERAL ABSORPTION AS RELATED TO RDA

Lewis base and acid interactions are at work in the intestine where mineral absorption takes place. Of all the elements needed by mammals, few enter the absorptive cell by passive diffusion. Several are carried into the body by proteins to which the minerals are loosely attached. Iron, zinc, and copper are imported via these transporters. Sodium and potassium enter (or are exchanged) by an ATPase specific for these ions. Chloride, iodide, and fluoride enter by way of an anion-cation

Table 7   Examples of Gene Products That Are Influenced by Minerals

Mineral	Gene Product
Selenium	Glutathione peroxidase
	5'-Deiodinase
Copper	Metallothionein
Zinc	Carbonic anhydrase
	Zinc fingers
	Zinc transcription factor
	Metallothionein
Iron	Ferritin
	Transferrin receptor
Calcium	Calbindin
Potassium	Aldosterone synthetase
Sodium	Cholesterol SCC, a P450 enzyme
	Endothelin I

exchange mechanism. The uptake of calcium and phosphorus (as phosphate) occurs by a protein-mediated process. It is known that optimal absorption occurs when the calcium:phosphorus ratio is between 1:2 and 2:1 and that an adequate vitamin D supply is essential. As discussed in the section on vitamin D (Unit 3, Section II), intestinal calcium uptake is mediated by a vitamin D-dependent calcium-binding protein. It is suspected that the uptake is also dependent on a phosphorylation/dephosphorylation process; hence, the importance of the calcium:phosphorus ratio.

Although all of these mechanisms of uptake are operative for the minerals, few of the minerals are 100% absorbable. The exceptions are sodium, potassium, chloride, selenium, and magnesium. For the others, the absorption process is dependent on a number of factors: the binding capacity of the transport protein (if needed), solubility, the composition of the diet, the mixture of elements present in the gut contents, and the presence of materials such as phytate and EDTA which bind specific elements thus changing the element mixture presented to the enterocyte, and the actual amount of the element to be absorbed. All of these factors contribute to the bioavailability of the anions and cations that are essential micronutrients. In addition, there are physiological factors (age, hormonal status, and health status) that also influence absorption and subsequent use. Those elements that are variable in terms of their absorption are those that are either divalent or multivalent, that is, ions that have more than one charged state. Iron, copper, and chromium fit into this category while calcium, magnesium, selenium, manganese, zinc, and molybdenum fit into the former category. The Food and Nutrition Board of the National Academy of Sciences took absorption into account when the RDAs for minerals were devised. For example, it has been estimated that between 12 and 50% of the adult calcium intake actually enters the enterocyte and subsequently is available for use. The RDA, therefore, is set at four times this (800 mg/day) to allow for losses in the feces due to incomplete uptake. Those elements where the database on absorption and need is large have an RDA. Those where the database is modest or small (or for the human, nonexistent) do not have an RDA. In some instances where scientists have strong evidence for need as well as evidence of the usual intake by healthy people, there is a recommendation that is defined as being generally agreed to be safe and adequate. A number of the microminerals are in this category.

How are the needs of humans for minerals determined? In contrast to the vitamins, which are not recycled, mineral intake adequacy is extremely difficult to determine. The end points for determining adequate intake are not particularly clear in most instances. Again, absorption is a critical factor. In times of inadequate intake, efficiency of absorption increases as a defense against deficiency. Recycling and retention is another compensatory mechanism that defends the body from an absolute lack of the mineral.

As in studies of the protein requirement, the use of the balance method has some merit. Careful measures of intake and excretion are made and, where possible and necessary, recycling is determined. The use of isotopes as markers has made the measurement of recycling possible. Calcium

Table 8 Elemental Analysis of the Human Body

Element	Serum (mg/ml)	Kidney (ppm)	Element	Serum (mg/ml)	Kidney (ppm)
AL	0.11–0.78	0.35–1.80	K	—	—
Ba	0.025–0.08	0.01[a]	Mn	0.00054–0.061	0.4–2.4
Ca	—	—	Mo	0.006–0.027	0.63,0.4[a]
Co	0.00022–0.062	0.008–0.071	Na	—	—
Cr	0.002–0.02	0.03–0.86	Pb	0.016–0.13	0.27–1.27
Cu	0.97–1.67	1.7–4.15	P	—	—
Fe	0.87–1.87	42–110	Se	0.098–0.327	0.1–3.5
I	0.045–0.100	0.03–0.04	Zn	0.67–1.83	25–67

[a] Only two analyses were available for this element.

and iron requirements have been studied in this way. The measurement of the mineral content of the diet, excreta, and body materials, while tedious and requiring great care to prevent contamination, is straightforward. Atomic absorption spectrometry, arc emission spectrometry, neutron activation, mass spectrometry, X-ray fluorescence spectrometry, and arc emission-flame spectrometry are used with excellent results. Each element has a characteristic electronic signature and thus can be quantitated using these very sophisticated technologies. Several publications have provided the mineral content of the human body. An example of mineral analysis of serum and renal tissue is shown in Table 8.

In the next unit the macrominerals will be discussed in terms of their functions. Microminerals needed in trace amounts will also be discussed.

SUPPLEMENTAL READINGS

Barton, J.C., Conrad, M.E., and Holland, R. 1981. Iron, lead, cobalt absorption: similarities and dissimilarities, *Proc. Soc. Exp. Biol. Med.,* 166:64-69.

Caster, W.O. and Wang, M. 1981. Dietary aluminum and Alzheimer's Disease — a review, *Sci. Tot. Environ.,* 17:31-36.

Fox, M.R.S. and Tao, S.H. 1981. Mineral content of human tissues from a nutrition perspective, *Fed. Proc.,* 40:2130-2134.

Koo, J.O., Weaver, C.M., Neylan, M.J., and Miller, G.D. 1993. Isotopic tracer techniques for assessing calcium absorption in rats, *J. Nutr. Biochem.,* 4:72-76.

Mertz, W. 1987. Use and misuse of balance studies, *J. Nutr.,* 117:1811-1813.

Mischler, E.H., Chesney, P.J., Chesney, R.W., and Mazeso, R.B. 1979. Demineralization in cystic fibrosis, *Am. J. Dis. Child,* 133:632–635.

Newberne, P.M. 1981. Disease states and tissue mineral elements in man, *Fed. Proc.,* 40:2134-2138.

Oster, M.H., Urin-Hare, J.Y., Trapp, C.L., Stern, J.S., and Keen, C.L. 1994. Dietary macronutrient composition influences tissue trace element accumulation in diabetic Sprague-Dawley rats, *J. Nutr.,* 207:67-75.

Pearson, R.G. 1968. Hard and soft acids and bases: fundamental principles, *J. Chem. Educ.,* 45:581-587.

Smith, J.C., Anderson, R.A., Ferritti, R., Levander, O.A., Moris, E.R., Roginski, E.E., Veillon, C., Wolf, W.R., Anderson, J.J.B., and Mertz, W. 1981. Evaluation of published data pertaining to mineral composition of human tissue, *Fed. Proc.,* 40:2120-2125.

Stika, K.M. and Morrison, G.H. 1981. Analytical methods for the mineral content of human tissues, *Fed. Proc.,* 40:2115-2120.

Strain, J.J. 1991. Disturbances of micronutrient and antioxidant status in diabetes, *Proc. Nutr. Soc.,* 50:591-604.

Williams, D.R. 1991. *The Metals of Life,* Van Nostrand Reinhold, New York.

UNIT **7**

Macrominerals

TABLE OF CONTENTS

I. OVERVIEW

The term macrominerals refers to those elements needed by the body in milligram quantities on a daily basis. The category includes sodium, potassium, chloride, calcium, phosphorus, and magnesium. While the body content of the first three is relatively small because of high turnover, the body content of calcium and phosphorus, by comparison, is relatively large. All of these serve as electrolytes and their critical use relates to this function. While they have a structural function as well, their roles as metabolic regulators is of primary importance. Each of these minerals will be discussed as they relate to each other.

II. SODIUM

Sodium is the major extracellular electrolyte. It has an atomic number of 23 and circulates as a fully dissociated ion due to its 1+ charge. It is thus fully water soluble. It has been estimated that the adult body contains 52 to 60 meq/kg (male) and 48 to 55 meq/kg (female). Thus, the average adult male would have about 83 to 97 g of sodium in his 70-kg body. Between 2/3 and 3/4 of this sodium is "fixed" in the mineral apatite of the bone. The remaining sodium comprises a pool which undergoes considerable flux as it participates in sodium-potassium exchange. The exchangeable sodium in the adult human body can be predicted using the following equation: Na_e (meq) = 163.2 (total body water) $-$ 69 $-$ Ke (meq). Ke is the exchangeable potassium which likewise can be predicted as follows: Ke (meq) = 150 (intracellular body water$_L$) + 4 (total body water $-$ intracellular body water). Total body water can be determined (see *Advanced Nutrition: Macronutrients*, Unit 2) or estimated using one of several prediction equations. Sodium is primarily an extracellular ion and, as such, the serum will contain 136 to 145 meq/l. Normal sodium intake varies from less than 2 g to 10 g/day. Most of this sodium comes from table salt, NaCl. Foods rich in added salt are usually the snack foods such as potato chips, salted nuts, pretzels, and so forth. Processed foods have more added salt than nonprocessed foods because salt not only improves the taste of the finished product but also serves as a preservative. Luncheon meats, cheese spreads, pickles, relishes, catsup, canned and frozen vegetables, crackers, breads, and frozen desserts are but a few of the foods that contain more sodium as a processed food than in their raw or nonprocessed state. Every living thing contains sodium and, except for pure fats and carbohydrates, no major food source lacks this element. There is no RDA figure for sodium but there is an estimated minimum intake for healthy adults of 500 mg Na per day. These estimates presume that the individual has a moderately active life style and lives in a temperate environment. Heavy work in a hot, dry environment and a variety of medical conditions (see Table 1) will affect the need for sodium.

Table 1   Causes of Hypernatremia and Hyponatremia

Hypernatremia (serum Na > 150 meq/l)	Hyponatremia (serum Na < 135 meq/l)
Dehydration — excess sweating, deficient water intake	Cachexia (any wasting disease, i.e., cancer)
Excess solute loading	Anorexia nervosa
Diabetes insipidus (too little ADH)	Ulcerative colitis
Brain stem injury	Liver disease
	Congestive heart failure
	Ascites, edema
	Major trauma
	Severe infection
	Excess water intake
	Inappropriate ADH release
	Diarrhea
	Certain drugs (chlorothiazide, mercurial diuretics, etc.)
	Adrenalectomy

Table 2 Hormones Involved in the Regulation of Serum Sodium

Hormone	Function
Vasopressin (ADH)	Serves to stimulate the reabsorption of water by the glomerulus and renal convoluted tubule.
Atrial natriuretic hormone	Counteracts vasopressin and thus induces water loss, sodium loss, and potassium loss. It also decreases blood pressure and increases the glomerular filtration rate. Suppresses renin release and aldosterone release. Antagonizes angiotensin II and norepinephrine.
Renin	Catalyzes the conversion of inactive angiotensin I to active angiotensin II.
Angiotensin II	At low serum sodium levels it conserves sodium by stimulating its reabsorption. At high serum sodium levels it has the reverse effect. Stimulates vasoconstriction which increases blood pressure. Reduces water loss, decreases the glomerular filtration rate. Stimulates aldosterone release.
Aldosterone	Conserves sodium by increasing sodium resorption by the kidney.

While sodium intake can be highly variable, serum sodium is not. As described above, the normal range of serum sodium is quite small. Values in excess of 150 meq/l (hypernatremia) and below 135 meq/l (hyponatremia) are considered abnormal and are of clinical concern. There are several reasons why hypernatremia or hyponatremia can develop. These are summarized in Table 1. In normal individuals, the level of sodium in the serum is tightly controlled and this control is intertwined with the control of potassium concentration, chloride concentration, and water balance.

A. Regulation of Serum Sodium

The system which regulates sodium levels in the blood also is involved in the regulation of water balance, pH, and osmotic pressure. Both hormones and physical/chemical factors are involved. Table 2 lists the hormones and their roles in sodium balance as well as in water balance. The hormones listed are all involved indirectly or directly because of the need to regulate the osmotic pressure within and around the cells. Osmolality, that is, the concentration of solutes on each side of a semipermeable membrane, is maintained by the passage of water through that membrane. This osmolality is maintained at roughly 270 to 290 mosmol. The proteins, many of which can not pass through the plasma membrane, are part of this solute load. In the well-nourished, healthy individual, the intracellular and extracellular proteins are maintained at fairly constant levels. This leaves the small, fully ionized solutes (Na^+, K^+, Cl^-) as major determinants of the osmotic pressure of the system. Osmotic pressure is the physical force required to keep the osmolality on both sides of the membrane approximately equal. If the solute load on one side exceeds that of the other, water and the small solutes (Na^+, K^+, Cl^-) will pass through the membrane to equalize the concentration of solutes.

Since the number of particles determines osmotic pressure, substances which ionize affect osmotic pressure according to the degree of dissociation. Thus, fully dissociated NaCl produces the ions Na^+ and Cl^- in such a fashion that at 0.154 M there are 1.85 particles each of Na^+ and Cl^- which exert a pressure of 286 mosmol. There are several ways to measure osmolality in the laboratory using rather simple instruments called osmometers. For example, the osmolality of a solution can be determined by using the effect of a solute on the freezing point. The addition of 1 osmol to 1 l of water will depress the freezing point by 1.86°C.

Several of the hormones listed in Table 2 are released in response to changes in sodium concentration or to signals generated by osmoreceptors located in the anterolateral hypothalamus. The sodium ion, of all the circulating ions, is the most potent of the solutes activating the osmoreceptors, which in turn signal the release of hormones which regulate osmolality. Vasopressin (ADH) is one of these; aldosterone is another. When the osmoreceptors sense a change (increase) in the solute load, ADH release is stimulated. This results in an increase in renal water resorption and thus dilution of the solute load. Aldosterone release is stimulated by low serum sodium-high

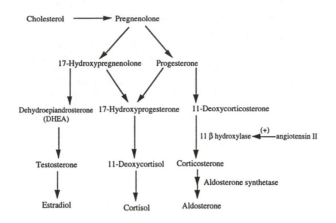

Figure 1 The steroid hormone biosynthetic pathway showing the synthesis of aldosterone.

potassium levels in the blood. Aldosterone, released by the adrenal cortex, functions in sodium conservation by increasing renal reabsorption of this ion. Of interest is the action of these ions at the level of the expression of the renin, angiotensin I, and aldosterone synthetase genes. At low sodium-high potassium levels, the transcription of these genes is stimulated. While more renin and angiotensin I synthesis has not been found with increasing mRNA, more aldosterone has been found. The reason for this difference in amounts of gene product has to do with the half-lives of these products. Renin and angiotensin I are made but are quickly degraded. Aldosterone does not disappear as readily. More messenger RNA is produced and more enzyme is synthesized.

The pathway for aldosterone synthesis (as part of the steroid hormone synthetic network) is shown in Figure 1. Aldosterone synthesis from corticosterone via the enzyme 11-β-hydroxylase (an enzyme that catalyzes 11-deoxycorticosterone conversion to corticosterone) is enhanced by angiotensin II. Angiotensin II release is stimulated by low sodium levels. Angiotensin II action requires the calcium ion and high potassium levels to facilitate calcium ion movement from outside to the inside of the cell. As aldosterone levels increase, the calcium ion facilitates its release by the cortex cell. Aldosterone then moves to the kidney where it stimulates electrolyte conservation. Figure 2 illustrates these hormone effects on electrolyte balance. Thus, the circle is completed. Sodium is regulated by several hormones and in turn regulates the synthesis of these hormones through effects on gene transcription. Sodium also stimulates the transcription of the genes for the cholesterol side chain lyase, a P450 enzyme, the gene for adrenodoxin and, in hypertensive animals, has been found to stimulate the transcription of the gene for endothelin 1. Endothelin 1 is an important vasoactive peptide that acts as a diuretic and as a natriuretic. It stimulates vasoconstriction and in genetic hypertension it seems to reduce sodium loss.

B. Function

Indirectly, the function of the sodium ion as a participant in the regulation of osmotic pressure has already been discussed as the regulation of serum sodium levels was presented. In addition to its function in this system, it also functions in nerve conduction, active transport both by the enterocyte and by other cell types, and plays a role in the formation of the mineral apatite of the bone (see Section VII.E.1). The common thread to its role in nerve conduction, active transport, and water balance is its function in the sodium-potassium ATPase. This enzyme, embedded in the plasma membrane of most cells, is perhaps the most thoroughly studied enzyme of the active transport systems. The cloning of the cDNAs encoding the subunits of this ATPase was achieved more than 10 years ago. The ATPase transmembrane protein was first isolated in 1957 and consists of two types of subunits: a 110-kDa nonglycosylated α-subunit that contains the enzyme's catalytic

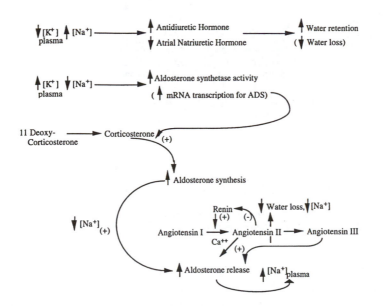

Figure 2   Schematic representation of how low-potassium high-sodium levels affect sodium conservation. Two systems are used. One involves the posterior pituitary which releases antidiuretic hormone (ADH). ADH stimulates water and sodium retention. The other system involves the adrenal cortex which is stimulated to release aldosterone, the mineralocorticoid responsible for Na⁺ retention.

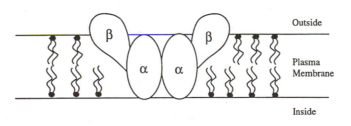

Figure 3   Structure of the Na⁺K⁺ ATPase.

activity and ion-binding site, and a 55-kDa glycoprotein β-subunit. The enzyme has two of each of these subunits. Figure 3 illustrates the structure of this enzyme. The glycoprotein probably plays a role in recognition of appropriate substrates, but this probable role is speculative. The ATPase is frequently called the Na⁺K⁺ pump because it pumps sodium out and, as potassium returns to the cell, there is a concomitant hydrolysis of ATP. The equation which describes this process is as follows:

$$3Na^+ \text{ (in)} + 2\ K^+ \text{ (out)} + ATP \leftrightarrow 3Na^+ \text{ (out)} + 2K^+ \text{ (in)} + ADP + Pi$$

The pump is an electrogenic system, illustrated in Figure 4, with the extrusion of three positively charged particles (the Na⁺) in return for two negatively charged ones (the K⁺). As an electrogenic system, the Na⁺K⁺ATPase generates an electrochemical potential gradient that is responsible for nerve action. Signal transmission along a nerve path occurs via a depolarization/repolarization scheme whereby potassium leaves the neuron and sodium enters (depolarization) and through ATPase activity the reverse occurs (repolarization). Much of the ATP that cells produce is used by this ATPase. In fact, in nerve cells up to 70% of their ATP production is consumed by the sodium pump as it functions in signal transmission.

Other cell types use the pump for other purposes. As mentioned, the active transport of needed nutrients into the enterocyte uses the pump. Muscle contraction/relaxation uses a Na⁺K⁺ ATPase

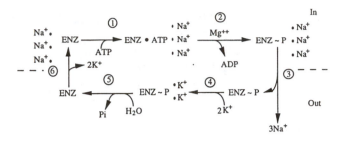

Figure 4 Mechanism of action of the Na⁺K⁺ ATPase. The ion exchange occurs via a series of reactions utilizing the α subunits of the enzyme which has an inward-facing high-affinity Na⁺ binding site which reacts with ATP to form the activated ENZ~P only when Na⁺ is bound to it. On the exterior aspect of the α subunit is a high-affinity K⁺ binding site which will hydrolyze, releasing inorganic phosphate only when K⁺ is bound to it. The obligatory sequence begins with the sodium ATP binding and ends with K⁺ import into the cell. This sequence is numbered on the figure.

or pump. In the muscle there is an additional pump, the Na⁺Ca²⁺ antiport system. This system pumps sodium out and allows calcium into the cell. Calcium triggers muscle contraction and so the two pump systems work together to regulate muscle action. When heart muscle degenerates, the clinician has several drugs that can be used to stimulate muscle action by inhibiting the Na⁺K⁺ ATPase. These drugs, called cardiac glycosides (digitalis, ouabain), inhibit the ATPase by binding to the α subunits (see Figure 2). This results in an increase in intracellular Na⁺ which in turn stimulates the Na⁺Ca²⁺ antiport system. The cell extrudes Na⁺ and the resultant influx of Ca²⁺ triggers an increase in the force of the cardiac muscle contraction. The drug dose must be carefully monitored because too much Ca²⁺ influx could be lethal unless counteracted. The regulation of intracellular calcium levels together with its role in metabolic regulation is a topic of intense interest by nutritionists, biochemists, and physiologists. This topic is addressed below (see pages 164–166).

III. POTASSIUM

Potassium is the major intracellular electrolyte. It has an atomic weight of 39. The healthy young adult male has between 42 to 48 meq K⁺ per kilogram of body weight or 2940 to 3360 meq in the 70-kg male. Persons with above average muscle mass, i.e., athletes, will have more body potassium than persons of average muscle mass. Virtually all the body potassium is exchangeable with the exception of small amounts that are irretrievably bound up in the bone mineral. Since potassium is primarily an intracellular ion, the number of cells in the body can be estimated using an infusion of the heavy isotope, K⁴⁰. The infused and exchangeable potassium equilibrates and by determining the dilution of the isotope one can determine cell number and mass while correcting for fat mass (see *Advanced Nutrition: Macronutrients*, Unit 2). The Na⁺K⁺ ATPase actively works to ensure that K⁺ stays within the cell and that very little (3.5 to 5.0 meq/l) is present in extracellular fluid.

Just as all living things serve as sources of sodium, so too are they sources of potassium. Only highly refined food ingredients, i.e., pure sugars, fats, and oils, lack this essential nutrient. Especially good sources are orange juice, avocados, fish, and bananas. There is no RDA for potassium but an intake deemed safe and adequate is 2000 mg/day. Potassium passes freely from the gastrointestinal system into the enterocyte and thence into the body. Potassium is distributed in response to energy-dependent Na⁺ redistribution. Almost all of the consumed potassium is excreted in the urine, with a very small amount found in the feces in healthy, normal adults. In persons experiencing diarrhea, however, the loss of potassium can be quite large and debilitating. If the diarrhea is of short duration (less than 12 hr) the body will compensate and the person will survive. However, should this condition persist, potassium supplementation will be needed. Such is the case with the disease,

Table 3   Causes of Hypokalemia and Hyperkalemia

Hypokalemia (Plasma Levels < 3.5 meq/l)	Hyperkalemia (Plasma Levels > 7 meq/l)
Vomiting in excess (loss of chloride)	Chronic renal failure
Diuretics that enhance K$^+$ loss	Addison's disease (no aldosterone)
Cushing's disease (excess steroids)	Major trauma, infection
Rehydration therapy without K$^+$	Metabolic acidosis
Chronic renal disease	
Metabolic alkalosis	
Diarrhea	

cholera, and for a number of the malabsorption syndromes. The plasma or serum level of potassium is not a reliable index of whole-body potassium status simply because potassium within the cell (not in the serum) is what is needed. Causes for concern with too little potassium (hypokalemia) or too much (hyperkalemia) have to do with muscle contractility. If hypokalemia persists the person could die of cardiac arrest. This occurs because too much K$^+$ has left the contractile unit and the heart muscle loses its ability to contract. Too much K$^+$ will have a similar effect; that is, the heart stops in diastole. Common causes of hypo- and hyperkalemia are listed in Table 3. The regulation of potassium balance follows that of sodium balance and its participation in the sodium potassium pump has already been discussed.

IV. CHLORIDE

Chloride (atomic weight 35.5) is the third leg upon which osmotic pressure and acid-base balance rests. Normal chloride levels in plasma are 100 to 106 meq/l and vary very little. The glomerular filtrate contains 108 meq/l and urine contains 138 meq/l. Sweat can contain as much as 40 meq/l but usually contains only trace amounts. The intracellular fluid contains very little Cl$^-$ (~4 meq/l) whereas intestinal juice contains 69 to 127 meq/l. In instances of secretory diarrhea, the chloride content of the excrement can be as high as 45 meq/l. Most of the chloride in the intestinal tract does not appear in the feces of normal individuals. Rather, this ion recirculates as sodium and potassium are carried into the body. The main excretory pathway is urine. This ion is a member of the halogen family of elements that includes fluoride, iodide, and bromide in addition to chloride. Although very reactive, chloride is passively distributed throughout the body. As mentioned, it moves to replace anions lost to cells via other processes. It is the other half of table salt, NaCl, and as such is found in abundance in most foods. Dietary intake is in excess of that of sodium yet the usual plasma Na$^+$:Cl$^-$ ratio is about 3:2. This imbalance is due to the passive nature of chloride transfer between water compartments and to the active system which serves to retain Na$^+$. As with Na$^+$ and K$^+$ there is no RDA, but an intake of 750 mg/day is deemed safe and adequate. Instances of below and above normal plasma levels of Cl$^-$ are not diet related but are due to metabolic reasons usually related to Na$^+$ and K$^+$ homeostasis. Listed in Table 4 are reasons why hypochloremia and

Table 4   Causes of Hypochloremia and Hyperchloremia

Hypochloremia	Hyperchloremia
Increased extracellular water volume due to trauma and/or cachexia	Dehydration
	Brain stem injury
	Diabetes insipidus
Vomiting with large loss of gastric HCl	
Overuse of diuretics	Ureterointestinal anastomoses due to reabsorption of Cl$^-$
Overuse of adrenal steroids with retention of Na$^+$	
Chronic respiratory acidosis (high CO_2, low pH)	
Chronic renal disease, renal failure	

hyperchloremia develop. Note the similarities between these causes and those listed for sodium in Table 1 and those for potassium in Table 3.

A. Function

As an electronegative element, Cl^- is a good oxidizing agent. In typical reactions it is reduced to its electronegative form. One of its main functions is as an essential ingredient of the gastric acid, hydrochloric acid. Gastric juice contains 120 to 160 meq Cl^-/l. This is completely dissociated into a strong electron donor (H^+) and a strong electron acceptor (Cl^-).

HCl is produced by the parietal cells of the gastric mucosa. This mucosa, consisting of a variety of secreting cells, also release pepsinogen, which is activated by HCl and is the intrinsic factor needed for vitamin B_{12} absorption, and mucus. The mucus is a necessary protectant of the mucosa. Without it, HCl and the various proteases of the gastric secretions would digest the organ itself. The main function of HCl, aside from its role in the conversion of pepsin from pepsinogen, is as a bactericide. In the absence of HCl bacterial overgrowth occurs, with subsequent deleterious effects on gastrointestinal function.

The function of chloride, aside from its passive participation in electrolyte balance, has to do with hemoglobin and its function as a carrier for oxygen and carbon dioxide. As hemoglobin exchanges oxygen for carbon dioxide, the enzyme carbonic anhydrase catalyzes the formation of HCO_3^-. This carbonate ion diffuses out of the red cell in exchange for Cl^-. The Cl^- is bound more tightly to deoxyhemoglobin than to oxyhemoglobin. Hence the affinity of hemoglobin is directly proportional to the concentration of Cl^-. As mentioned, the carbonate ion, HCO_3^-, freely permeates the erythrocyte membrane so that once formed it equilibrates with the plasma. The need for charge neutrality on both sides of the red cell membrane requires that Cl^- flow into the erythrocyte to replace HCO_3^- as it leaves. This is called the chloride shift. Cations (Na^+, K^+) can not do this shifting, but Cl^- and HCO_3^- can. Because of the shift, the Cl^- ion in the venous blood erythrocyte is higher than in the arterial blood erythrocyte.

V. CALCIUM

A. Overview

Calcium is the fifth most abundant element in the body, exceeded only by carbon, hydrogen, oxygen, and nitrogen. It has an atomic weight of 40 and is the primary mineral in bones and teeth where it is present as hydroxyapatite [$3Ca_3(PO_4)_2 \cdot Ca(OH)_2$]. On a dry weight basis, bone contains about 150 mg calcium per gram. By comparison, soft tissue such as liver, muscle, or brain contains less than 35 μg calcium per gram. A normal 70-kg man will have about 22 g calcium per gram of fat-free tissue or a total of 1.54 kg. While the calcium in the teeth is seldom mobilized, that which is in the skeletal muscle is mobilized and replaced at a range of about 0.5 g/day. This daily turnover of calcium is essential to the maintenance of metabolic homeostasis because not only does calcium serve as a structural element, it also serves, in its ionized form, as an essential element in signal transduction. Of the total body calcium, 1% serves as an intracellular/intercellular messenger/regulator. Calcium mobilization and deposition change with age, diet, hormonal status, and physiological state. Bone calcium homeostasis is related to bone strength, and if mobilization exceeds deposition the bones will become porous (osteoporosis) and break easily.

B. Sources

The average daily calcium intake for adults in the U.S. ranges from 500 to 1200 mg. The range is quite broad because it depends on the percent of the diet that comes from dairy products. Milk,

Table 5 Food Sources of Calcium

Source	Calcium (mg/100 g)	Weight of Average Serving (g)
Skim milk	123	245
Whole milk	119	244
Ice cream	129	66
Yogurt	120	227
Oysters	45	84
Cheddar cheese	728	28
Spinach	135	90
Mustard greens	74	70
Broccoli	48	44
White bread	125	24
Whole wheat bread	72	25
Carrots	26	72
Potatoes	10	202
Winter squash	14	102
Egg	50	50
Hamburger	10	100
Hot dog	19	57

cheese, ice cream, yogurt, sour cream, buttermilk, and other fermented and nonfermented milk products can provide as much as 72% of the daily calcium intake. Nuts and whole grain products are also good sources of calcium while other foods are relatively poor sources of this mineral. Shown in Table 5 are a number of foods and their calcium content.

Some foods contain calcium-binding agents that reduce the availability of the calcium to the enterocyte. For example, some plant foods contain calcium in measurable quantities but these same foods also contain phytate, a six-carbon anomer of glucose having six phosphate groups. Phytate will bind calcium, reducing its availability for absorption. Phytate can be degraded by the enzyme phytase which, in turn, releases the bound calcium so that it is once again available for absorption. Unfortunately, this release occurs in the lower third of the intestine and in the large intestine, areas which are less active in terms of calcium absorption. Phytate binds other divalent ions (Zn, Fe, and Mg) as well, and has a similar effect on their absorption. In addition, oxalate and some tannins can have this effect.

1. Food Mixtures

Milk and milk products are excellent sources of calcium, as mentioned earlier. The reason why milk calcium absorption is so good is because of the type of carbohydrate (lactose) and protein found in these foods. Lactose favors calcium absorption. Casein, the main protein in milk, is a relatively small protein (23,000 Da) having numerous phosphorylated serine residues. These residues are negatively charged, thus enabling the protein to bind the calcium ions. Lactalbumin, another milk protein, is also a calcium-binding protein. In addition to calcium, it will also bind zinc. This is true for a number of proteins; those that bind one divalent ion will also bind other divalent ions. Hence, there could be a competition for binding that would affect the availability of the minerals involved. As the proteins are degraded by the digestive enzymes, these protein-bound minerals become available for uptake by the enterocyte. In mixtures of foods this availability can be enhanced or compromised, depending on the food mixture. As mentioned, cereal foods and green leafy vegetables contain oxalates or phytate that bind calcium. When these foods are mixed with dairy foods, one could anticipate a reduction in the availability of the calcium in the dairy food. In contrast, foods that are rich in vitamin C enhance calcium availability, probably due to the redox nature of ascorbic acid. This vitamin readily changes from an oxidized to a reduced form and assists not only calcium absorption but also assists in the absorption of iron.

Table 6   Food Components That Affect Calcium Absorption

Component	Effect
Alcohol	↓
Ascorbic acid	↓↑
Cellulose	↓
Fat[a]	↑↓
Fiber	↓
Lactose	↑
Medium-chain triglycerides	↑
Oxalates	↓
Pectin	↑↓
Phytate	↓
Protein[b]	↑↓
Sodium alginate	↓
Uronic acid	↓

[a] In cases of steatorrhea, calcium absorption is reduced.
[b] Certain proteins, e.g., those in milk, enhance calcium availability while others, e.g., those in plants, reduce it.

Foods and food mixtures that provide calcium and phosphorus together in a ratio of 2:1 to 1:2 optimize calcium absorption. Both minerals are actively transported and yet do not share a single transport mechanism (see below). When the food mixtures are unbalanced with respect to this ratio then calcium uptake will be impaired. Table 6 summarizes the influence of food components on calcium availability.

C. Bioavailability, Absorption

In contrast to the macronutrients, the vitamins, and the electrolytes sodium, potassium, and chloride, not all of the calcium that is consumed is absorbed. The fraction which is absorbed can vary depending on the food source, the mixture of foods consumed, and the physiological status of the individual. That which is actually involved in biological processes is the bioavailable fraction. The determination of calcium bioavailability and absorption efficiency is a complicated process that involves careful food analysis to determine calcium content: careful measurements of the food consumed followed by feces and urine analysis of calcium excretion, corrected for calcium recycling. While the amount of calcium in the urine reflects the calcium that is absorbed, it does not reveal the amount of calcium that has been recycled. Likewise, the calcium in the feces reflects not only the calcium that was not absorbed from the food but also the calcium that was secreted into the intestine and not reabsorbed. The use of the calcium balance technique also does not measure the amount of calcium deposited in the bones and teeth, nor does it provide an estimate of the amount of calcium that is mobilized from these depots. However, the balance technique can be combined with tracer techniques which provide reasonably good estimates of absorption and bioavailability.

Bioavailability estimates can be obtained using isotopes of calcium as tracers. The heavy isotope Ca (^{46}Ca, ^{48}Ca) or the radioisotope calcium (^{45}Ca, ^{47}Ca) can be incorporated into a food and its presence in blood, urine, and feces monitored over time (flux). Flux is a term used to provide a time dimension to the movement of calcium. It can refer to a loss or a gain in concentration in a given volume or mass. If a plant food, the plant can be grown in a calcium isotope-enriched growth medium and the edible portions provided to the subject or animal. If an animal food, the animal either consumes an isotopically labeled feed or is infused with a solution of labeled $CaCl_2$. Knowing the total food calcium and the percent that was isotopically labeled will then allow for calculations of intestinal uptake, recycling, excretion, storage, and use. The double isotope technique involves the consumption of a ^{45}Ca-enriched food followed by an infusion of ^{47}CaCl in the vein. ^{47}Ca has a short half-life (~4.7 days) while ^{45}Ca has a much longer one (~163.5 days). The stable isotopes (^{48}Ca, ^{49}Ca) can be substituted for the radioisotopes. The infused ^{47}Ca will be diluted in the blood by the calcium mobilized from the depots as well as by the absorbed calcium which also dilutes the food ^{45}Ca. The fraction that is absorbed is calculated as follows:

$$J_{ms} = \frac{J_{max}\left[Ca_L^{2+}\right] + A\left[Ca_L^{2+}\right]}{K_T + \left[Ca_L^{2+}\right]} \tag{1}$$

where: J_{ms} = the amount of calcium that has entered the body from the lumen; it is equal to the appearance of ^{45}Ca (corrected for nonlabeled calcium) in the blood
J_{max} = maximum saturable flux
Ca_L^{2+} = lumen, $J_{max}/2$ is observed
A = diffusion constant

In practice, absorption = the fraction of oral ^{45}Ca in urine/fraction of ^{47}Ca in urine. The use of ^{47}Ca assumes that the infused calcium will behave as though it had been absorbed. In each instance the measurement is a single time point. Urine is collected for 24 hr after isotope administration. To obtain an estimate of recycling the investigator will collect blood, urine, and feces at intervals over a 2- to 4-day period, monitor the dilution of the consumed and infused labels, and using this information calculate rate constants for each calcium pool. Absorption can also be calculated from the feces using the loss of the consumed label to estimate the absorption. However, since there is considerable individual variation in gut passage time which can influence calcium absorption, feces must be collected for periods of up to 12 days. Given the shorter half-life of ^{47}Ca that is infused to provide the estimate of recycling, this method for determining apparent absorption is not as popular.

Combining the use of both radioactive and stable isotopes also has some problems. The stable isotope ^{48}Ca degrades to ^{49}Ca with the emission of a γ-ray. ^{49}Ca has a half-life of 8.8 min. ^{46}Ca converts to ^{47}Ca which has radioactivity. The use of heavy isotopes require the use of mass spectrometry to detect their presence while liquid scintillation or gamma counters are needed for detecting the radioisotopes. Small animals such as the rat, mouse, and chicken with their smaller body sizes, faster rates of growth, and faster metabolic rates, reduce the expense and increase the number of measurements as well as the validity of these measurements due to their genetic homogeneity.

1. Apparent Absorption

Apparent absorption is the fraction of the consumed calcium that disappears from the gastrointestinal tract. Thus, it is the net movement of calcium from the lumen into the animal. This movement can be tracked *in vitro* using an intestinal segment and a calcium isotope. Phenol red is used as a marker of absorbing cells. The apparent absorption can be calculated using the following equation:

$$\text{Apparent Absorption} = \frac{V\left[^{40}Ca_i - \left(^{40}Ca_f\right)(PRR)\right]}{L \text{ or } W} \tag{2}$$

The subscripts i and f refer to initial and final concentrations of calcium in micromoles per milliliter. PRR is the ratio of phenol red in the initial and final samples. L is the length and W is the weight

**Table 7   Apparent Absorption of Calcium *In Vitro*
by Duodenal Loops from Normal Rats**

Volume perfused	240 ml
Duration of perfusion	2 hr
Concentration of calcium	0.8 mM
Concentration of ^{45}Ca (specific activity, 2000 µCi/mg)	12 µCi/l
Length of intestine, cm	87
Weight of intestine, g	5.4
Mucosal dry weight, mg/cm	7.2
Net absorption, µmol/hr	
Per cm segment length	0.140
Per g dry weight mucosa	20.1
Lumen to plasma flux	
Per cm segment length	0.196
Per g dry weight mucosa	27.6

of the intestinal segment, and V is the volume perfused in milliliters. The lumen to plasma flux is unidirectional and can be calculated as follows:

$$\text{Lumen to Plasma Flux} = \frac{V\left[{}^{45}Ca_i - \left({}^{45}Ca_f\right)(PRR)\right]}{\left[(SA_i - SA_f)/2\right]W} \tag{3}$$

In this calculation SA refers to the specific activity of the calcium isotope and W is the dry weight of the intestinal segment. All the other definitions are the same as in Equation 2. These equations have been successfully used to calculate calcium absorption in normal rats, as shown in Table 7.

2. Physiological Status

Absorption efficiency is greater in the young, growing individual than in the mature adult, which in turn is greater than in the aged individual. As well, there are gender differences due in part to hormonal status. Postmenopausal females have a less efficient calcium absorption than premenopausal females. Men, both young and mature, have a greater calcium absorption efficiency than females of the same age. Testosterone has been shown to enhance calcium absorption. Calcium absorption is impaired in vitamin D-deficient individuals as well as in persons with insulin-dependent diabetes mellitus. Clearly the endocrine status of the individual has effects on calcium uptake and this, in turn, can influence calcium status in terms of bone structure and calcium content.

3. Mechanisms of Absorption

Only 20 to 50% of ingested calcium is absorbed yet this mineral is so important to metabolism that two mechanisms exist for its absorption. One of these is vitamin D dependent while the other is not. The latter is one that uses passive diffusion as the means for calcium entry into the enterocyte. However, once in the enterocyte the mechanism for its disposal is vitamin D dependent. The former is an energy-dependent active transport system and is illustrated in Figure 5. This is a saturable system which operates actively when calcium is in short supply in the diet. Thus, when the diet is rich in calcium this system is far less active than when a calcium-poor diet is consumed. Because both systems are operative, a wide range of apparent calcium absorption exists. In the active system, calcium diffuses across the brush border down its thermodynamic gradient into the cell as free unbound Ca^{2+}. This calcium is then bound by an intracellular protein called calbindin D_{9k} which serves to maintain the level of calcium in the cell at a low, nontoxic level. Calcium released from

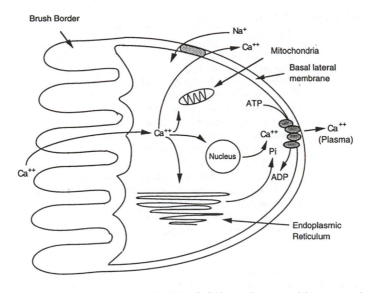

Figure 5   Calcium absorption by the enterocyte. Both the $Ca^{2+}Na^+$ exchange and the energy-dependent systems are shown.

calbindin enters and leaves the subcell compartments such as the mitochondria. This occurs in an orderly oscillatory manner. The calcium ion leaves the enterocyte either in exchange for sodium or is extruded from the cell by a calcium-activated ATPase. This ATPase has been found in both the brush border and at the basal-lateral membrane. As calcium is extruded, ATP is cleaved to ADP and Pi. Hence the energy dependence of this system. Because the sodium that is exchanged for calcium must be actively removed from the intracellular compartment by the Na^+K^+ ATPase, this process is also part of this energy-dependent system.

Absorption of calcium by the enterocyte is but one of the roles of vitamin D. Other roles include renal calcium conservation, intracellular calcium movement, bone calcium deposition, as well as bone calcium mobilization. Calcium homeostasis is thus one of the main functions of vitamin D. Vitamin D or 1,25-dihydroxycholecalciferol, has these effects on calcium homeostasis due to its effects on the synthesis of calcium-binding proteins (Table 8). In the intestine the protein of interest is calbindin D_{9k}. Vitamin D binds to its cognate receptor in the enterocyte and this steroid-receptor complex migrates to the nucleus where it binds to a specific DNA sequence which encodes the protein, calbindin D_{9k}. Studies of vitamin D-deficient animals have shown a rapid induction of calbindin mRNA transcription when the missing vitamin was provided. This was followed by a restoration of normal calcium absorption in these repleted animals. In addition to the rapid increase in transcription was an effect of the vitamin on calbindin mRNA half-life. There was an increase in this half-life which indicates a vitamin effect on mRNA stability. Thus, the vitamin both stimulates transcription and has a post-transcriptional effect on calbindin synthesis.

Vitamin D is not the only hormone involved in calbindin synthesis. Testosterone, growth hormone, progesterone, insulin-like growth factor 1, and estrogen augment, while glucocorticoids inhibit the synthesis of calbindin D_{9k}. Calbindin D_{28k}, another vitamin D-dependent calcium-binding protein in the enterocyte and renal cell, has its synthesis regulated by retinoic acid. In the brain this calcium-binding protein is not regulated by vitamin D. The multiplicity of hormonal controls of calbindin synthesis explains in part the gender and age differences in calcium absorption, and indeed help to elucidate the reasons why postmenopausal females are more at risk for calcium inadequacy than are young, growing males and females. Those hormones that have a positive effect on calbindin D synthesis are the same hormones that are missing (or in short supply) in the postmenopausal female. Should calbindin D_{9k} synthesis be inadequate, calcium absorption will decline. As well, calbindin D_{28k}, an important calcium-binding protein in the renal cell responsible

Table 8   Calcium Binding Proteins

Protein	Function
α-Lactalbumin	Carries calcium in milk
Casein	Carries calcium in milk
Calmodulin	Serves as major intracellular calcium receptor; activates cyclic nucleotidephosphodiesterase
Calbindin D_{9k} and D_{28k}	Facilitates intracellular Ca^{2+} translocation
Osteocalcin	Essential for calcium deposition in bone
$Ca^{2+}Mg^{2+}$ ATPase	Essential to movement of calcium across membranes
Prothrombin	Essential to blood clot formation
Calcitonin	Inhibits osteoclast-mediated bone resorption
	Regulates blood calcium levels by preventing hypercalcemia
Parathyroid hormone	Stimulates calcitonin synthesis, bone Ca resorption, renal Ca conservation
Albumin	Carries calcium in the blood
Globulin	Carries calcium in the blood
Osteopontin	Essential for calcium mobilization from bone
Troponin C	Muscle contraction
Alkaline phosphatase	Mineralization of bone
Sialoprotein	Embryonic bone growth
GLA-rich clotting proteins	Binds calcium in the coagulation cascade (see vitamin K)
Villin, gelsolin	Cytoskeleton stabilization

for renal calcium reabsorption, could also be synthesized at a reduced rate and thus calcium conservation is reduced. The two calbindins are subject to nearly the same hormonal influences. With decreased calcium absorption and conservation bone calcium mobilization increases, with the result of an age/gender-related loss in bone calcium, osteoporosis.

D. Calcium Transport, Blood Calcium Regulation

The concentration of calcium in the plasma is the result of three processes which are integrated so as to maintain a constancy of calcium in the circulation. Blood calcium is regulated at 100 mg/l (2.50 mmol/l) across the life span, although in late adulthood there may be a small (10%) decline due to an age related decline in the total calcium-binding capacity of the serum proteins. Most (80%) of the blood calcium bound to protein is carried by albumin; the remainder is bound to a variety of globulins. About 60% of blood calcium circulates as the free ion or as an ion complex. Calcium levels in the blood are regulated mainly by three hormones: active vitamin D (1,25-dihydroxycholecalciferol), calcitonin, and parathyroid hormone (PTH), a hormone released by the parathyroid glands. These glands are embedded in the thyroid gland and are stimulated by falling calcium levels to release PTH. PTH acts on the bone and the kidneys. In the kidneys PTH reduces calcium loss by stimulating its reabsorption. In the bone PTH stimulates calcium release. It also inhibits collagen synthesis by osteoblasts. Osteoblasts, through the synthesis of collagen, provide the organic matrix on which the minerals of the bone are deposited. Osteoclasts, in contrast, are those bone cells responsible for bone resorption. PTH stimulates osteoclast activity indirectly because PTH stimulates renal inorganic phosphate loss. Since phosphate is the counterion of Ca^{2+} in the bone, phosphate loss causes $Ca_5(PO_4)_3OH$ to leach out of the bone and thus raise serum calcium levels. Finally, PTH has one other effect. It stimulates the synthesis of 1,25-dihydroxycholecalciferol which in turn stimulates intestinal calcium uptake. This active form of vitamin D, in turn, enhances the PTH effect on bone calcium mobilization. Thus, PTH has a major role in blood calcium regulation and it has its effects at several different sites.

Counteracting PTH is calcitonin. Calcitonin, a single chain of 32 amino acids, is synthesized by C cells in the thyroid gland. The gene for its synthesis has been localized to chromosome 11 and the expression of this gene is tissue specific. Calcitonin inhibits osteoclast-mediated bone resorption. Calcitonin also inhibits the activation of vitamin D and renal calcium conservation.

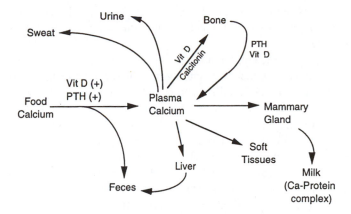

Figure 6 Pathways of calcium use.

Altogether, PTH, vitamin D, and calcitonin regulate blood calcium levels such that there is little variation in normal individuals. Should blood levels fall below the 2.2 to 2.5 mmol/l level, calcium tetany will occur. In newly lactating females this is called "milk fever." It can quickly be reversed with an infusion of a calcium lactate or gluconate. Milk fever develops because of a great demand for calcium by the mammary gland. When the demand exceeds the elasticity of the blood calcium homeostatic system, hypocalcemia results. As mentioned, this can be temporary and reversible with appropriate treatment. Failure to treat can be fatal.

Hypocalcemia due to underactive parathyroid glands or to chronic renal failure, vitamin D deficiency, or hypomagnesemia, is more difficult to manage because the underlying causes are more difficult. Hormone replacement, renal transplant, or correction of blood magnesium levels are the usual strategies followed. With respect to the low blood magnesium, this is one of the consequences of alcoholism. Excess ethanol intake can interfere with the intake and use of magnesium, which in turn results in a loss of responsiveness of osteoclasts to PTH. This interrupts or interferes with the homeostatic mechanisms needed to control blood calcium levels. The pathways of calcium use are illustrated in Figure 6.

E. Function

1. Bone Mineralization

About 99% of the total body calcium is found in the bones and teeth. This calcium is part of a mineral complex that is deposited on an organic matrix comprised primarily of type I collagen. This collagen has a unique amino acid composition consisting of large amounts of glycine, proline, and hydroxyproline. A single molecule of type I collagen has a molecular mass of ~285 kDa, a width of ~14 Å and a length of ~300 Å. There are at least 17 different polypeptides that comprise the collagen molecule. The polypeptides used vary throughout the body and each collagen uses at least three of them. Collagen is about 30 to 33% glycine with another 15 to 30% of the amino acid residues as proline and 3-, 4-, or 5-hydroxyproline. Collagen is a left-handed triple helix stabilized by hydrogen bonding. These bonds may involve bridging water molecules between the hydroxy-prolines. The collagen fibrils are also held together by covalent cross linking. These cross links are between the side chains of lysine and histidine and the linkage is catalyzed by the copper-dependent enzyme, lysyl oxidase. Up to four side chains can be covalently bonded to each other. All in all, the collagen provides a network of fibers upon which the crystals of hydroxyapatite [$Ca_3(PO_4)_3OH$] are deposited. The hydroxyapatite is by no means pure calcium phosphate. Some ions (magnesium, iron, sodium, and chloride) are adsorbed onto the surface of the hydroxyapatite crystallites while other ions (strontium, fluoride, and carbonate) are incorporated into the mineral lattice. The presence of these other ions affects the chemical and physical properties of the calcified tissue. Solubility, for example, is decreased when strontium and fluoride ions are present. Hardness is enhanced by the presence of fluoride.

Bone formation begins in the embryo and continues throughout life. The nature of the process and the cells involved change as the individual ages. Osteoprogenitor cells in early development synthesize the extracellular matrix described above and also regulate the flux of minerals into that matrix. As the calcified tissue begins to form, osteoclasts appear on the surface of this tissue, and osteoblasts connected to one another by long processes are totally surrounded by mineralizing matrix. Each type of mineralized tissue has some unique properties but all share several histologic features in the early mineralization process. Hunziker has described this process in the epiphysial growth plate during the ossification of the endochondral cartilage as it becomes bone.

Initial mineral deposition occurs at discrete sites on membrane-bound bodies (matrix vesicles) in the extracellular matrix. These initial deposits are diffuse and lack orientation. The mineral crystals proliferate and mineralization proceeds filling the longitudinal, but not the transverse, septa. Changes in the activities of enzymes which catalyze the hydrolysis of phosphate esters and those which catalyze certain proteolytic reactions follow or accompany this mineralization. These reactions are a prerequisite to vascular invasion. Following vascular invasion, lamellar bone is formed by osteoblasts directly on the surface of the preexisting mineralized cartilage. These osteoblasts secrete type I collagen with very little proteoglycan and few extracellular matrix vesicles. This process is repeated over and over until the bone has finished growing. At this point the growth plate closes and the mature length and shape of the bone is apparent. The bone, however, is not at all metabolically inert. It continues to lose and gain mineral matter; that is, it is continuously remodeled through the action of the osteoblasts which synthesize the collagen matrix, and the osteoclasts which are stimulated by PTH to reabsorb calcium (and other minerals) in times of need. While the number of osteoblasts declines with age, the number of osteoclasts increases, especially in postmenopausal females. This helps to explain some of the age-related loss in bone mineral that occurs in aging females. Osteoclasts act first during bone remodeling by producing cavities on either the cortical or cancellous (trabecullar) bone surfaces. When these cavities develop osteoblasts are recruited for bone remineralization, thereby filling (or refilling) the cavities. The bone matrix reforms and remineralizes as described above, resulting in new bone formation. The remodeling process is an ongoing one with rates of resorption equaling the rates of new bone formation as long as the hormones controlling each process are in balance and as long as the nutrients needed to support this ongoing process are provided. Figures 7 and 8 illustrate calcium turnover in bone and the influence of hormones on this process.

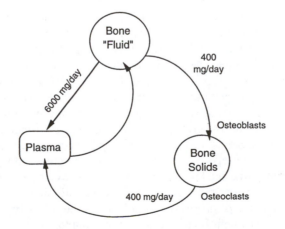

Figure 7 Calcium turnover in bone.

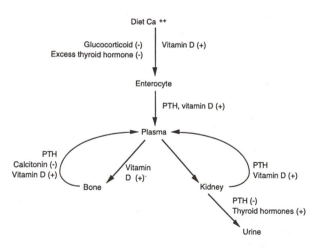

Figure 8   Hormones that influence bone remodeling.

Bone mass can remain constant for many decades. However, once the hormone balance changes this constancy changes. In females, bone mass declines by an estimated 1 to 2% per year after menopause. In senile men, bone mass loss also occurs. In fact, both senile males and females experience about a 1% loss per year. Not only is there a loss in bone mass but there is a loss in structural integrity. The bones lose their mineral apatite and become porous (osteoporosis) and as well lose the architecture upon which the mineral has rested. The very compact cortical portions of the bone disappear, leaving a fragile, largely trabecular bone. The result of these changes is a fragile skeletal system subject to nontrauma-related fracture.

While the importance of appropriate hormone balance (PTH, calcitonin, active vitamin D, and estrogen) can not be overemphasized, it should also be recognized that dietary calcium (as well as phosphorus and other nutrients) plays an important role in the maintenance of bone mass. Intakes at or exceeding 800 mg/day have been shown to counteract the age-related loss in bone mass.

2.   Cell Signaling

Metabolic regulation and the integration of a variety of metabolic pathways and cell systems depend largely on the communications the cells, and the organelles within cells, have within and between each other. Signaling systems exist that orchestrate this communication. An integral part of these signaling systems is the calcium ion. Although less than 1% of the total body calcium store serves this function, its importance can not be overemphasized. The flux of calcium from one compartment to another plays a vital role in metabolic regulation. This flux is facilitated by an intracellular calcium-binding protein called calmodulin. Calmodulin contains four Ca^{2+}-binding sites with affinities in the micromolar range. It is ubiquitous in all eukaryotic cells and mediates many of calcium's effects. Among these are the activation of phosphodiesterase, a component of the cAMP second messenger system and the stimulation of renal Ca^{2+}, Mg^{2+} ATPase. Phosphodiesterase catalyzes the conversion of cAMP to 5′-AMP and requires calcium as a cofactor. Calcium is translocated from its storage site on the endoplasmic reticulum by calmodulin to the interior aspect of the plasma membrane, whereupon it is released to serve as a cofactor for phosphodiesterase. This is illustrated in Figure 9.

A similar mechanism exists for the action of calcium in another cell second messenger system, the phosphatidylinositol system (see Unit 5, Section III for a diagram of this system). In this instance, phospholipase C, a membrane-bound protein, is activated by the binding of an external compound, for example, a hormone, to its cognate receptor. Phospholipase C catalyzes the release of inositol-1,4,5-phosphate from phosphatidylinositol, one of the plasma membrane's phospholipids.

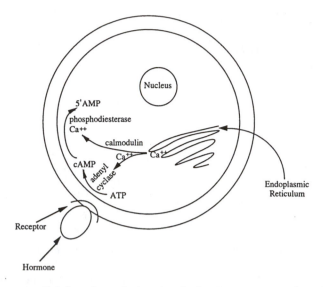

Figure 9 Calmodulin moves Ca^{2+} from the endoplasmic reticulum to serve as a cofactor in reactions catalyzed by phosphodiesterase and adenyl cyclase in the cyclic AMP second messenger system.

Diacylglycerol (DAG) and inositol-1,4,5-phosphate then migrate forward into the cytoplasm. DAG binds to protein kinase C and activates it with the help of the calcium ion. Inositol-1,4,5-phosphate, in the meantime, migrates to the endoplasmic reticulum, stimulating the release of more calcium which in turn further stimulates protein kinase C. Protein kinase C catalyzes the phosphorylation of a variety of proteins. Some of these are enzymes that must be phosphorylated to increase or decrease their metabolic activity whereas others are necessary for secretion processes, i.e., gastric acid release or hormone release, or for substrate uptake such as glucose transport, or for any of a number of energy-driven processes.

Calcium and the cAMP signaling system together with the phosphatidylinositol signaling system have been shown to explain the action of many hormones and cell regulators. Figure 10 illustrates these two systems. Angiotensin, cholecystokinin, acetylcholine, insulin-like growth factors, insulin, and glucagon are but a few hormones whose mode of action involve the calcium ion in one or the other of these signaling systems. There is considerable cross talk between these systems as a result of their mutual need for Ca^{2+}.

In addition to its role in these second messenger systems, Ca^{2+} flux between the cytoplasm and mitochondria regulates mitochondrial activity. Ca^{2+} uptake by mitochondria is energetically less demanding than its export. Uptake followed by active export is an oscillatory process. Ca^{2+} flows in until a 200 μM concentration is reached, whereupon it is actively pumped out using the energy of ATP. This active system costs about 63% of the ATP hydrolysis energy. There are three separate Ca^{2+} transport mechanisms at work (Figure 11). One is the calcium uniporter. The uniporter rapidly sequesters external Ca^{2+} into the mitochondrial matrix and in a similar fashion also sequesters Fe^{2+}, Sr^{2+}, Mn^{2+}, Ba^{2+}, and Pb^{2+}. (Mg^{2+} uptake is much slower than Ca^{2+} and probably is not mediated by this uniporter system.) The other two Ca^{2+} transport mechanisms facilitate Ca^{2+} efflux rather than influx. There is a sodium-independent and a sodium-dependent mechanism. The latter is the more powerful of the two for facilitating Ca^{2+} efflux. Its velocity is much higher than the sodium-independent mechanism. Altogether, these three mechanisms function to control Ca^{2+} flux and hence mitochondrial metabolism, particularly oxidative phosphorylation.

The mitochondrial Ca^{2+} cycle is designed to regulate intramitochondrial Ca^{2+} levels and to relay changes in cytosolic Ca^{2+} to the mitochondrial matrix. Surges in cytosolic Ca^{2+} via the cell signaling systems activate a variety of ATP-requiring reactions. In turn, as ATP is used, its metabolic end

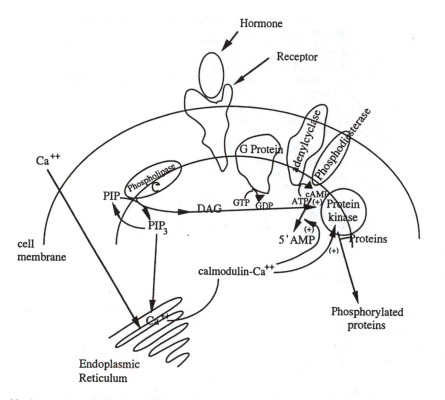

Figure 10 Integration of cAMP and PIP second messenger systems showing the role of Ca²⁺ in both.

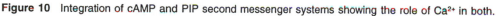

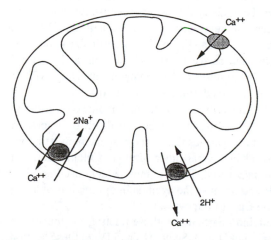

Figure 11 Ca²⁺ flux in the mitochondrial compartment.

product, ADP or AMP, is transported back into the mitochondria whereupon it is rephosphorylated to ATP and exported (along with the Ca^{2+}) to the cytosol. This multifaceted system provides flexibility and responsivity to changing cellular environments and has considerable control strength with respect to the balance of catabolic and anabolic metabolic pathways. In this instance, Ca^{2+} is more than a mere signal, it is a key element in metabolic control. Shown in Table 9 are some of the many reactions or reaction sequences activated by Ca^{2+}.

Table 9   Ca²⁺ as a Metabolic Regulator: Reactions or Reaction Sequences Stimulated by Ca²⁺

Fatty acid oxidation
Amino acid transport into hepatocytes
Citric acid cycle (isocitrate dehydrogenase, α-ketoglutarate dehydrogenase)
Pyruvate dehydrogenase
ATP-Mg/Pi carrier (mitochondrial carrier)
Glucose-stimulated insulin release
Phosphodiesterase
Stimulation of olfactory neurons
Trypsinogen conversion to trypsin
Pancreatic α-amylase activation
Pancreatic phospholipase A₂
Hydrolysis of troponin in muscle to tropomyosin
Phospholipase C
Blood clotting (binding of calcium to GLA-rich proteins)

3. Calcium and Cell Death

Just as Ca^{2+} is important to the regulation of cell metabolism, it has another role: it can mediate the death of a cell or a group of cells. When the integrity of the cell's membrane is breached through injury, sepsis, chemical insults, or anoxia, the normal flux of Ca^{2+} from storage depots to sites of use and return is interrupted. Just as the extracellular Ca^{2+} is carefully regulated so as not to exceed that very narrow range of 2.2 to 2.5 mmol, so too is the intracellular Ca^{2+} concentration. As described above, Ca^{2+} flows into the mitochondria but is actively exported. If the injury to the cell interrupts this active, energy-driven export, the Ca^{2+} will continue to flow into the mitochondria and raise the ionic concentration of the mitochondrial matrix. This has negative effects on oxidative phosphorylation and the stage is set for a downward spiral towards mitochondrial dysfunction. Ca^{2+} influx into the cytosol as well as the nucleus also occurs because it is energetically downward under these conditions. When sufficient calcium accumulates, the cell dies. While the loss of one cell is not devastating, the loss of many cells can be and is. Of particular concern is the accumulation of Ca^{2+} by interconnected muscle such as the heart. Muscle contraction is a Ca^{2+}-mediated event. Ca^{2+} flows into the myocyte mitochondria and is pumped out using ATP. If Ca^{2+} accumulates in the myocyte and is not actively pumped out, the myocyte dies.

Counteracting this Ca^{2+} movement in cells under duress is a class of pharmaceutical agents called calcium blockers. These drugs postpone cell death by interfering with Ca^{2+} influx. Since their discovery, they have been very useful in the management of hypertension and heart disease, and have been found useful in several other settings. Calcium ionophores, agents that facilitate Ca^{2+} flux, have also been discovered. The one most widely used is A23187. Two molecules of this compound surround Ca^{2+} and because the agent is lipophilic it is able to passively cross the plasma membrane and deliver the Ca^{2+} to the cytosol.

Other functions of calcium, particularly those relating to clot formation and embryonic development, have been discussed in Unit 3, Sections I and IV. In these sections, the synthesis of specific proteins that bind calcium and that perform specific roles in the processes of interest are described.

4. Muscle Contraction

The muscle cell has a unique calcium storage site called the sarcoplasmic reticulum. This reticulum is similar to that found in other cell types but is highly specialized. It contains ribosomes and many of the same enzymes found in the endoplasmic reticulum of other cell types but, in addition, also contains large quantities of calcium-activated ATPase. Approximately 75% of the sarcoplasmic reticulum is ATPase. The ATPase also requires magnesium as its name indicates:

$Ca^{2+}Mg^{2+}$ATPase. It serves as a calcium pump using the energy released by ATP to drive the calcium ion from the cytosol to the sarcoplasmic reticulum. There the calcium resides until needed for muscle contraction. Upon receipt of a signal to contract, a Ca^{2+} channel in the sarcoplasmic reticulum is opened and Ca^{2+} flows into the cytoplasm of the muscle cell, whereupon it binds to troponin, a contractile protein of skeletal and cardiac muscle. This protein is a long, rod-like structure that extends over the length of the muscle fiber. When Ca^{2+} binds to it, it changes its shape, becoming shorter. The muscle cell contains two other filaments, actin and myosin, which interact when troponin shortens due to Ca^{2+} binding. When troponin is in the relaxed state these two filaments are too far apart to interact.

Muscles are signaled to contract by a wave of depolarization-repolarization flowing down the muscle fiber from its point of contact at the neuromuscular junction. During depolarization of skeletal muscle, extracellular Na^+ flows into the cell and potentiates the Ca^{2+} release from the sarcoplasmic reticulum. In the heart muscle, with its slightly different muscle fiber organization, the signal for contraction is generated by the AV sinus node on the right side of the heart. This signal is regularly spaced and results in depolarization-repolarization just as happens in skeletal muscle. However, with depolarization Ca^{2+} flows into the cytosol from the extracellular fluid as well as from the sarcoplasmic reticulum. This has the result of increasing the strength of the contraction because more calcium is present. During repolarization Ca^{2+} is then pumped via the $Ca^{2+} Mg^{2+}$ pump back into the sarcoplasmic reticulum. In heart muscle there are many more mitochondria providing ATP than are found in skeletal muscle, hence the need for Ca^{2+} by the heart muscle is greater than that of skeletal muscle.

In contrast to the heart and skeletal muscle, smooth muscle does not contract and relax strongly. These muscles can sustain contraction for a longer period of time and are far less dependent on calcium for contractile strength. Rather, the chief role of calcium in this muscle type is that of serving in the various hormone-mediated cell signaling systems.

F. Deficiency

Considering the vital role of vitamin D and other micronutrients in determining calcium status, it is truly difficult to produce a "pure" calcium-deficient state. Calcium deficiency does occur but it is usually due to other factors: lack of vitamin D activation, loss of estrogen production, adrenal dysfunction, parathyroid gland dysfunction, and so forth. If any of these conditions develop then signs of calcium deficiency do indeed occur. These signs include inadequate bone calcification and growth in children and weak porous bones in adults (osteoporosis). Rickets in children and osteomalacia in adults, characterized by malformed, poorly calcified bones, is more of a disease of inadequate vitamin intake than one of inadequate calcium intake. Should blood calcium levels fall acutely, calcium tetany will result, and unless calcium is provided quickly by the intravenous route, death will ensue.

G. Recommended Dietary Allowance

Because calcium absorption is dependent on so many different factors there has been vigorous discussion among experts as to what the recommended intake of calcium should be. In addition, there are a number of dietary factors (excess protein, calcium:phosphorus ratio, calcium:magnesium ratio, oxalates, and phytates) that increase calcium loss from the system and these are hard to quantitate such that an age-appropriate recommendation can be made. Several diseases stem from or affect calcium use and these must be considered. For example, hypertension has been linked to inadequate dairy calcium intake. Critical experiments that would irrefutably support such a linkage have yet to be conducted, nonetheless there are suggestions arising from population studies that those who consume calcium by way of dairy foods have less hypertension than those who avoid dairy foods. Follow-up studies in hypertensive rats have shown that increasing the dietary calcium reduces the hypertensive state. Calcium supplementation studies of pregnant women have shown

Table 10   Recommended Dietary Allowances for Calcium

Group		Intake (mg/day)
	Birth–6 months	400
	6–12 months	600
	1–3 years	800
	4–6 years	800
	7–10 years	800
Males	11–14	1200
	15–18	1200
	19–24	1200
	25–50	800
	51+	800
Females	11–14	1200
	15–18	1200
	19–24	1200
	25–50	800
	51+	800
Pregnancy	1200	
Lactation	1200	

a significant benefit with respect to a reduction in systolic and diastolic blood pressure and pre-eclampsia. Pregnancy-associated hypertension appears to be ameliorated by such supplementation.

As mentioned above, vitamin D and the estrogen status affect calcium use. Increasing the calcium intake can compensate for a reduction in absorption efficiency and thus the postmenopausal female could benefit. Note that older people have a larger RDA for calcium than young adults. Physical activity is another factor influencing calcium retention. Bedridden individuals tend to lose calcium, whereas the person who maintains a moderately active life style optimizes his/her calcium retention.

On the basis of the information currently available, the NIH Consensus Conference estimated the following optimal intakes for humans:

Birth–6 months, 400 mg/day
6–12 months, 600 mg/day
1–5 years, 800 mg/day
6–10 years, 800 to 1200 mg/day
Adolescents and young adults, 1200 to 1500 mg/day
Females age 25–50, 1000 mg/day
Postmenopausal females on hormone replacement therapy, 1000 mg/day
Postmenopausal females without hormone replacement therapy, 1500 mg/day
Males age 25–65, 1000 mg/day
After age 65, both males and females, 1500 mg/day.

These guidelines were based on calcium in the diet plus that provided by supplements. These recommendations differ from the 1989 RDAs in that for older people the intake recommendation is higher and postmenopausal women are divided into two groups: those having estrogen replacement and those without. Table 10 provides the RDAs of the Food and Nutrition Board, National Academy of Sciences.

VI. PHOSPHORUS

A. Overview, Recommended Dietary Allowance

Calcium and phosphorus are essential minerals that are usually considered together because the formation of bone and the uptake of calcium for this purpose is closely tied to an optimal

Table 11   Recommended Dietary Allowances for Phosphorus

Group		Intake (mg/day)
	Birth–6 months	300
	6–12 months	500
	1–3 years	800
	4–6 years	800
	7–10 years	800
Males	11–14	1200
	15–18	1200
	19–24	1200
	25–50	800
	51+	800
Females	11–14	1200
	15–18	1200
	19–24	1200
	25–50	800
	51+	800
	Pregnancy	1200
	Lactation	1200

calcium:phosphorus ratio of 1:2 to 2:1. However, phosphorus, like calcium, has other functions in addition to bone formation. Since bone formation was discussed in the preceding section concerning calcium, this section will present information about other aspects of the need for phosphorus.

Phosphorus is a member of Group V in the 4th period of the periodic table. It has an atomic number of 15 and an atomic weight of 31. There are no heavy isotopes but there are some useful radioisotopes. ^{32}P is the radioisotope most frequently used in biological systems. It has a short half-life (14.3 days).

Little free phosphorus is found in the living body. Most phosphorus is in the form of phosphate PO_4^{3-}. Phosphate is comprised of a central atom of phosphorus surrounded by four atoms of oxygen. At pH 7, hydrogen is joined to the phosphorus and oxygen to form HPO_4^{2-}. At low pH it is phosphoric acid, H_3PO_4. Other phosphates include H_3PO_4, $H_2PO_4^-$, and PO_4^{3-}. Phosphate in the free form is called inorganic phosphate with the abbreviation Pi. Phosphates are widely distributed in nature and, thus, a deficiency due to inadequate intake is highly unlikely. Soft drinks, processed foods, and foods of animal origin are excellent sources of phosphate. The usual intake of humans consuming a mixed diet is about 1 g/day for females and 1.5 g/day for males. Even though a deficiency is unlikely, a recommended dietary allowance very close to that of calcium is available, as shown in Table 11.

Symptoms of deficiency have been observed in premature infants fed a low-phosphorus milk. These symptoms include anorexia, muscle weakness, rickets, impaired growth, and bone pain. Adults consuming large amounts of aluminum oxide antacids and a low-phosphate diet can also develop some of these same symptoms. Rickets, of course, is only seen in the young. There is a genetic disease related to phosphate deficiency carried on the X chromosome that phenotypes as phosphate deficiency (X-linked hypophosphatemia). It is a dominant trait that is more severe in males than in females since males have only one X chromosome while females have two. The above symptoms can be ameliorated by phosphate supplements, and it is clear from biochemical studies using tissues from these patients that many of their symptoms are due to phosphate-related deficits in intermediary metabolism. The bone pain, poor skeletal growth, and mineralization are due to a lack of phosphate and hence hydroxyapatite for deposition in the bone matrix. Phosphates are readily absorbed with little loss except that which is tightly bound in indigestible portions of food. Phytic acid, a hexose containing six phosphate groups that is a component of some plant foods, can form insoluble salts with calcium, magnesium, and iron, rendering these minerals unavailable for absorption. However, there is a phytase lower in the intestinal tract that will

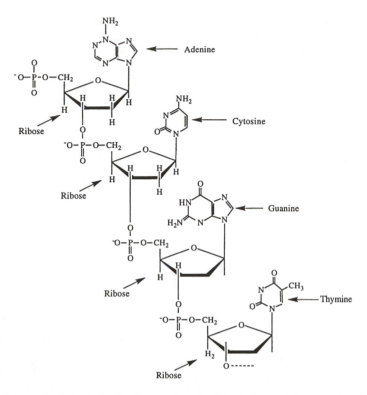

Figure 12 The bases which comprise the DNA polynucleotide chain are joined together by phosphodiester bonds using ribose as the common link between the bases.

dephosphorylate phytic acid, and when this happens these minerals are released. Usually, this happens too far away from their absorption sites to be of benefit.

Phosphorus as phosphate is readily absorbed via an active, saturable, sodium-dependent mechanism. Calcitriol (active vitamin D) facilitates the absorption as it facilitates calcium uptake. Of the total body pool of phosphorus (~750 g), about 600 g is found in the bones and teeth; 1 g is found in the extracellular compartment while the remainder (~150 g) is found within the cells. Excretion is via the urine although up to 25% of the food phosphorus can appear in the feces. Renal conservation of phosphorus is the main mechanism for phosphorus homeostasis. Vitamin D, glucocorticoids, and growth hormone enhance, while estrogen, thyroid hormones, parathyroid hormones, and elevated plasma Ca^{2+} levels inhibit renal phosphate conservation.

B. Function

A principal use for phosphorus is as the anion in hydroxyapatite used in bone mineralization. However, more important is the role of phosphate in intermediary metabolism. It is a crucial part of the genetic material DNA and RNA, of phospholipids, phosphoproteins, the adenine nucleotides (ATP, ADP, AMP), guanine nucleotides (GTP, GDP, GMP), and of the second messenger systems, and it plays a critical role in all anabolic and catabolic pathways. In the genetic material the purine and pyrimidine bases are linked together by deoxyribose or ribose and phosphate groups as shown in Figure 12.

In this structure the phosphate group serves as the links between the bases and because of the polarity of the phosphate group it serves to stabilize the structure. The DNA polymer is a very stable structure under nonenzymatic conditions. It owes its stability to the fact that the phosphate group can bind the bases yet still have sufficient polarity to retain a negative charge, thus repelling other negatively charged molecules such as peroxides. Of course, the phosphate group is not the

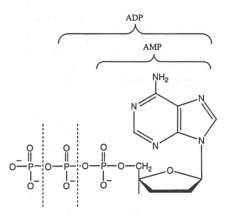

Figure 13 Structure of ATP. AMP has only one phosphate group; ADP has two.

only negatively charged group in the DNA molecule. Hydrogen bonding leaves some atoms vulnerable to attack but, overall, the phosphate group is the important group when nonenzymatic degradation is considered.

The ATP molecule (Figure 13) is another important use of phosphate. The bonds that hold the phosphate groups to the ribose and thence to the adenine are called high-energy bonds represented by the symbol ~. When broken, these bonds release about twice the energy of a normal bond. As such, ATP and its related high-energy compounds GTP and CTP are the keystones of energy transfer from one metabolite to another. A full discussion of ATP synthesis and degradation can be found in Unit 3 in the first volume of this text, *Advanced Nutrition: Macronutrients*.

The phosphorylates of intermediates in both catabolic and anabolic pathways are important uses of phosphate. Again, because of its unique structure it provides a necessary electronegative charge that creates a vulnerable position in the molecule to which it is attached. For example, glucose could not be metabolized to pyruvate unless it was phosphorylated. The glucokinase (or hexokinase) using the high-energy phosphate group from ATP phosphorylates glucose at carbon 6. In so doing the molecule becomes somewhat unstable such that in the next few steps it can be rearranged to form fructose-6-phosphate (a five-member ring).

This structure now has a vulnerable carbon at position 1 and the next step is to attach another phosphate group at this position. With two strong electronegative centers, one at each end of the molecule, this six-carbon structure can be split in half to form two phosphorylated three-carbon structures, and on it goes. The phosphate group is reused over and over and in each use it provides a means for subsequent reactions in metabolism, only to be discarded by the resultant metabolic product. Its highly charged structure thus is its reason for use and reuse.

Use and reuse also applies to the role of phosphate in the structure and function of the membrane phospholipids. Phospholipids have both a lipophilic and a lipophobic portion in their structure. The lipophilic portion (see Figure 14) is the fatty acid portion while the phosphatidylated compounds provide the lipophobic (or hydrophilic) portion. This structure is absolutely required for the functional attributes of the phospholipids that are part of the lipid-carrying blood proteins and that are

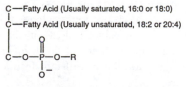

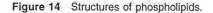

R = choline, ethanolamine, inositol, serine

Figure 14 Structures of phospholipids.

important components of the membranes. The membranes (see *Advanced Nutrition: Macronutrients,* Unit 6) serve as geographical barriers around the cells and organelles. As such, some materials are refused entry into the cell or organelle while other materials are either embedded in these phospholipids and held there or are allowed to pass into or out of the cell or organelle. Lipid-soluble materials can diffuse through the lipophilic portion of the phospholipid while lipophobic materials are excluded unless carried through by one of the embedded proteins. The charge contributed by the phosphate group in the phospholipid is what holds the proteins in place and allows it to permit entry or exit of lipophobic metabolites and substrates. It should be noted, however, that highly charged metabolites such as the phosphorylated intermediates do not cross membranes. They are repelled by the phosphate group of the phospholipids.

From the above discussion of the function of phosphorus in living systems it is easy to understand why phosphorus is so widely distributed in the food supply. Every living thing must have phosphorus in its cells or it would not survive. It is as essential to life as oxygen, carbon, and nitrogen.

VII. MAGNESIUM

A. Overview

Magnesium is an alkaline earth metal with an atomic number of 12 and an atomic weight of 24. It is in Group II of the 3rd period of the periodic table. Magnesium has two naturally occurring isotopes, Mg^{25} and Mg^{26}, and seven radioisotopes. Mg^{28} is the most commonly used radioisotope with a half-life of 21 hr.

Magnesium is a very abundant divalent cation in living systems. As such its distribution in the food supply is broad. Both vegetables and meats are good sources of magnesium while milk and milk products are relatively poor sources of this mineral. Magnesium stabilizes mammalian membranes and in plants this mineral is ionically bound in the center of the chlorophyll molecule. In addition, magnesium is a cofactor in almost all phosphorylation reactions involving ATP. Because of the universality of its presence in the food supply, deficiency states are unlikely to develop in persons consuming a variety of foods.

B. Absorption, Metabolism, Excretion

Magnesium is absorbed by both passive diffusion and active transport. While there are two systems for Mg^{2+} uptake, neither is particularly efficient. Between 30 and 70% of that consumed in food is absorbed. When food is supplemented with Mg^{2+} the percent absorbed falls. Thus, a meal containing 40 mg in food will result in 28 mg actually entering the enterocyte and appearing in the blood, whereas in an enriched Mg^{2+}-containing meal (40 mg + 920 mg magnesium salt) only 11 to 14% will be absorbed, or 105 to 134 mg. The usual 300 mg Mg^{2+} intake has an apparent absorption of about 100 mg, a 33% efficiency.

Magnesium is recirculated via biliary secretion into the intestinal contents. The recirculated mineral can be reabsorbed and in times of need this reabsorption can be very efficient. If not reabsorbed this magnesium will be excreted via the feces. The usual excretory route for absorbed magnesium is via urine. In fact, the renal absorption mechanism is the main means for regulating magnesium status. About 100 mg of magnesium is lost via the urine per day by normal adults consuming about 300 mg/day in the food. In times of need, magnesium reabsorption by the renal tubules will occur and urinary magnesium levels will fall. In the deficient state the level will fall to zero as the deficiency proceeds.

After magnesium is absorbed, it circulates throughout the body; about 30 to 35% of the circulating magnesium is protein bound while the remaining circulates as magnesium salts (13% as citrate or

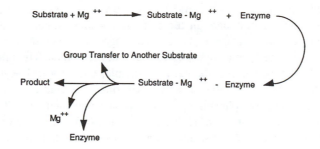

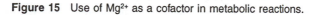

Figure 15   Use of Mg^{2+} as a cofactor in metabolic reactions.

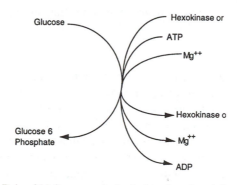

Figure 16   Role of Mg^{2+} as a cofactor in the phosphorylation of glucose.

phosphate complexes) or as free magnesium (~55%). Magnesium is principally an intracellular ion occupying a central role in intermediary metabolism, as described in the next section.

C. Function

More than 300 metabolic reactions require magnesium as a cofactor. The role of magnesium is one of forming a labile association with a substrate, allowing the enzyme to complex with it, and then once a product is formed, the product, the magnesium, and the enzyme separate for further use. This is illustrated in Figure 15.

Mg^{2+} reduces the high negative charge of the substrate (usually ATP) by chelate formation with two phosphate groups (the β and γ P). The adenine ring is not involved. Actually, the above reaction sequence occurs concurrent with the transfer of the liberated phosphate group to another substrate such as glucose. This coupled reaction sequence is facilitated by the enzymes hexokinase or glucokinase. Any kinase, however, will use this same reaction sequence, as will a number of other reactions involving cleavage of a high-energy bond and the use of that energy to activate via attachment of a reactive electronegative group to a formerly inactive metabolic substrate or intermediate. An example of this is shown in Figure 16 which illustrates the role of Mg^{2+} in the phosphorylation of glucose. Some coupled reactions use more than one Mg^{2+}. Enolase, for example, uses four Mg^{2+}. The Mg^{2+} ion binds to enolase and activates it by keeping it in its active conformation. Magnesium is probably binding to the sulfur group of sulfur-containing amino acids, thus favoring the reaction by polarizing the P-O bonds. Conformational change likely explains the Mg^{2+} in many of the enzymes in which it is a required cofactor for activation. In contrast, Mg^{2+} can be an inhibitor; it can bind with tyrosyl residues. If these residues are part of the active site of an enzyme then the enzyme will be less active. Actually, the binding of Mg^{2+} to the tyrosyl residue of albumin accounts for its transport in the blood. Much (32%) of the magnesium in the blood is carried by albumin.

Phospholipids form complexes with both Mg^{2+} and Ca^{2+}. These phospholipid complexes are integral parts of the various membranes in the cell (plasma membrane, endoplasmic reticulum, mitochondrial membrane, and nuclear membrane). The degree to which these minerals are held by the membrane depends on the type of phospholipid in that membrane. The phospholipids are not uniformly distributed. The plasma membrane, for example, has very little cardiolipin, while the mitochondrial membrane has very little phosphatidylserine (see Unit 6 in *Advanced Nutrition: Macronutrients*). Highly negative phospholipids will attract and bind more Ca^{2+} and Mg^{2+} than phospholipids having a lesser charge. In addition, Ca^{2+}, due to its stronger charge, will be more attracted than will Mg^{2+}. Nonetheless, the attraction of these minerals lends a stabilizing effect to an otherwise labile and mobile membrane constituent.

Bone accounts for 60 to 65% of the total magnesium in the body. It is deposited in the bone matrix along with calcium phosphate as part of the mineral apatite. Hormones which affect calcium deposition and mobilization also affect magnesium deposition and mobilization.

D. Deficiency

Deficiency states have been produced in animals under stringent magnesium exclusion conditions. As early as 1926 mice were shown to develop magnesium deficiency by use of a magnesium-deficient diet. Cattle, and later, rats, were also made deficient. The first clinical evidence in humans appeared in 1934 and subsequent studies have shown that persons experiencing prolonged malabsorption, renal dysfunction or failure, alcoholism, and a number of endocrine disorders, can become magnesium deficient. This deficiency is characterized by very low blood levels of magnesium and neuromuscular symptoms such as muscle spasms, twitching, muscle fasciculations, tremor, personality changes, anorexia, nausea, and vomiting. Acutely deficient individuals may have convulsions and lapse into coma. In almost every instance of clinically evident magnesium deficiency there has been a clinically important predisposing condition as cited above. Marginally deficient states have also been suggested in patients with normal serum or blood levels but depleted tissue levels of magnesium. In these patients the symptoms are varied and it may be difficult to assign magnesium deficiency as their cause unless tissue samples (muscle) are obtained and assayed. A positive magnesium balance of 1 meq/kg can be demonstrated in such individuals. Persons at risk are those with renal disease or malabsorption syndrome which, in turn, reduces magnesium conservation in the former and decreases magnesium absorption in the latter. Chronic ulcerative colitis and chronic granulomatous enteritis are the most common causes of the diarrhea of the malabsorption syndrome. Other causes are gluten-induced enteropathy, celiac disease, and unrecognized lactose intolerance. Frequently, magnesium deficiency is accompanied by hypocalcemia. This appears to be due to a failure of bone to exchange calcium for magnesium. The osteoclast receptor for PTH loses its responsiveness to this hormone with the resultant loss in active bone resorption. This means that there is a failure in the system used to maintain blood calcium levels and also that magnesium is a key feature in the PTH-calcium regulatory pathway. Once magnesium is restored, the sensitivity of the osteoclast receptor to PTH is reinstated and the serum calcium returns to normal levels.

Magnesium deficiency also has effects on the vitamin D-calcium relationship. Active 1,25-dihydroxycholecalciferol is not as active in promoting intestinal calcium uptake in the absence of magnesium. Even though neither ion is absorbed very efficiently, this efficiency is further reduced when one or the other is absent or in short supply. Both are poorly absorbed in vitamin D-deficient states because vitamin D mediates the uptake of both.

The use of mercurial or thiazide diuretics in the management of hypertension can result in excess magnesium loss. These diuretics interfere with renal magnesium conservation. They also enhance potassium loss as do some other drugs, e.g., furosemide, ethacrynic acid, goutamicin, cabenicillin, cisplatin, and amphotericin B. Many of these are cytotoxic drugs used in cancer

Table 12   Recommended Dietary Allowances for Magnesium

Age Group		Magnesium (mg/day)
	Birth–6 months	40
	7–12 months	60
	1–3 years	80
	4–6 years	120
	7–10 years	170
Males	11–14 years	270
	15–18 years	400
	19–24 years	350
	25–50 years	350
	51+ years	350
Females	11–14 years	280
	15–18 years	300
	19–24 years	280
	25–50 years	280
	51+ years	280
Pregnancy		320
Lactation	1st 6 months	355
	7–12 months	340

chemotherapy and, as such, are used over a short time span. While minerals are lost through the use of these drugs, they can be replaced from the body store or through supplementation. Many physicians using these therapies may elect to supplement the patient's diet after the chemotherapeutic regimen is complete, anticipating that the cancer cell also needs magnesium. Chemotherapy consists of using highly toxic materials, anticipating that the fast-growing cancer cell will be more likely to take up the drug and die than will the normal cell. Part of the drug action is to interfere with cell replication which, in turn, requires magnesium. If the cancer cell becomes magnesium deficient then the drug will be a more effective chemotoxic agent.

Magnesium deficiency in rats has been shown to result in elevated blood lipids as well as in proliferation of smooth muscle cells. These responses are key elements in the atherogenic process and it has been proposed that a relative magnesium deficiency in humans could pave the way for atherosclerosis or other degenerative diseases. However, other studies of alcoholism, renal disease, and various endocrinopathies have shown that these conditions must be in place prior to the development of magnesium deficiency. Thus, atherosclerosis could occur as a secondary complication of alcoholism or renal disease or diabetes, etc. and this secondary complication might develop as a result of an induced magnesium deficiency.

E. Recommended Dietary Allowance

As mentioned, magnesium is widely distributed in the food supply and thus a deficiency in an individual having access to a variety of foods is unlikely. Nonetheless, the Food and Nutrition Board of the National Academy of Sciences has recommended intakes based on age and gender of 40 to 400 mg/day, as detailed in Table 12. As mentioned in Section D, above, certain predisposing diseases may affect either magnesium absorption or reabsorption by the kidney. In these circumstances magnesium status may be negatively affected and an intake above that recommended as desirable may be needed. Assessment of that need, however, is imperative before an increased intake is undertaken. Excess intake can be toxic, with symptoms similar to those of uremia (nausea, vomiting, hypotension). Other responses to excess intake include changes in heart action (bradycardia, vasodilation) and CNS function.

SUPPLEMENTAL READINGS

Sodium

Austic, R.E. and Calvert, C.C. 1981. Nutritional interrelationships of electrolytes and amino acids, *Fed. Proc.,* 40:63-67.

Esther, C.R., Howard, T.E., Marino, E.M., Goddard, J.M., Capecchi, M.R., and Bernstein, K.E. 1996. Mice lacking angiotensin-converting enzyme have low blood pressure, renal pathology and reduced male fertility, *Lab. Invest.,* 74:953-965.

Feron, O., Salomone, S., and Godfraind, T. 1995. Influence of salt loading on the cardiac and renal preproendothelin-1 mRNA expression in stroke-prone spontaneously hypertensive rats, *Biochem. Biophys. Res. Commun.,* 209:161-166.

Holland, O.B. and Carr, B. 1993. Modulation of aldosterone synthase mRNA levels by dietary sodium and potassium and by adrenocorticotropin, *Endocrinology,* 132:2666-2673.

Kirby, R.F., Page, W.V., Johnson, A.K., and Robillard, J.E. 1996. Dietary sodium effects on renin and angiotensinogen gene expression in preweanling WKY and SHR Rats, *Am. J. Physiol.,* 27:R1439-R1446.

Pressley, T.A. 1996. Structure and function of the Na$^+$ K$^+$ pump: ten years of molecular biology, *Miner. Electrolyte Metab.,* 22:264-271.

Potassium

Bieri, J.G. 1977. Potassium requirement of the growing rat, *J. Nutr.,* 107:1394-1398.

Dow, S.W., Fettman, M.J., Smith, K.R., Hamar, D.W., Nagode, L.A., Refsal, K.R., and Wlke, W.L. 1990. The effects of dietary acidification and potassium depletion on acid-base balance, mineral metabolism and renal function in adult cats, *J. Nutr.,* 120:569-578.

Mann, M.D., Bowie, M.D., and Hansen, J.D.L. 1975. Total body potassium, acid-base status and serum electrolytes in acute diarrhoeal disease, *S. Afr. Med. J.,* 49:709-711.

Chloride

Simopoulos, A.P. and Bartter, F.C. 1980. The metabolic consequences of chloride deficiency, *Nutr. Rev.,* 38:201-205.

Kays, S.M., Greger, J.L., Marcus, M.S.K., and Lewis, N.M. 1991. Blood pressure, fluid compartments and utilization of chloride in rats fed various chloride diets, *J. Nutr.,* 121:330-337.

Calcium

Anon. 1994. Optimal calcium intake. NIH Consensus Statement, National Institutes of Health, Washington, D.C., 12:1-31.

Allen, L.H. 1982. Calcium bioavailability and absorption: a review, *Am. J. Clin. Nutr.,* 35:783-808.

Anderson, J.B. 1991. Nutritional biochemistry of calcium and phosphorus, *J. Nutr. Biochem.,* 2:300-307.

Ayachi, S. 1979. Increased dietary calcium lowers blood pressure in the spontaneously hypertensive rat, *Metabolism,* 28:1234-1238.

Broess, M., Riva, A., and Gerstenfeld, L.C. 1995. Inhibitory effects of 1,25(OH)$_2$ vitamin D$_3$ on collagen type 1, osteopontin, and osteocalcin gene expression in chicken osteoblasts, *J. Cell. Biochem.,* 57:440-451.

Bronner, F. 1984. Role of intestinal calcium absorption in plasma calcium regulation of the rat, *Am. J. Physiol.,* 246:R680-683.

Bronner, F. 1994. Calcium and osteoporosis, *Am. J. Clin. Nutr.,* 60: 831-836.

Bronner, F. and Peterlik, M. (Eds.) 1995. Proc. Int. Conf. Progress in Bone and Mineral Research, *J. Nutr.,* Suppl. 125:1963S-2037S.

Bucher, H.C., Guyatt, G.H., Cook, R.J., Hatala, R., Cook, D.J., Lang, J.D., and Hunt, D. 1996. Effect of calcium supplementation on pregnancy-induced hypertension and preeclampsia. A meta analysis of randomized controlled trials, *J. Am. Med. Assoc.,* 275:1113-1117.

Bygrave, F.L. and Benedetti, A. 1993. Calcium: its modulation in liver by cross-talk between the actions of glucagon and calcium mobilizing agonists, *Biochem. J.,* 296:1-14.

Bygrave, F.L. and Roberts, H.R. 1995. Regulation of cellular calcium through signaling cross-talk in intricate interplay between the actions of receptors g-proteins and second messengers, *FASEB J.,* 9:1297-1303.

DeGrazia, J.A., Ivanovich, P., Fellows, H., and Rich, C. 1965. A double isotope method for measurement of intestinal absorption of calcium in man, *J. Lab. Clin. Med.,* 66:82-829.

Duflos, C., Bellaton, C., Baghdassarian, N., Gadoux, M., Pansu, D., and Bronner, F. 1996. 1,25 Dihydroxy-cholecalciferol regulates rat intestinal calbindin D_{9k} posttranscriptionally, *J. Nutr.,* 126:834-841.

Farber, J.L. 1981. The role of calcium in cell death, *Life Sci.,* 29:1289-1295.

Foletti, D., Guerini, D., and Carafoli, E. 1995. Subcellular targeting of the endoplasmic reticulum and plasma membrane. Ca^{2+} pumps: a study using recombinant chimeras, *FASEB J.,* 9:670-680.

Fujita, T. 1992. Vitamin D in the treatment of osteoporosis, *Proc. Soc. Exp. Biol. Med.,* 199:394-399.

Garlid, K.D. 1994. Mitochondrial cation transport: a progress report, *J. Bioenerg. Biomembr.,* 26:537-542.

Grauer, A., Ziegler, R., and Raue, F. 1995. Clinical significance of antibodies against calcitonin, *Endocrinol. Diabetes,* 63:345-351.

Gunter, K.K. and Gunter, T.E. 1994. Transport of calcium by mitochondria, *Am. J. Physiol.,* 267:C313-C339.

Hamet, P. 1995. Evaluation of the scientific evidence for a relationship between calcium and hypertension, *J. Nutr.,* Suppl. 125:311S-400S.

Hiraoka, Y., Segawa, T., Kuwajima, K., Sugai, S., and Murai, N. 1980. α Lactalbumin: calcium metalloprotein, *B.B.R.C.,* 95:1098-1104.

Hope, W.G., Bruns, M.E.H., and Thomas, M.L. 1992. Regulation of duodenal insulin-like growth factor 1 and active calcium transport by ovariectomy in female rats, *Proc. Soc. Exp. Biol. Med.,* 200:528-535.

Hope, W.G., Ibarra, M.J., and Thomas, M.L. 1992. Testosterone alters duodenal calcium transport and longitudinal bone growth rate in parallel in the male rat, *Proc. Soc. Exp. Biol. Med.,* 200:536-541.

Hunziker, E.B., Herrmann, K.W., Schenk, R.K., Mueller, M., and Moor, H. 1984. Cartilage ultrastructure after high pressure freezing, freeze substitution and low temperature embedding. 1. Chondrocyte ultrastructure-implications for the theories of mineralization and vascular invasion, *J. Cell. Biol.,* 98:267-276.

Jaros, G.G., Belonje, P.C., van Hoorn-Hickman, R., and Newman, E. 1984. Transient response of the calcium homeostatic system: effect of calcitonin, *Am. J. Physiol.,* 246:R693-697.

Koo, J.O., Weaver, C.M., Neylan, M.J., and Miller, G.D. 1993. Isotopic tracer techniques for assessing calcium absorption in rats, *J. Nutr. Biochem.,* 4:72-76.

Sneyd, J., Keizer, J., and Sanderson, M.J. 1995. Mechanisms of calcium oscillations and waves: a quantitative analysis, *FASEB J.,* 9:1463-1472.

Trump, B.F. and Berezesky, I.K. 1995. Calcium mediated cell injury and cell death, *FASEB J.,* 9:219-228.

Walker, B.E. and Schedl, H.P. 1979. Small intestinal calcium absorption in the rat with experimental diabetes, *Proc. Soc. Exp. Biol. Med.,* 161:149-152.

Wang, Y.-Z. and Christakos, S. 1995. Retinoic acid regulates the expression of the calcium binding protein, calbindin D_{28k}, *Mol. Endocrinol.,* 9:1510-1521.

Wasserman, R.H. 1981. Intestinal absorption of calcium and phosphorus, *Fed. Proc.,* 40:68-72.

Weaver, C.M. 1994. Age related calcium requirements due to changes in absorption and utilization, *J. Nutr.,* 124: 1418S-1425S.

Wimalawansa, S.J. 1996. Calcitonin gene-related peptide and its receptors: molecular genetics, physiology, pathophysiology and therapeutic potentials, *Endocrinol. Rev.,* 17:533-585.

Phosphorus

Berner, Y.N. and Shike, M. 1988. Consequences of phosphate imbalance, *Annu. Rev. Nutr.,* 8:121-148.

Knochel, J.P. 1977. Pathophysiology and clinical characteristics of severe hypophosphatemia, *Arch. Intern. Med.,* 137:203-220.

Westheimer, F.H. 1987. Why nature chose phosphates, *Science,* 235:1173-1178.

Whyte, M.P., Schranck, F.W., and Armamento-Villareal, R. 1996. X-linked hypophosphatomia: a search for gender, race, anticipation, or parent of origin effects on disease expression in children, *J. Clin. Endocrinol. Metab.,* 81:4075-4080.

Magnesium

Bussiere, L., Mazur, A., Gueux, E., and Rayssigiuer, Y. 1994. Hypertriglyceridemic serum from magnesium deficient rats induces proliferation and lipid accumulation in cultural vascular smooth muscle cells, *J. Nutr. Biochem.*, 5:585-590.

Corica, F., Ientile, R., Allegra, A., Romano, G., Cangemi, F., DiBenedetto, A., Buemi, M., Cucinotta, D., and Ceruso, D. 1996. Magnesium levels in plasma, erythrocyte, and platelets in hypertensive and normotensive patients with type II diabetes mellitus, *Biol. Trace Element Res.*, 51:13-21.

Flink, E.B. 1981. Magnesium deficiency. Etiology and clinical spectrum, *Acta Med. Scand.*, Suppl. 647:125-137.

Forbes, R.M. and Parker, H.M. 1980. Effect of magnesium deficiency on rat bone and kidney sensitivity to parathyroid hormone, *J. Nutr.*, 110:1610-1617.

Rayssiguier, Y. 1981. Magnesium and lipid interrelationships in the pathogenesis of vascular diseases, *Magnesium Bull.*, 12:165-177.

Rivlin, R.S. 1994. Magnesium deficiency and alcohol intake: mechanisms, clinical significance and possible relation to cancer development, *J. Am. Coll. Nutr.*, 13:416-423.

Robeson, B.L., Martin, W.G., and Freedman, M.H. 1980. A biochemical and ultrastructural study of skeletal muscle from rats fed a magnesium deficient diet, *J. Nutr.*, 110:2078-2084.

UNIT **8**

Trace Minerals

TABLE OF CONTENTS

I. OVERVIEW

In addition to the minerals already described as members of the macromineral class of nutrients, there are two groups of minerals needed in far smaller amounts. These groups fall into the general class of microminerals. One of these is the trace mineral group that includes iron, copper, and zinc, while the other group, the ultratrace minerals, includes chromium, manganese, fluoride, iodide, cobalt, selenium, silicon, arsenic, boron, vanadium, nickel, cadmium, lithium, lead, and molybdenum. Of these minerals, only four, iron, zinc, iodide, and selenium, have been studied sufficiently to provide a database upon which a recommended dietary allowance (RDA) has been made. Table 1 gives the RDAs for these elements.

Table 1   Recommended Dietary Allowances (RDA) for Iron, Zinc, Iodide, and Selenium

Group	Age	RDA			
		Iron (mg)	Zinc (mg)	Iodide (mg)	Selenium (μg)
Infants	0–6 months	6	5	40	10
	7–12 months	10	5	50	15
Children	1–3 years	10	10	70	20
	4–7 years	10	10	90	20
	8–11 years	10	10	120	30
Males	12–14 years	12	15	150	40
	15–18 years	12	15	150	50
	19–24 years	10	15	150	70
	25–50 years	10	15	150	70
	51+ years	10	15	150	70
Females	12–14 years	15	12	150	45
	15–18 years	15	12	150	50
	19–24 years	15	12	150	55
	25–50 years	15	12	150	55
	51+ years	10	12	150	55
Pregnancy		30	15	175	65
Lactation	0–6 months	15	19	200	75
	7–12 months	15	16	200	75

Table 2   Safe and Adequate Intakes
for Selected Minerals

Mineral	Intake
Copper (Cu)	1.5–3.0 mg/day
Fluoride (F)	1.4–4.0 mg/day
Manganese (Mn)	2.0–5.0 mg/day
Chromium (Cr)	50–200 µg/day
Molybdenum (Mo)	75–250 µg/day

For some of the elements listed above we have an intake recommendation that is "generally recognized as safe and adequate" — abbreviated GRSA. GRSA recommendations (Table 2) have been made for copper, fluoride, manganese, chromium, and molybdenum. While cobalt is known to be needed for microbial synthesis of vitamin B_{12}, an essential micronutrient (see Unit 4, Section IX), an intake recommendation for this mineral has not been made. No intake recommendations have been made for the remaining minerals and it should be acknowledged that many of these are toxic when large exposures occur. Table 3 summarizes these minerals, some of which will be discussed in detail later in this chapter.

Almost all of the trace and ultratrace minerals can be found in the bones and teeth. These minerals are deposited in the organic matrix of these structures as is calcium phosphate. Mineralization is not solely a macromineral event, but one which also involves the other 18 minerals known to be consumed by humans and other animals. These minerals are present in far lower amounts, but nonetheless they comprise part of the mineral apatite that characterizes the skeletal system. These minerals can be mobilized from the bones but the extent of this mobilization is variable. To a large degree, the mobilization of the trace elements is very slow indeed. This results in a long residence time and long half-life. When coupled with a low absorption efficiency, this could be regarded as part of a system designed to protect the body from excess mineral exposure, i.e., mineral toxicity. For many of the trace elements, their discovery as essential nutrients was preceded by their recognition as toxic elements.

II. TOXICITY OF MICROMINERALS

Inadvertent exposure to a variety of minerals, whether it be via inhalation, absorption through the skin, or ingestion with food or drink, can elicit a toxic response. The first line of defense is offered by the gastrointestinal system: vomiting and diarrhea. Through vomiting, contaminated food is expelled. Through diarrhea, malabsorption as well as excretion of a recirculated (via bile) mineral is facilitated, reducing the intestinal exposure and subsequent uptake of the mineral. Failing to ablate the toxic state, the kidney tubules will attempt to reduce the body load; however, some minerals, e.g., copper, iron, zinc, and lead, are not as subject to renal filtration as are other minerals such as magnesium, calcium, molybdenum, etc. Reduction of the body load that is in circulation then is accomplished by depositing the excess mineral in the bones. Bone mineral content has been used to document cases of suspected toxicity. Accidental or intentional poisoning can sometimes be masked by other nonspecific symptoms, but bone analysis can provide the documentation needed to support or deny a supposition of toxicity.

To a lesser extent, hair analysis together with blood analysis can reveal the mineral status of an individual. The difficulty in using these analyses is that the mineral content can be transient. That is, blood levels of trace minerals represent the immediate mineral intake rather than long-term exposure, whereas hair mineral content can represent not only food or drink mineral but also airborne mineral. Hair mineral can be contaminated by shampoos and other hair treatments.

The adverse effects of trace minerals are as diverse as the minerals themselves. Each mineral has its preferred target in the body. For some, the target is DNA. Certain minerals (copper, arsenic,

Table 3   Trace Elements and Their Key Features

Micromineral	Function	Remarks
Trace Minerals		
Copper	Essential cofactor for a variety of enzymes involved in iron use, collagen synthesis, energy metabolism, and antioxidants.	Wilson's disease and Menckes disease are genetic disorders characterized by disturbed copper homeostasis.
Iron	Essential for hemoglobin synthesis, cytochrome activity, urea cycle activity, lipogenesis, and cholesterogenesis.	Hemochromatosis results from excess intake. Anemia is the major sign of inadequate intake.
Zinc[a]	Essential to the function of over 70 enzymes; important component of DNA binding proteins.	Poor growth in children with renal disease due to excess zinc loss during dialysis. Deficiency may occur with use of diuretics. Zinc loss is increased in traumatized patients.
Ultratrace Minerals		
Arsenic	Needed for growth and optimal iron use.	Toxic; well-known metabolic poison.
Chromium	Needed for optimal action of insulin at target tissue.	Widely dispersed in a variety of foods. Brewer's yeast and beer are good sources. Deficiency is unlikely.
Cobalt	Important component of vitamin B_{12}.	Deficiency symptoms are those of B_{12} deficiency.
Fluorine	Increases the hardness of bones and teeth, activates adenylate cyclase.	Fluorosis (mottling of teeth) results from excess intake.
Iodine[a]	Needed for thyroid hormone synthesis.	Goiter and cretinism result from inadequate intake.
Manganese	Cofactor in a wide variety of enzymes; essential to reactions using ATP or UTP.	Widely distributed throughout the body. Deficiency is unlikely.
Molybdenum	Activates adenylate cyclase; cofactor in sulfite oxidase and xanthine oxidase.	Widely distributed in the food supply. Deficiency is unlikely.
Nickel	The need for this element has not been shown for humans.	Widely distributed in the food supply. Deficiency is unlikely.
Selenium[a]	Essential to glutathione peroxidase and thyroxine deiodinase.	Toxicity and need are influenced by environmental factors.
Silicon	The need for this element has not been shown for humans but has been shown for animals.	Widely distributed in the food supply. Deficiency is unlikely.
Vanadium	The need for this element has not been shown for humans but has been shown for animals.	Widely distributed in the food supply. Deficiency is unlikely.

[a] An RDA has been set for this mineral (see Table 1).

nickel, chromium) bind to DNA in a cross-link fashion. The binding is a covalent one and produces either a nonfunctional DNA or a DNA which can not repair itself. Evidence of this cross-linking has been demonstrated *in vitro* using a variety of cell types. Chinese hamster cells were used to show copper-induced, chromium-induced, and nickel-induced DNA cross-linking, while human fibroblasts and epithelial cells have been used to show arsenic-induced cross-linking.

The concept of chemically induced cross-linkage of DNA as a factor in carcinogenesis has been proposed to explain the role of asbestos and the development of mesothelioma. Mesothelioma is a malignant growth of the pleural and peritoneal cavities. These tumors are stimulated to grow by the presence of asbestos fibers which act as artificial linkers of DNA, resulting in mutations within the pleural and peritoneal cells. Changes in the CDKN2 (p16) gene seem to be involved. This gene is either lost or mutated. Its gene product is a regulator of the phosphorylation of protein 105, a tumor suppressor. Unphosphorylated p105 can inhibit passage from the G1 to the S phase of the cell cycle whereas phosphorylated 105 permits this passage. Passage inhibition is a common feature of cancer cell initiation. Thus, any substance that interferes with this passage could be regarded as a carcinogen. Minerals in excess can have this effect and excess intakes of some have been linked

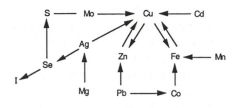

Figure 1 Trace mineral interactions.

with certain forms of cancer. Iron for example has been linked to colon cancer. The mechanism whereby excess iron has its effect is far from clear. It may induce DNA cross-linking as described above, but it may also act as an ion that stimulates free radical formation and attacks cells and their DNA, causing them to mutate. In either scenario, excess iron and colon cancer are associated.

III. ANTAGONISMS AND INTERACTIONS AMONG TRACE MINERALS

No general discussion of trace minerals would be complete without mention of mineral interactions. Numerous antagonisms and synergisms have been reported. This should be expected as one realizes that many of the trace minerals have more than one charged state and that living cells have preferences with respect to these states. For example, the uptake of iron is much greater when the iron is in the ferrous (2+) state than when in the ferric (3+) state. Minerals that keep iron in the ferric state will interfere with its absorption and use. Minerals that do the reverse will enhance iron uptake. Such is the beneficial action of copper on iron. The copper ion (Cu^{2+}) keeps the ferrous ion from losing electrons and becoming the ferric ion. The interactions of essential minerals are best illustrated in Figure 1. To the nutrition scientist seeking to design a purified diet providing all the known nutrients in needed amounts, these mineral interactions can be quite a problem. Sometimes, the so-called purified ingredients contain (or fail to contain) minerals unknown to the producer or user. This is especially a problem in the protein portion of the diet. Proteins can bind minerals (as described in the sections on each of the minerals) and these minerals can be found in the proteins. Soybean protein can contain phytate-bound phosphorus and magnesium; casein and lactalbumin, depending on origin, contain variable amounts of calcium, magnesium, and selenium. Unless the investigator determines the mineral content of the diet ingredients there is the possibility that an unexpected mineral imbalance could occur which could affect the outcome of the experiment. The specifics of these imbalances and interactions will be detailed as each of the minerals is discussed.

IV. IRON

A. Overview

Iron, element 26 in the periodic table, is the fourth most prevalent mineral in the earth's crust. It has an atomic weight of 56. Neolithic man learned to mine iron and to forge tools from iron. The Romans used iron preparations as tonics but the clinical recognition of iron as an essential nutrient was not accomplished until the seventeenth century. Sydenham was the first to propose that chlorosis (a sickness in adolescent females, characterized by a pale skin color) was due to iron deficiency anemia. He showed that iron salts were an effective treatment.

In 1713, Remmery and Jeffrey demonstrated the presence of iron in the mineral matter of blood and in 1852 Funke showed that this mineral was contained by the red cell. Thus, it was learned that iron and the number of red cells were related and that the red cell's function of carrying oxygen depended on its hemoglobin content.

Iron is present in a variety of inorganic salts in the environment. It exists mainly in a trivalent form as ferric oxide or hydroxide or its polymers. Absorption of these salts is very limited unless they can be solubilized and ionized by the intestinal contents. Both ferric and ferrous salts are present in the diet but only the ferrous salts are absorbed from the gastrointestinal tract. Ferric compounds must be reduced in the gastric juice in order to be absorbed.

The availability of iron from food depends on its source. Soybean protein, for example, contains an inhibitor of iron uptake. Diets such as those in Asia contain numerous soybean products and iron absorption is adversely affected by this soybean inhibitor. Tannins, phytates, certain fibers (not cellulose), carbonates, phosphates, and low-protein diets also adversely affect the apparent absorption of iron. In contrast, ascorbic acid, fructose, citric acid, high-protein foods, lysine, histidine, cysteine, methionine, and natural chelates, i.e., heme, all enhance the apparent absorption of iron. Zinc and manganese reduce iron uptake by about 30 to 50% and 10 to 40%, respectively. Excess iron reduces zinc uptakes by 13 to 22%. Stearic acid, one of the main fatty acids in meat, also enhances iron uptake.

In foods, as well as in animal tissues, iron is present in a variety of metalloproteins which include hemoglobin, myoglobin, cytochromes, transferrin, ferritin, and a variety of other iron-binding proteins. In the heme proteins, iron is coordinated within a tetraporphyrin moiety which, in turn, is bound to a polypeptide chain. Hemoglobin is a tetramer with a molecular weight of 64,500 Da and which contains two α-subunits and two β-subunits that give the protein allosteric properties in the uptake and release of oxygen. Each polypeptide subunit contains 1 atom of ferrous iron which amounts to 0.34% of the protein by weight.

B. Absorption, Metabolism, Excretion

Iron uptake by the gut, iron use and reuse, and iron loss comprises a system that for all intents and purposes is a closed system. The gain through the gut is very inefficient and there is virtually no mechanism aside from blood loss that rids the body of its iron excess. This system is shown in Figure 2. The total iron content of the body averages 4.0 g in men and 2.6 g in women. As shown in Table 4, there are two groups of iron-containing compounds that are considered essential to life. Essential iron compounds in the body include hemoglobin, myoglobin, and the cytochromes. In addition, there are a number of enzymes whose active site has an iron-sulfur center. Hemoglobin is the most abundant and easily sampled of the heme proteins and accounts for greater than 65% of body iron. The second group of molecules are those involved in iron transport (transferrin) and storage (ferritin, hemosiderin).

Transferrin is the iron-transport protein that carries ferric iron between the sites of its absorption, storage, and utilization. It is a β-glycoprotein of 76,000 Da which binds 2 atoms of ferric iron per mole. Iron is transferred from the intestinal mucosa to transferrin and is carried through the blood to peripheral tissues containing receptor sites for transferrin. Transferrin is synthesized in the liver, brain, and testes as well as other tissues. The regulation of the gene for transferrin varies from cell type to cell type and each cell type has its own array of promoters and transcription factors that control the amount of transferrin synthesized. The amount of transferrin synthesized is inversely related to the iron supply. In times of low intake, more transferrin is produced so as to optimize iron availability.

Once iron enters the cell it is chelated to a protein which is called ferritin. The enzyme that catalyzes this chelation is called ferrochelatase. This reaction then represents the ultimate destination for the majority of the iron that enters the cell. Chelation of iron to its storage protein occurs at the outer aspect of the mitochondrial membrane. Ferritin has a molecular weight of 450,000 Da. It is composed of 24 subunits which form an outer shell within which there is a storage cavity for polynuclear hydrous ferric oxide phosphate. Over 30% of the weight of ferritin may be iron. It is present in the liver, gut, reticuloendothelial cells, and bone marrow. Its synthesis is highly regulated

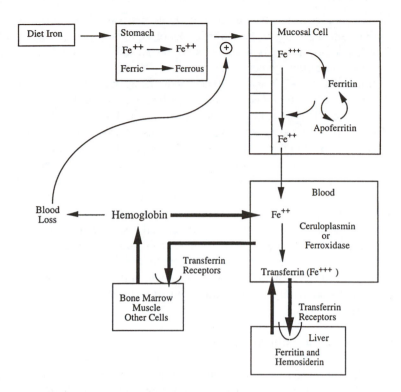

Figure 2 Overview of iron uptake and use showing the apparently closed system which indicates the recycling and conservation of iron once absorbed from the gut.

Table 4 The Body Content of Iron

Types of Iron	Male (70 kg)	Female (60 kg)
Essential Iron	3.100 g	2.100 g
Hemoglobin	2.700	1.800
Myoglobin, cytochromes, and other enzymes	0.400	0.300
Storage and transport iron	0.900	0.500
Ferritin, Hemosiderin	0.897	0.407
Transferrin	0.003	0.003
Total iron	4.000	2.600

by iron at the level of translation. When iron is present, the mRNA is available for translation. In the absence of iron the mRNA folds up on itself such that the start site for translation is covered up. Hemosiderin is a form of denatured ferritin which contains significantly less (~66%) iron.

1. *Iron-Containing Materials in the Body*

The cytochromes are enzymes involved in the electron transport system which is located principally in the mitochondria. Cytochrome P-450, a specialized cytochrome, is used to oxidize organic compounds. This cytochrome is located in the endoplasmic reticulum. While the cytochrome P-450 enzymes are active in the detoxification of drugs and chemicals, these enzymes also activate carcinogens. Cytochrome P-450 I has this function while P-450 IIE has a propensity to form oxygen radicals which are both cytotoxic and carcinogenic. Other cytochromes generate oxygen radicals by futile cycling. In some respects, the ability to generate peroxides has a protective effect in that peroxides will kill invading pathogens. Peroxide formation is, in fact, the first line of defense against such an invasion. Other enzymes in which iron is not bound to heme include iron-sulfur proteins, metalloflavoproteins, and certain glycolytic enzymes.

Since the lifetime of a red cell is about 120 days in humans, the flow of iron through the plasma space amounts to about 25 to 30 mg/day in the adult (about 0.5 mg per kilogram of body weight). This amount of iron corresponds to the degradation of about 1% of the circulating hemoglobin mass per day. Iron is conserved in males and postmenopausal females to a great degree; only 10% being lost per year in normal males, or about 1 mg/day. This loss of 1 mg/day has to be made up by absorption of iron from the diet, which is only about 10% efficient, thus requiring about 10 mg of dietary iron per day. In menstruating females the loss is increased to 2 mg/day during the menstrual period of the estrus cycle. This means that the intake and absorption of iron must be increased to avoid iron deficiency anemia.

In contrast to the turnover of hemoglobin in the red cell, tissue iron compounds which include the cytochrome enzymes and a variety of other nonheme enzymes, are heterogeneous in respect to the life span. Furthermore, these compounds are subject to degradation at exponential rates similar to the rate of turnover of the subcellular organelle with which they are associated. For example, in rats, mitochondrial cytochrome C has a half-life of about 6 days, whereas hemoglobin has a half-life of about 63 days.

C. Recommended Dietary Allowance

The apparent absorption of iron, i.e., the amount absorbed from food, can vary from less than 1% to more than 50%. The percentage that is absorbed depends on the nature of the diet, on the type of iron compound in the diet, and on regulatory mechanisms in the intestinal mucosa that reflect the body's physiological need for iron.

Two types of iron are present in the food: namely, heme iron which is found principally in animal products and nonheme iron which is inorganic iron bound to various proteins in plants. Most of the iron in the diet, usually greater than 85%, is present in the nonheme form. The absorption of nonheme iron is strongly influenced by its solubility in the upper part of the intestine. Absorption of nonheme iron depends on the composition of the meal and is subject to enhancers of absorption such as animal protein and by reducing agents such as vitamin C. On the other hand, heme iron is absorbed more efficiently. It is not subject to these enhancers. Although heme iron accounts for a smaller proportion of iron in the diet, it provides quantitatively more iron to the body than dietary nonheme iron.

The regulation of iron entry into the body takes place in the mucosal cells of the small intestine. Its iron gate is very sensitive to the iron stores, so if the iron stores are low, which is true for most women and children, the intestinal mucosa increases its iron uptake efficiency, particularly that of the nonheme iron. On the other hand, if the body is replete with iron, as is typical of healthy men and postmenopausal women, then the percentage of iron absorbed is low. This mechanism offers some protection against iron overload. In infancy, lactoferrin, an iron-binding protein in human milk, promotes the absorption of iron through lactoferrin receptors on the surface of the intestinal mucosa of infants. This may explain why the small amount of iron that is in milk is well absorbed by breast-fed infants. Milk is not usually considered a good source of iron, but for the breast-fed infant this lactoferrin-iron mechanism is important. As the infant grows, however, this mechanism may be inadequate. Iron deficiency can develop, particularly if the hepatic iron stores are insufficient at birth. This can happen in infants of malnourished mothers who themselves are iron deficient.

On the average, only about 10% of dietary iron is absorbed. In order to be absorbed the iron must be in the ferrous state, but upon entry into the enterocyte it is incorporated into ferritin as ferric ion. When the iron is transported from the mucosal to the serosal side of the enterocyte it is transported in the ferrous state, probably bound to cytoplasmic proteins. When the iron is pumped out of the enterocyte it must be oxidized to the ferric state in order to bind to transferrin. This is accomplished by ceruloplasmin (160,000 Da) which contains 8 copper ions in the divalent state. Ceruloplasmin copper is reduced by the iron, resulting in the formation of cuprous ions in ceruloplasmin and ferric iron in transferrin.

As mentioned earlier, transferrin is recognized in the periphery by cells that have transferrin receptors. The transferrin receptors vary, depending on the tissue and the condition. Tissue such as erythroid precursors, placenta, and liver have a large number of transferrin receptors and have a high uptake of iron. When these cells are in an iron-rich environment, the number of receptors decreases and, conversely, when they are in an iron-poor environment the number of receptors increases. The up- and down-regulation of transferrin receptors is accomplished at the genetic level. Measurements of messenger RNA for the transferrin receptors indicate that there can be as much as a 20-fold change in messenger RNA and, presumably, as much as a 20-fold difference in transcription of the transferrin receptor gene. The change in mRNA and its transcription is related to the concentration of iron.

After iron is delivered to an erythroid precursor cell in the bone marrow, the ferric iron has again to be reduced to the ferrous state in order to be incorporated into the heme prosthetic group. This reduction is accomplished by an NADH-dependent reductase and the insertion of iron in the heme ring is accomplished by another enzyme known as chelatase. When the ferrous iron is inserted into heme associated with specific subunits in hemoglobin, the various subunits polymerize to form the tetramer of hemoglobin A.

The presence of oxygen, of course, tends to oxidize a certain small percent of the iron each day and the formation of ferric iron in the hemoglobin molecule results in its conversion to methemoglobin, which has no capacity to take up and release oxygen. In order to minimize this effect of the oxidation of ferrous iron in hemoglobin by cellular oxygen concentrations, methemoglobin reductase, which is also an NADH-dependent enzyme, reduces the ferric iron in methemoglobin back to the ferrous state which, in turn, regenerates the oxygen-carrying hemoglobin.

1. Iron Needs

A normal red cell lasts for about 120 days in the human circulation and is then taken up by the reticuloendothelial system and degraded. The hemoglobin is degraded into bile pigments to which iron is attached. These pigments are secreted via the bile into the intestinal lumen, contributing iron to the intestinal pool. Iron is recirculated to the extent of about 25 mg/day. Thus, the turnover of iron within the body is 10 to 20 times the amount absorbed. A similar small amount, about 1 mg/day is lost by the sloughing of GI cells and by skin cells. Fecal losses of iron are about 0.6 mg/day. Urinary losses are essentially nil.

In menstruating women, or in individuals with hemorrhage, the iron losses can be considerable and anemia can occur as a result of menstrual losses or bleeding. This is the basis for chlorosis in adolescent girls, who were first identified as iron-deficient in the seventeenth century.

During the childbearing years, females must replace the iron lost in menstrual blood, which over a month amounts to about 1.4 mg/day. During infancy and childhood, about 40 mg of iron are required for the production of essential iron compounds associated with the gain of 1 kg of new tissue. Obviously, the iron needs are great in infants and adolescents. The needs of pregnant women are also great; a total of about 1.0 g of iron is needed to cover both fetal and maternal needs during the course of pregnancy and delivery. It is difficult to obtain this amount of iron from the usual diet. It is estimated that about 30 mg/day of elemental iron is needed in the diet to provide 4 mg/day for absorption.

The RDA for iron varies between 10 and 15 mg/day for different groups, except in pregnancy when it is 30 mg/day. Table 1 gives the RDAs for various groups of males and females.

D. Deficiency Disease

Iron deficiency is probably the most common nutritional deficiency present in the world population. This is true because iron is poorly absorbed and because many diets, especially those consumed by Third World populations, are iron poor. Diets which contain whole grain cereals and legumes contain only nonheme iron which is poorly absorbed. Furthermore, women and children are at constant risk for iron deficiency. Assessment of deficiency includes the determination of levels of tissue and serum ferritin, transferrin, transferrin receptor activity, heme iron, red cell number and size (mean corpuscular volume), hematocrit, and hemoglobin levels.

Clinical iron deficiency anemia occurs in three stages: the first involves depletion of iron stores as measured by a decrease in serum ferritin which reflects the ferritin supply (iron stores) in the body, without loss of essential iron compounds and without any evidence of anemia. The second stage is characterized by biochemical changes that reflect the lack of iron sufficient for the normal production of hemoglobin and other iron compounds. This is indicated by a decrease in transferrin saturation levels and an increase in erythrocyte protophyrin — so-called iron deficiency without anemia. In the final stage, iron deficiency anemia occurs, with depressed hemoglobin production and a change in the mean corpuscular volume of the RBC to produce a microcytic hypochromic anemia. This is expressed clinically as pallor and weakness. There are also changes in the nails, which take on a spoon shape when the iron-deficient state is severe.

In rats made iron deficient, several changes in intermediary metabolism have been reported. These include an increase in peripheral tissue sensitivity to insulin, an increase in hepatic glucose production (gluconeogenesis), a decrease in the conversion of thyroxine to triiodothyronine, decreased heat production, impaired fatty acid oxidation and ketogenesis, an increased need for carnitine, evidence of oxidative damage to the erythrocyte membrane, abnormal monoamine metabolism in the brain (increased dopamine synthesis and down-regulation of dopamine receptors), increased serum triglycerides and cholesterol, and slightly less pentose shunt activity. In addition to these metabolic changes, iron-deficient rats had an impaired immune response to a pathogen challenge. There was a decrease in antibody production and a decrease in the natural killer cell population. Whether these same responses also exist in iron-deficient humans is not certain; however, it is likely that there are numerous similarities.

E. Pharmacological Action

The treatment of iron deficiency anemia is a pharmacologic activity and involves giving large doses of iron, usually equivalent to 60 mg of elemental iron or 300 mg of ferrous sulfate, once or twice a day. It is usually given with meals to minimize gastrointestinal side effects and maximize uptake. Fortunately, the more severe the anemia, the greater will be the percentage of iron absorbed. Iron supplementation is usually continued for 2 to 3 months to normalize hemoglobin levels and iron stores. These should be monitored until satisfactory values are obtained.

F. Toxicology

Iron toxicity is a result of excess iron intake. This can occur acutely in children who ingest iron pills or iron-vitamin supplements, not realizing that they can be toxic. Severe iron poisoning is characterized by damage to the intestine with bloody diarrhea, vomiting, and sometimes liver failure. Systemic effects include hemorrhage, metabolic acidosis, and shock. Lethality occurs at doses in excess of 200 to 250 mg/kg. Effective treatment includes induced emesis (vomiting), food and electrolyte treatment to prevent shock, and the use of iron-chelating agents to bind the iron. This treatment has substantially decreased the mortality from about 50% in 1950 to less than a few percent in recent years.

Chronic overload of iron can result either from chronic excess intake (hemosiderosis, abnormally high levels of hemosiderin) or from a genetic disorder, hemochromatosis. This is the most common form of chronic iron overload. It is a genetic disorder carried on chromosome 6. The disorder is characterized by an increased iron absorption with damage to the pancreas, liver, and heart, and which results in diabetes, liver failure, and heart failure. There is evidence that heterozygous individuals also have increased iron absorption but tissue pathology does not result. The frequency of the homozygous condition is about 0.3 to 0.4% while that of the heterozygous condition is about 10%. Certain populations in the African sub-Saharan regions have a higher percentage of their population with the disorder. The symptoms can vary widely depending both on diet and on whether one or two copies of the aberrant gene are present. Transferrin saturation is a helpful screening test. Greater than 60% saturation is a good indication of the disorder. Phlebotomy on a regular basis can be helpful in reducing tissue damage.

Chronic iron overload has also been found in the South African Bantu tribesmen. In this instance it was of dietary origin. Their traditional maize beer is very high (40 to 80 mg/l) in iron due to the iron containers used to make the brew. Bantu may also be genetically susceptible to iron overload but the possibility requires further study.

Frequent blood transfusions can also lead to iron overload. One unit of blood contains about 200 to 250 mg of iron in its hemoglobin. This is roughly equivalent to 150 to 200 times the usual daily intake; thus 6 to 12 transfusions could lead to iron overload. Persons with hemochromatosis are at greater risk for hepatocellular carcinoma.

In addition to the development of hemochromatosis, there is a growing body of evidence that suggests that chronically high iron intakes are associated with the development of cancer, in particular, colon cancer. Two lines of evidence have been put forth that support this suggestion. The first line concerns the production of free radicals. Iron, in excess, can catalyze the production of free radicals which in turn can damage cell membranes as well as act as mutagens through damaging DNA. At low exposures to mutagens the DNA can repair itself, but free radical damage could be so great that such repair might be inadequate. Free radical damage to circulating lipid-protein complexes, especially the low-density lipoproteins, has also been proposed as a response to iron overload. The second line concerns the fact that cancer cells, like normal cells, require iron as an essential ingredient of metabolism. Having a surplus of iron in the system could increase the survival and proliferation of the cancer cell. Several population studies have provided support for this line of thought. In these studies a dose-response relationship, that is, a correlation of iron intake, ferritin levels, and the development of colon cancer, was found that was highly suggestive of a causal role for excess iron intake in colon cancer development.

Carcinogenesis can also be instigated by other minerals. Nickel subsulfide, for example, is a potent carcinogen having the renal tissue as a target. In the presence of high to moderate iron levels, the activity of the nickel compound is increased. In copper excess due to a genetic disorder involving the protein that transports copper, hepatic cancer develops and is potentiated by high iron levels. It would appear in these last examples that the role of iron is that of a cancer promoter rather than that of an initiator as described for colon cancer.

Although high iron intakes can be harmful, it should be noted that optimal iron intakes can protect against lead toxicity. Lead competes with iron for uptake by the enterocyte. If the transporter is fully saturated by its preferred mineral, iron, then the lead will be poorly absorbed and excreted in the feces. Well-nourished individuals with respect to iron nutriture are at less risk for lead toxicity than are those whose iron intake is marginal or deficient. Unfortunately, humans at risk for lead toxicity are frequently those whose diets are less than optimal. Lead intoxication has anemia as a characteristic because lead substitutes for iron in the hemoglobin molecule and kills the red cell. As the heme is being synthesized lead competes with iron for placement yet does not have the divalent characteristic of the iron so the heme is nonfunctional. Lead-induced anemia therefore is a direct effect of the lead, not a sign of iron deficiency per se. Nonetheless, lead toxicity and iron deficiency frequently coexist.

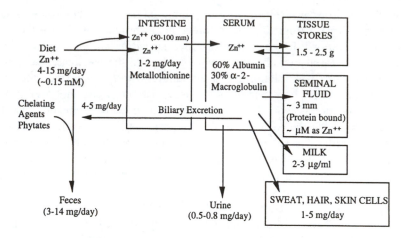

Figure 3   Zinc balance in normal adult humans.

V. ZINC

A. Overview

Zinc is the last transition element in the series of the fourth period of the periodic table. It has an atomic number of 30 and an atomic weight of 65.4. There are 15 isotopes of which ^{65}Zn is the most useful. This radioisotope has a half-life of 245 days.

Zinc is a good reducing agent and will form stable complexes with other ions as well as form a wide range of salts with members of the halogen family as well as with carbonates, phosphates, sulfates, oxalates, and phytate.

B. Absorption, Metabolism, Excretion

Like iron, zinc absorption is relatively poor. Of the approximately 4 to 14 mg/day consumed, only 10 to 40% is absorbed. Absorption is decreased by the presence of binding agents or chelating agents which render the mineral unabsorbable. Zinc binds to ligands that contain sulfur, nitrogen, or oxygen. Zinc will form complexes with phosphate groups (PO_4^{2-}), chloride (Cl^-), and carbonate groups (HCO_3^-) as well as with cysteine and histidine. Buffers such as N-2-hydroxyethyl-pyserazine-N′-2-ethanesulfonic acid (HEPES) have little effect on zinc binding to these ligands. Clay, a mixed mineral soil fragment, for example, can render zinc unavailable. So too can fiber, phosphate, and phytate (inositol hexaphosphate). Zinc bound in this fashion is excreted via the feces. People who are geophagic (pica) and/or who consume large amounts of phytate-containing foods (mainly cereal products) are at risk for developing zinc deficiency. Oberleas has calculated that diets having a phytate to zinc ratio greater than 10 will induce zinc deficiency regardless of the total zinc content in these diets.

Unlike iron, zinc exists in only one valence state: Zn^{2+}. The normal 70-kg human absorbs 1 to 2 mg/day (Figure 3) using both a nonsaturable and a saturable process. The former is passive diffusion while the latter may involve the zinc-binding metallothionein protein and/or a cysteine-rich intestinal protein. Studies on the mechanisms of zinc absorption by the enterocyte have shown that fast zinc uptake is attributable to extracellular binding of zinc followed by internalization of the zinc ligand mediated by an unknown molecular entity. After entry into the enterocyte the zinc is bound to a cysteine-rich intestinal protein (CRIP) which in turn transfers the zinc to either metallothionine or through the serosal side of the enterocyte to albumin which carries it to its site

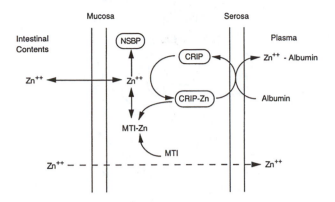

Figure 4 Intestinal zinc absorption. Passive diffusion is shown at the lower part of the diagram while mediated transport involving metallothionen I (MTI), the cysteine-rich protein (CRIP), and the nonspecific binding proteins (NSBP) is shown in the upper portion of the diagram.

Table 5   Enzymes Requiring Zinc as a Cofactor. These Are Representative of the Many Requiring Zinc for Activity

Alcohol dehydrogenase	δ-Aminolevulinate dehydrase
Lactate dehydrogenase	Fructose-1,6-bisphosphatase
Alkaline phosphatase	Transcarboxylases
Angiotensin converting enzyme	Reverse transcriptase
Carbonic anhydrase	Leukotriene hydrolase
Carboxypeptidase A, B, and DD	Phosphodiesterase
Cytoplasmic superoxide dismutase (also requires copper)	Elastase
DNA and RNA polymerases	Adenosine deaminase
Pyruvate dehydrogenase	5′-Nucleotidase
Proteases and peptidases	Glyoxalase
Aspartate transcarbamylase	Transcription factor Sp1
Thymidine kinase	Thymulin

of use. Figure 4 shows this proposed uptake system. Vitamin D enhances zinc uptake probably due to an effect on the synthesis of metallothionein. From the enterocyte it is transferred to the plasma where ~77% is loosely bound to albumin, ~20% is tightly bound to an α-2-macroglobulin, and 2 to 8% is ultrafilterable. This ultrafiltrate is excreted either in the urine (0.5 to 0.8 mg/day) or in the feces via biliary excretion.

The liver appears to be a major site of Zn^{2+} uptake after it has been absorbed. There is both rapid uptake ($t_{1/2} = 20$ s) and a slower linear uptake.

C. Function

Zinc has two important functions. One is that of serving as an essential cofactor for more than 70 enzymes. Table 5 provides a partial list of these enzymes. In this role, zinc binds to the histidine and cysteine residues of the enzyme proteins and in so doing stabilizes and exposes the active sites of these enzymes such that catalysis of the reaction in question can take place. Figure 5 illustrates this binding. Even though these enzymes require zinc as a cofactor, these enzymes appear to function at near normal levels in deficient animals. In part, this occurs because these enzymes are intracellular enzymes and tenaciously retain the zinc so as to continue to function. There obviously is a hierarchy of zinc need by the living body. Tissue stores of zinc are raided well before the intracellular zinc stores needed by these enzymes. Furthermore, deficient states are characterized by an increase in zinc absorption efficiency, further protecting the system from self destruction.

active site

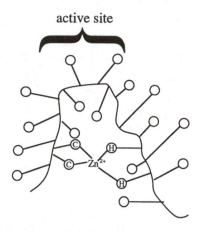

Figure 5   Zinc binds to cysteine (C) and histidine (H) residues of an enzyme protein stabilizing it so as to expose its active catalytic site. The rods and balls are used to represent the various amino acid residues sticking out of the amino acid chain.

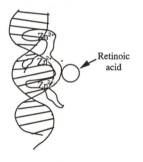

Figure 6   A zinc-DNA binding protein in action. In this instance retinoic acid bound to its zinc-containing DNA binding receptor protein is shown.

Equally important is the binding of zinc to specific DNA binding proteins found in the nucleus. In this role, zinc binds again to histidine and cysteine residues in the same fashion as shown above in Figure 5. This binding to the linear portions of the molecule give it a shape like a string of sausages or a bunch of fingers. These proteins, with zinc attached, are called zinc finger proteins or simply zinc fingers. More than one zinc is attached so that the DNA binding protein can envelop the DNA on both sides. Up to 37 zinc fingers can be part of these transcription factors. Figure 6 provides a visual representation of a zinc finger as it binds to both sides of the double-stranded DNA helix.

A number of nutrients, e.g., vitamin A and vitamin D, and hormones such as the steroids, insulin-like growth factor I, growth hormone, and others have their effects on the expression of specific genes because they can bind to very specific zinc fingers which in turn bind to very specific DNA regions. These DNA binding proteins (transcription factors) also contain leucine in sequence so as to form a hydrophobic region around the binding site for the DNA. Because more than one transcription factor is usually involved in turning on (or turning off) the synthesis of new messenger RNA, the hydrophobic regions allow these factors to associate along the DNA without interacting yet enhancing or suppressing RNA polymerase II action in mRNA synthesis. Each of these transcription factors has a preferred base sequence on the DNA. Retinoic acid as well as steroid hormones bind to factors that prefer the GGTCA sequence. This is the sequence that these proteins recognize and bind. Other transcription factors similarly have preferred base sequences.

If there is a mutation in the genes which encode these DNA binding proteins such that they lack the requisite two residues each of histidine and cysteine in the linear part of their structure, then the functional attributes of these vitamins and hormones at the genetic level will be ablated. Instances of such mutations have been published as well as instances where these zinc fingers have been purposely modified as a therapeutic approach to disease control. Zinc-containing transcription factor Zif268 has been modified with the result of a loss in sequence-specific recognition of DNA by viruses, thus ablating the viral invasion and takeover of their target cells. Although this modification was done *in vitro* and not tested in whole animals, this approach might have therapeutic application in the future as a means to avert the consequences of viral diseases such as AIDS.

Zinc as part of a zinc finger or by itself stimulates the expression of its own transporter protein, metallothionein. Metallothionein exists as two distinct yet related compounds termed MT-1 and MT-2. These proteins are hydrophilic, low molecular weight proteins (6 to 7 kDa) containing a high percentage of cysteine residues (23 to 22 mol%). The function of the cysteine is to bind heavy metals via clusters of thiolate bonds. The synthesis of metallothionein is regulated by zinc through its action on the expression of the genes for these proteins. The level of MT-1 is a very sensitive indicator of zinc deficiency. The metallothionein gene was identified by Palmiter et al. By combining the results of DNA sequence information with the results of deletion mapping studies, unique short sequences of DNA were found that mediated the role of zinc in metallothionein gene expression. The metal response elements were sites for trans-acting transcription factors that bind and enhance the basal rate of transcription of the genes for metallothionein. In the absence of dietary zinc, gene transcription is impaired and metallothionein levels are low. In addition, in zinc-deficient animals numerous breaks in single-strand DNA have been observed. This can be reversed when dietary zinc is restored. Incidentally, transgenic mice that overexpress metallothionein I are very resistant to zinc deficiency. The overexpression of metallothionein increases the absorption efficiency of these mice thus compensating for inefficient absorption.

The cytokine, interleukin 1, has been shown to direct and regulate zinc metabolism in the traumatized or septic individual as well as in normal persons. Interleukin 1 increases the expression of the metallothionein gene thereby increasing zinc uptake through the gut and its transport to, and uptake by, bone marrow and thymus, with relatively less zinc taken up by other body components. Trauma and sepsis both require zinc for new protein synthesis for tissue repair and both conditions are characterized by a rise in interleukin 1 levels in the blood.

Zinc is stored in the β cells of the islets of Langerhans in the pancreas. There, zinc is incorporated into the hormone insulin. Insulin contains two to four atoms of zinc as part of its crystalline structure. Zinc may play a role in insulin release but the details of this role have not been completely elucidated. Pharmaceutical preparations of insulin needed by diabetics for hormone replacement therapy contain zinc. It should be noted that not all species incorporate zinc in the insulin structure.

Zinc can sometimes be displaced on the zinc fingers by other divalent metals. Iron, for example, has been used to displace zinc on the DNA binding protein that also binds estrogen. This protein binds to the estrogen response element of the DNA in the promoter regions encoding estrogen-responsive gene products. When this occurs in the presence of H_2O_2 and ascorbic acid, damage to the proximate DNA, the estrogen response element, occurs. It has been suggested in this circumstance of an iron-substituted zinc finger that free radicals are more readily generated, with the consequence of genomic damage. This suggestion has been offered as an explanation of how excess iron (iron toxicity) could instigate the cellular changes that occur in carcinogenesis.

In excess, cadmium can also substitute for zinc in the zinc fingers. In this substitution, the resultant fingers are nonfunctional. Because of the importance of these fingers in cell survival and renewal, a cadmium substitution is lethal. Cadmium toxicity is an acute illness with little lag time needed for the symptom of cell death to manifest itself.

In addition to its function in metallothionein transcription and as a component of numerous enzymes and in the zinc fingers, zinc also is important for the stabilization of membranes and provides structural strength to bone as part of the bone mineral apatite. Excess zinc intake can adversely affect copper absorption and also affect iron absorption. Further, excess zinc can interfere with the function of iron as an antioxidant and can interfere with the action of cadmium and calcium as well. Ferritin, the iron storage protein, can also bind zinc. In zinc excess, zinc can replace iron on this protein. Other interactions include the copper-zinc interaction. Copper in excess can interfere with the uptake and binding of zinc by metallothionein in the enterocyte. In humans consuming copper-rich diets the apparent absorption of zinc is markedly reduced. In part this is due to a copper-zinc competition for enterocyte transport and in part due to a copper effect on metallothionine gene expression. Metallothionein has a greater affinity for copper than for zinc and thus zinc is left behind while copper is transported to the serosal side of the enterocyte for export to the plasma, whereupon the copper rather than the zinc is picked up by albumin and transported to the rest of the body. Fortunately, excess copper in the normal diet is not common. Zinc is usually present in far greater amounts and this interaction is of little import in the overall scheme of zinc metabolism.

The metallothionein protein, in addition to binding zinc and copper, also binds other heavy metals such as lead, mercury, and cadmium. This occurs when the individual is acutely exposed to toxic levels of these metals.

D. Deficiency

Until the early 1960's, zinc had not been demonstrated as an essential nutrient for humans. Prasad in 1961 and Halsted in 1958 and 1963 described conditions in humans later found to be due to inadequate zinc intake. Among the symptoms were growth failure, anemia, hypogonadism, enlarged liver and spleen, rough skin, and mental lethargy. These features can be attributed both to the loss of zinc as a cofactor in many enzymatic reactions *and* to the loss of zinc as an essential component of the DNA binding zinc fingers. Detailed studies of populations having these symptoms among its members revealed the custom of clay eating as well as diets that were very low in animal protein and high in cereal products. Geophagia (clay eating) can affect the bioavailability of not only zinc, but also iron and other minerals needed for optimal growth and development. In Iran, Prasad and Halsted found that the provision of iron and protein supplements corrected the anemia and the enlarged spleen and liver. Pubic hair and the gonads also began to develop. It was difficult to explain all of the clinical features (and their reversal) solely on the basis of iron deficiency and/or protein deficiency since other investigators had not reported the features of hypogonadism as part of the iron- or protein-deficient state. However, studies in animals showed that this feature is characteristic of zinc deficiency.

Later, Prasad in Egypt reported on growth retardation and testicular atrophy in young men. Geophagia was not a custom in this group nor were there signs of enlarged spleens and livers. The dietary patterns were similar to those found in Iran in that they were high in cereals and low in animal protein. Zinc concentrations in hair, plasma, and red cells were lower than normal. Zinc turnover using ^{65}Zn was increased above normal and the 24-hr exchangeable pool of zinc was smaller than expected. There were no signs of liver disease or any other chronic disease that would affect zinc status except that the Egyptian subjects were infected with schistosomiasis and hook-worms. Studies of populations in Egypt where these infections were absent but where the diets were similar lead to the conclusion that the growth failure and hypogonadism were indeed signs of zinc deficiency. This was proven without a doubt when zinc supplements were provided and these signs were reversed.

The zinc deficiency signs of growth failure and sexual immaturity are the result of an individual's inability to support cell division and hence tissue growth. The skin symptoms are the most obvious because skin cells turn over very rapidly (~7 days). These symptoms include a moist eczematoid dermatitis found in the nasolabial folds and around other body orifices. There is a failure in zinc-deficient individuals to replace these routinely desquamated cells. In infants and young children, inadequate zinc intake can result in abnormal CNS development as well as impaired skeletal development. In the latter instance, zinc deficiency results in an impaired calcium uptake probably due to a decreased synthesis of intestinal calbindin. Impaired immune response and impaired taste sensitivity also characterize the deficient state. These features again relate to the role of zinc in cell turnover. Immunity requires antibody synthesis involving zinc fingers while the taste sensation involves short-lived epithelial cells on the surface of the tongue and oral cavity. The features of zinc deficiency have been reported in infants having an autosomal recessive mutation in one of the genes which encode the zinc-carrying metallothionein found in the enterocyte (acrodermatitis enteropathica). This condition is treated with oral zinc supplements which, through mass action, provides enough zinc to the enterocyte by passive diffusion. Because only one of the metallothionine genes has mutated, this strategy overcomes the inherent zinc-deficient state.

Other zinc-deficient states have been reported in severely traumatized individuals and in patients with end-stage renal disease with or without dialysis. In renal disease, more zinc is lost via the kidneys than normal. In renal failure, excess zinc is lost through the dialysate when patients are maintained on regular dialysis treatment. Children who are anephric and on dialysis must be monitored with respect to their zinc status. Failure to do so will result in growth failure and lack of sexual maturation. Again, a zinc supplement can reverse these symptoms.

E. Status

Zinc status can be difficult to assess sensitively. Plasma and neutrophil zinc levels can give a static measure of status; however, these blood levels can only evaluate the amount of zinc in transport, not the functional state of the individual. Measurement of alkaline phosphatase, carbonic anhydrase, or 5′-nucleotidase activity is quite useful because these are zinc-requiring enzymes and are sensitive to zinc deprivation more so than the level of metallothionein I in blood. Hair zinc levels have been suggested as indicators of chronic zinc status; however, hair samples are frequently contaminated by zinc-containing shampoos or zinc-containing water. Hair growth rate could also influence hair zinc content. Hence, assessing zinc status using hair samples probably is not very useful. Currently, the intake recommendation is set at 15 mg/day (see Table 1). Assuming that the individual consumes a wide variety of foods and that the intake recommendation for good quality protein is met, the average individual should be well nourished with respect to zinc.

F. Toxicity

Zinc toxicity is not a common occurrence. In some instances it has occurred as a result of food contamination from galvanized food containers. Food or drink can pick up significant quantities of zinc as it leaches from the container into the food. This is particularly a problem when the food or drink is slightly acidic and the storage is prolonged. Symptoms of acute toxicity include nausea, vomiting, epigastric pain, abdominal cramps, and diarrhea. In severe cases the diarrhea can be bloody. Central nervous system symptoms (lethargy, light-headedness, staggering gait, and difficulty with fine finger movement) have been reported in an individual consuming elemental zinc in large quantities.

Chronic excess zinc ingestion in the range of 100 to 300 mg/day in the absence of adequate copper intake can also result in symptoms of toxicity that more nearly replicate those of copper deficiency. These symptoms include low blood copper levels, anemia, leukopenia, and neutropenia. The use of a copper supplement will reverse the condition. Interestingly, once the zinc supplements were discontinued the copper supplement was no longer necessary. At risk for this zinc-copper imbalance are those persons medicating themselves with zinc supplements. Even small supplements (15 to 100 mg zinc per day) may elicit adverse symptoms which may include not only anemia as described above but also disturbances in the serum lipoprotein profile. Decreases in high-density lipoprotein have been reported in such individuals and these decreases were reversed when the supplement was withdrawn. The mechanism of this zinc-copper interaction probably involves the metallothionein in the mucosal cell. This metal-binding protein has a higher affinity for copper than for zinc, and it may sequester this mineral in preference to zinc, creating a mineral imbalance.

VI. COPPER

A. Overview

Since the Bronze Age, copper alloyed with tin has been used to fabricate a vast array of useful items. However, it has only been in the last few decades that it was recognized as an essential nutrient for humans and other animals. In the 1920s it was recognized that copper, in addition to iron, was needed for hemoglobin synthesis. This came about when anemic animals supplemented with iron did not improve unless copper was also provided. The pioneering work of Cartwright and associates showed the relationship between the two metals in heme biosynthesis. Other roles for copper have since been elucidated.

Copper is a transition metal in the fourth period of the periodic table. It has a molecular weight of 63.4 Da, an atomic weight of 29, and two oxidation states, cuprous (Cu^+) and cupric (Cu^{2+}). The 2+ form is biologically active and found in most living systems. There are two naturally occurring isotopes, Cu^{63} and Cu^{65} and two radioisotopes, ^{64}Cu and ^{67}Cu. The former has a half-life of 12.7 hr while the latter has a half-life of 62 hr.

Copper is present in nearly all foods in varying amounts. Dairy products are poor sources of copper while legumes and nuts are rich in this mineral. Raisins, whole grains, beef liver, shellfish, and shrimp are excellent sources as well. Surveys of foods consumed by a variety of population groups in the U.S. indicate a range of intake from 0.7 to 7.5 mg/day. On low intakes, absorption is markedly more (56% of intake) than when intake is high (12% of intake). High levels of zinc, tin, ascorbic acid, and iron adversely affect copper absorption.

B. Absorption, Metabolism, Excretion

Copper absorption takes place in the small intestine and to a limited extent in the stomach. Copper status affects absorption; where need is great, uptake is high. The amount absorbed also depends on the food mixture consumed and on the presence of other divalent minerals which may compete for uptake. Absorption efficiency is low, with an average uptake of 12%. Copper absorption is not affected by phytate. That which is not absorbed is excreted in the feces. Also excreted in the feces is copper transported to the intestine from the liver via the bile. About 2 mg/day is excreted via the biliary route. Copper is also excreted in the urine and lost through the skin and hair. The percent lost via the urine, feces, skin, and hair is between 12 and 43% of the intake. The daily urinary copper is quite small, amounting to 10 to 50 µg/day.

Once copper is absorbed by the enterocyte, it passes to the blood where it is bound to either albumin or transcuprein. The half-life of albumin-bound copper is on the order of 10 min. The copper is then delivered to the liver whereupon it is incorporated into an α-globulin transport protein called ceruloplasmin. Ceruloplasmin can carry six atoms of copper. It has been estimated that from 60 to 95% of plasma copper is transported by this protein. A computer-based prediction model suggests that, in humans, 62 to 72% of the plasma copper is carried by ceruloplasmin. Blood levels of copper are about 1 µg/ml while ceruloplasmin varies from 15 to 60 mg/dl. Ceruloplasmin is not only useful in transporting copper to all parts of the body but also has enzyme activity as a ferroxidase, an amide oxidase, and as a superoxide dismutase. As a ferroxidase it is an active participant in the release of iron from its liver storage sites to transferrin in the plasma. It is active in the conversion of iron from the ferrous to ferric state and in the linkage of the ferric iron to

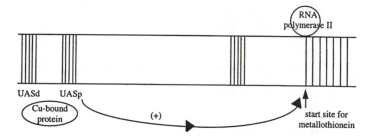

Figure 7   Copper plays a role in the expression of the gene for the cysteine-rich metallothionein by being a part of a DNA binding protein. This protein has several zinc fingers which attach to the UASd and UASp sites. When bound it stimulates transcription.

apotransferrin to form transferrin which, in turn, transports the iron to the reticulocyte for hemoglobin synthesis.

Although ceruloplasmin may indeed be the most active of the copper transporters, other transporters also participate in the delivery of copper to the cells which use and/or store this mineral. Albumin, as mentioned, can serve in this function as can a recently discovered 270-kDa protein (transcuprein) and certain of the amino acids, notably histidine. The liver is the major user and repositor of copper. The copper levels in the liver remain relatively constant. Biliary excretion and ceruloplasmin release are the major mechanisms used to maintain copper levels in this tissue. Ceruloplasmin has a high copper content and accounts for 70 to 90% of the approximately 1 μg/ml copper in the plasma.

Transcuprein has been shown to compete for copper with albumin in the intestine, yet functions in the portal circulation as a donor of copper to albumin. The existence and function of transcuprein in the maintenance of copper status has not been fully explored.

While the transport of copper in the blood has received considerable attention, its transport into the cell has not been as well studied. Copper passes through the plasma membrane via fixed membrane transporter proteins. These membrane proteins may either reversibly bind the copper or form channels through which the copper passes. The kinetics of copper transport have been studied. The Km values are uniformly in the low micromolar range, whereas the Vmax is highly variable depending on cell type, incubation conditions, and media used.

C. Function

Copper, zinc, and iron are all involved in the regulation of the expression of the genes for the metal-binding proteins, the cysteine-rich metallothioneins. These genes have metal response elements that are specific for each of these metals. The one for copper is called CUPI. The gene it affects is the one that encodes metallothionein, a 6570-Da protein which binds heavy metals, particularly copper. The promoter region for this gene does not respond directly to copper. Rather, it responds to an upstream activating sequence (UAS) present as a tandem sequence designated UASp and UASd located between −105 and −108 bp from the transcription start site. It is this sequence that is bound by the zinc and copper DNA binding protein. It would appear that transcription of the metallothionine is a function of both copper and zinc since this metal-binding protein can only be synthesized in the presence of both. This cascade-like process for the expression of the copper-responsive metallothionein is illustrated in Figure 7.

Using the messenger RNA differential display method, ten other genes have been shown to have a copper response element needed for expression. Seven of these had substantial homology with ferritin mRNA, fetuin mRNA, mitochondrial 12S and 16S rRNA, and with mitochondrial tRNA for phenylalanine, valine, and leucine. These homologies suggest roles for copper in mitochondrial gene expression which in turn relate to the observation of decreased oxidative phosphorylation in

Table 6   Enzymes Requiring Copper as a Cofactor

Cytochrome c oxidase
Lysyl oxidase
Tyrosinase
Dopamine-β-hydroxylase (DOPA-4-monoxygenase)
Tyrosine oxidase
Cytoplasmic superoxide dismutase (Cu/Zn SOD)
Amine oxidase
Diamine oxidase
Monoamine oxidase
α-Amidating enzyme
Ferroxidase II
Ascorbate oxidase
Phenylalanine-4-monooxygenase
Metallothionein
Ceruloplasmin

copper-deficient rats. This observation has also been related to the requirement for copper by one of the mitochondrial respiratory enzymes, cytochrome c oxidase. Of the remaining RNAs identified as having a copper response element, no gene product has yet been found. It is possible that these products might be enzymes requiring copper as a cofactor (Table 6) or may be copper transport proteins. This would follow the paradigm of gene expression found with zinc and iron.

D. Deficiency

Copper deficiency is rare in humans consuming a wide variety of foods. One of the major characteristics of copper deficiency is anemia and poor wound healing, similar to that observed in vitamin C deficiency. The anemia is not responsive to iron supplementation. Weakness, lassitude, joint ache, osteoporosis, small petechial hemorrhaging, and arterial aneurysms can all be attributed to the vital role of copper in the synthesis of connective tissue and, in particular, collagen synthesis. Hypertrophy of the heart followed by rupture is a frequently reported feature of copper-deficient rats. Central nervous system degeneration can be related to a decline in respiratory chain activity and ATP synthesis that is essential to neural activity. Reduced immune response has also been reported. Copper-deficient animals have been shown to have decreased T lymphocyte and neutrophil activities.

Other signs of the deficient state include elevated levels of plasma cholesterol, neutropenia, achromatism, twisted kinky hair, and hemacytic hypochromic anemia. Adrenal steroidogenesis is impaired as is catecholamine synthesis. The latter is due to a deficiency of the copper-containing enzyme dopamine beta hydroxylase. Chronic diarrhea and malabsorption have been reported in infants fed copper-deficient formulas. In male rats fed purified diets, the use of pure sugars (mono- and disaccharides) in a high-carbohydrate diet accelerate the development of the copper-deficient state. Probably this has to do with the purity of this dietary ingredient rather than on any copper-sugar interaction at the cell or subcellular level.

E. Abnormal Copper Status

In normal humans, copper intake excess is rare. Although copper toxicity can develop if the exposure is high enough and long enough, the body can protect itself from occasional excess intake by lowering its absorption and increasing excretion via bile and urine. The normal human should consume 1.5 to 3.0 mg/day of copper to maintain an optimal nutritional status. There is some discrepancy between the figure given in the RDA table as an estimated safe and adequate dietary intake (Table 2) and the population studies which indicate that the usual intake is between 1 and 1.5 mg/day. At intakes of 1 to 1.5 mg/day no signs of deficiency have been observed. Turnlund has reported that young men consuming between 0.75 to 7.53 mg/day were able to attain positive copper balance regardless of intake. Likely, the figure given for optimal intake is a little high because of the paucity of data on copper status under controlled conditions.

There are two rare genetic disorders that have assisted scientists in understanding the function and metabolism of copper. These two disorders affect copper status in opposite directions. In one, Menkes syndrome, copper absorption is faulty. This is an X-linked genetic disorder. Patients with Menkes disease have the symptoms of copper deficiency, i.e., depigmentation of skin, kinky hair, brain damage, muscle and connective tissue abnormality in the absence of anemia, and neutropenia. Intestinal cells absorb the copper but can not release it into the circulation. Parenteral copper can overcome intestinal malabsorption but cannot correct the problem with respect to neural tissue uptake. Infants with Menkes disease are characterized by cerebral degeneration and rarely survive infancy.

Another genetic disorder in copper status is Wilson's disease. This disease is an autosomal recessive disorder associated with premature death and associated excess copper accumulation. It is due to an impaired incorporation of copper into ceruloplasmin and decreased biliary excretion of copper. The genetic defect, like that of Menkes disease, involves the P-type ATPase cation transporters. These transporters play a role in the intracellular transport of copper. Human and mouse gene mapping studies have placed the ATPase cation transporter defect associated with Wilson's disease on chromosome 8 for the mouse and chromosome 13 for the human. This results in an accumulation of copper in the liver and brain. Early signs of Wilson's disease include liver dysfunction, neurological disease, and deposits of copper in the cornea manifested as a ring that looks like a halo around the pupil. This lesion is called the Kayser-Fleischer ring. Renal stones, renal aciduria, neurological deficits, and osteoporosis also characterize Wilson's disease. Wilson's disease can be managed by providing copper-chelating agents such as D-penicillamine and by increasing the intake of zinc which interferes with copper absorption.

F. Copper Need

There is no RDA for copper. However, there are sufficient data that document the need for this mineral. Thus there is a recommendation for an intake that should be safe and adequate. This is shown in Table 2.

VII. SELENIUM

A. Overview

Selenium is one of the "newer" minerals discovered during this century as being both required and toxic, with a relatively narrow range of intake between the two. The existence of selenium as a metal was first reported by Berzelius in 1817 and can occur in nature in a variety of forms and colors. In nature, selenium is frequently found in combination with lead, copper, mercury, and silver. These combinations are called selenides. Its chemistry is similar to that of sulfur. Selenium is an allotropic metal in group 6 of the fourth period of the periodic table. Its molecular weight is 78.96 Da and its atomic weight is 34. Although selenium has 26 isotopic forms, only five of these are naturally occurring: Se^{76}, Se^{78}, Se^{77}, Se^{80}, Se^{82}. Of the radioisotopes, ^{75}Se is the most useful, having a half-life of 118 days. Selenium has three valence states: Se^{2+}, Se^{4+}, and Se^{6+}. It can form selenides, as described above, and selenate. Because it will react with sulfur and oxygen it will form selenomethionine, selenocystine, methylselenocysteine, and dimethylselenide. These compounds are volatile.

Although the presence of selenium in the earth's mineral matter was known, its recognition as an essential nutrient did not occur until Schwarz and Foltz showed that a form of liver necrosis in

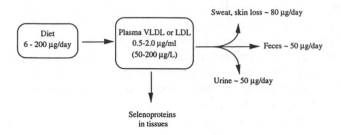

Figure 8   Daily selenium flux in a 70-kg man.

rats could be cured if either vitamin E *or* selenium were administered. This report and others showed that for some purposes these two nutrients were interchangeable. It was this interchangeability that interfered with the identification of selenium as an essential nutrient. In hindsight, we now realize that selenium and vitamin E both play important roles in the detoxification of peroxides and free radicals.

B. Absorption, Metabolism, Excretion

Absorption is very efficient, with most of the ingested selenium absorbed readily from a variety of foodstuffs. The source of the mineral can have effects on its absorption. Figure 8 provides an overview of the daily selenium flux in a normal human.

Selenium is transported from the gut on the very-low- and low-density lipoproteins. Red cells, liver, spleen, muscle, nails, hair, and tooth enamel all contain significant quantities of this mineral. Normal blood values for adults range from 55 to 72 µg/l. People with disorders that are characterized by increased oxidative stress to the red cell, i.e., β-thalassemia, diabetes, and/or smoking tend to have slightly higher blood selenium levels, whereas pregnant and lactating women tend to have lower selenium levels. Excess (greater than 10 ppb in water or 0.05 ppm in food) intake is toxic, but unlike iron and copper which have inefficient excretory pathways, selenium is actively excreted in the urine. The urinary system functions to maintain optimal selenium status.

Figure 9 shows how selenium is utilized. The metabolic use of selenium follows that of sulfur. It involves the formation of a selenium-sulfur bond using the SH group of either cysteine or methionine. From there it is incorporated into one of a group of proteins called selenoproteins. Under normal intake conditions (50 to 200 µg Se per day), about 50 µg can be found in the feces

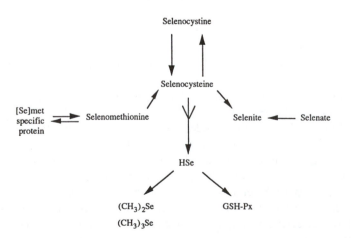

Figure 9   General scheme for selenium metabolism. Selenium is used by almost all cell types because of its vital role in glutathione peroxidase.

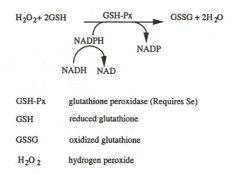

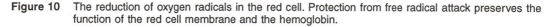

GSH-Px	glutathione peroxidase (Requires Se)
GSH	reduced glutathione
GSSG	oxidized glutathione
H_2O_2	hydrogen peroxide

Figure 10   The reduction of oxygen radicals in the red cell. Protection from free radical attack preserves the function of the red cell membrane and the hemoglobin.

and a similar amount is excreted in the urine. Sweat and desquamated skin cells account for another 80 µg/day. These losses can vary depending on dietary conditions. When intakes are low, losses are low, and when intakes are high there are corresponding rises in fecal and urine losses. Diets which include whole grain products, seafood, and organ meats will provide an optimal amount of selenium. In addition to these rich food sources, selenium in lesser amounts can be found in a wide variety of foods. In the U.S., selenium deficiency is rare. This is not the case in China or in some parts of New Zealand and perhaps other parts of the world where the variety of foods available for consumption is severely constrained or reduced to those items produced locally. If the locality is a selenium-poor area, humans as well as domestic animals may become deficient.

C. Function

Selenium is an essential element in a group of proteins called the selenoproteins. The synthesis of these selenoproteins involves sulfur-containing amino acids and selenium. These are joined via selenophosphate to form selenocysteine. The reaction is catalyzed by the enzyme selenophosphate synthetase. Vitamin B_6 serves as a coenzyme in this synthetic reaction.

Of the selenoproteins, glutathione peroxidase (GSH-PX or GPX, EC 1.11.1.9) has been the most widely studied. Glutathione peroxidase catalyzes the reduction of various organic peroxides as well as hydrogen peroxide. This reaction is shown in Figure 10. Glutathione furnishes the reducing equivalents in this reaction. Since membranes contain readily oxidizable unsaturated fatty acids, the stability of these membranes (and hence their function) is dependent on the activity of the antioxidant system of which this selenium-containing enzyme is a part.

If the diet is marginal in selenium but adequate in copper, iron, and vitamins A, E, and C, which also serve as antioxidants, then cell damage by free radicals will be minimized. These other antioxidants can and do suppress free radical formation. While vitamin E serves an important role in suppressing free radical production, its site of action is separate from that of selenium in its role as an essential component of glutathione peroxidase. Studies of selenium-deficient rats given a vitamin E supplement showed that these rats had no change in enzyme activity. Similarly, vitamin E-deficient rats show little improvement in red cell fragility with selenium supplements despite the overlap in antioxidant function of the two nutrients. The antioxidant properties of these cell components, however, are of particular interest to the pharmacologist because many drugs are, in themselves, oxidizing agents that work by disrupting the membranes of invading pathogens.

The aging process as well as carcinogenesis may well be related to the adequacy of the body's antioxidant system. Since free radicals damage cells, these cells may not be replaced at the same rate as the rate of destruction or the damage. That, in turn, may make the cell vulnerable to invasion by cancer-producing viruses or agents that initiate cancer growth. Anticancer drugs, as mentioned, may be strong oxidizing agents. Normal as well as infected cells of the host will be affected by drug treatment. Should the host's antioxidant system be compromised either by nutritional deficiency or because of some genetically determined deficiency in the maintenance of intracellular redox states, cell survival and normal function will be compromised. Other enzymes shown in Figure 10 include catalase and superoxide dismutase (SOD). Superoxide dismutase is found in both cytoplasm and mitochondria and requires different divalent ions as cofactors. Manganese, zinc, copper, and magnesium function in this respect. Glutathione peroxidase is of major importance to the maintenance of red blood cell redox state. The red cell lacks mitochondria (found in other cell types) which function in these cells in the maintenance of an optimal redox state. The red cell, because it contains the oxygen-carrying hemoglobin, must regulate the redox state so that this hemoglobin can release oxygen in exchange for CO_2. In this exchange, there are opportunities for peroxide formation. These must be suppressed, and glutathione peroxidase does just this.

Glutathione peroxidase is less active in deficient animals than in normally nourished animals. In fact, a decline in enzyme activity is a sensitive indicator of selenium status. At least four isozymes exist and these have been isolated and characterized. The four enzymes are numbered 1 through 4 as GPX1, GPX2, GPX3, and GPX4. Two of these, GPX1 and GPX4, are expressed in most tissues. GPX1 is found in large quantities in red blood cells, liver, and kidney, whereas GPX4 is found largely in testes. GPX2 is found mainly in the gastrointestinal tract and GPX3 is expressed mainly in kidney, lung, heart, breast, and placenta. There are species differences in the expression of these isozymes. In humans, GPX2 and 3 are expressed in the liver. In rodents this is not the case. Rodent liver expresses only GPX1, not GPX2 or 3.

Selenocysteine in proteins is encoded by either a UGA opal codon or the TGA triplet which is normally a stop codon. In order to read the TGA codon as selenocysteine there must be a stem-loop structure in the 3′-untranslated region of the selenoprotein genes. Although this stem-loop structure appears to be absolutely required for the incorporation of selenocysteine into a protein, documentation of this requirement is not fully complete. The active site of the selenium dependent glutathione peroxidase contains a selenocysteine encoded by a UGA opal codon. However, not all of the isozymes are selenium dependent. There is an androgen-induced epididymal cell enzyme that shares sequence homology with GPX3 but is not selenium dependent nor does it have the UGA codon in its mRNA. The GPX2 maps to chromosome 14 while GPX3 and GPX4 map to chromosomes 5 and 19, respectively. GPX1 maps to human chromosome 3 and has sequences which are homologous to those found in chromosome 21 and the X chromosome.

Several drugs have been developed that have antiinflammatory properties and that also contain selenium. They work by catalyzing the degradation of peroxides, much like glutathione peroxidase, or by reducing the production of leukotriene B. Both actions serve to reduce inflammation.

Although approximately 36% of the total selenium in the body is associated with glutathione peroxidase, a number of other proteins in the body also contain this mineral. Table 7 provides a list of these proteins. There are 13 different selenoproteins ranging in weight from 10 to 71 kDa that have been identified. Several of these are glutathione peroxidase isozymes and several have been isolated from a variety of cell lines. One, having thioredoxin reductase activity, has been isolated from human lung adenocarcinoma cells. Another, selenoprotein W, is thought to be responsible for white muscle disease when this protein is not made due to deficient selenium intake.

Table 7   Selenoproteins of Biological Importance

Cytosolic glutathione peroxidase
Phospholipid hydroperoxide glutathione peroxidase
Gastrointestinal glutathione peroxidase
Extracellular glutathione peroxidase
Selenoprotein W
Selenoprotein P
Iodothyronine deiodinase
Sperm capsule selenoprotein

Selenoprotein P, a protein that accumulates in plasma, may be a selenium transport protein but its true function has yet to be elucidated.

Selenium is an integral part of the enzyme, type 1 iodothyronine deiodinase (DI, EC 3.8.1.4) which catalyzes the deiodination of the iodothyronines, notably the deiodination of thyroxine (T_4) to triiodothyronine (T_3), the most active of the thyroid hormones. This deiodination is also catalyzed by type II and type III deiodinases, which are not selenoproteins. While all the deiodinases catalyze the conversion of thyroxine to triiodothyronine, there are differences in the tissue distribution of these enzymes. The pituitary, brain, central nervous system, and brown adipose tissue contain types II and III, whereas type I is found in liver, kidney, and muscle. These two isozymes (II, III) contribute very little triiodothyronine to the circulation except under conditions (i.e., starvation) that enhance reverse triiodothyronine (rT_3) production. In selenium-deficient animals type I synthesis is markedly impaired and this impairment is reversed when selenium is restored to the diet. Under these same conditions, the ratio of T_3 to T_4 is altered. There is more T_4 and less T_3 in the deficient animals and the ratio of the two is reversed when selenium is restored. Because type II and III deiodinase also exist, these enzymes should increase in activity so as to compensate for the selenium-dependent loss of function. However, they do not do this because their activity is linked to that of the type I. When T_4 levels rise (as in selenium deficiency), this rise feeds back to the pituitary, which in turn alters (reduces) TSH release. The conversion of T_4 to T_3 in the pituitary is catalyzed by the type II deiodinase yet TSH release falls. T_4 levels are high because the type I deiodinase is less active. Whereas the deficient animal might have a T_3/T_4 ratio of 0.01 the sufficient animal has a ratio of 0.02, a doubling of the conversion of T_4 to T_3.

The effect of selenium supplementation on the synthesis and activity of the type I deiodinase probably explains the poor growth of deficient animals. Sunde and co-workers have reported significant linear growth in selenium-deficient rats given a single selenium supplement. This growth was directly related to the supplement-induced increase in type I deiodinase activity and to the conversion of thyroxine to triiodothyronine. In turn, the observations of changes in selenium status coincident with changes in thyroid hormone status provided the necessary background for establishing the selenium-iodide interaction that today is taken for granted. Selenium as part of type I deiodinase clearly explains the selenium-iodide interaction. Humans lacking both selenium and iodine show impaired thyroid gland function which in turn results in poor growth, poor mental capacity, and shortened life-spans. In this situation the deficiencies have cumulative effects on the patient. Of interest is the observation that in this dual state there is no thyroid gland enlargement as is typical of simple iodide deficiency.

Other trace mineral interactions also exist. Copper-deficient rats and mice have been shown to have reduced glutathione peroxidase activity. Copper deficiency increases oxidative stress yet oxidative stress affects all of the enzymes involved in free radical suppression. Even though glutathione peroxidase does not contain copper, the expression of the genes for this enzyme and for catalase is reduced in the copper-deficient animal. Other trace minerals are also involved as required components for SOD. Copper, zinc, magnesium, and manganese are part of the antioxidant system as is NADPH and NAD (niacin-containing coenzymes). The NAD, although not usually shown as part of the system, is involved because it can transfer reducing equivalents via the transhydrogenase cycle to NADP. Clearly, there are numerous nutrient interactions required for the maintenance of the optimal redox state in the cell. This is important not only because it stabilizes the lipid portion of the membranes within and around the cells but also because it optimizes the functional performance of the many cellular proteins.

D. Deficiency

Selenium deficiency can develop in premature infants and in persons sustained for long periods of time by selenium-free enteral or parenteral solutions. Symptoms characteristic of deficiency in humans include a decline in glutathione peroxidase activity in a variety of cell types, fragile red

Table 8   Signs and Symptoms of Selenium Deficiency in Animals

Poultry	Exudative diathesis, skeletal myopathy, encephalomalacia, pancreatic necrosis, reduced growth, reduced egg production, reduced fertility, reduced feather growth.
Bovines	Reduced growth, skeletal and cardial myopathy, embryonic death, retained placenta.
Equines	Skeletal myopathy, reduced performance, foals also have muscle steatitis.
Ovines	Skeletal and cardial myopathy, poor growth, reduced fertility, embryonic death.
Porcines	Poor growth, skeletal myopathy, "mulberry heart disease", gastric ulcers, hepatic dysfunction.
Rodents	Skeletal myopathy, erythrocyte hemolysis, testicular degeneration, fetal death and resorption, increased hepatic malic enzyme and glutathione reductase activity.

blood cells, enlarged heart, cardiomyopathy, growth retardation, cataract formation, abnormal placenta retention, deficient spermatogenesis, and skeletal muscle degeneration. Some of these characteristics are shared with other species as shown in Table 8. In China, selenium deficiency is called Keshan disease. It appears mainly in children and is marked by degenerative changes in the heart muscle (cardiomyopathy). This develops in children whose intakes are less than 17 µg/day. Selenite-enriched salt has been shown to reverse this deficiency and the time needed for this reversal in all cells depends on the half-life of the affected cells. Those cells that turn over rapidly will quickly show signs of deficiency and just as quickly show signs of reversal. Should cells that are not normally replaced quickly be affected by the deficient state, that effect will not be quickly reversed by selenium supplementation.

E. Toxicity

Selenium intake in excess of 750 µg/day is toxic. Toxicity does not usually occur unless the individual is exposed not only to high diet levels but also to industrial conditions (smelters, selenium-rich smoke, etc.) that increase entry of the mineral into the body. Selenium toxicity in farm animals has been observed when the food supply for these animals consists of selenium-rich pastures and grain. Selenium toxicity in these animals is characterized by hoof loss and a neuro-muscular condition known as "blind staggers." Damage to the liver and muscle is observed as well. Excess selenium intake interferes with zinc absorption and use, reduces tissue iron stores, and increases copper level in heart, liver, and kidney. Clearly, selenium excess upsets the normal trace element balance in the body.

F. Recommended Dietary Allowance

Data are still being gathered for the establishment of the human requirement for selenium. There are, however, sufficient reports in the literature that support the essentiality of its intake. Thus, the NAS-NRC has recommended that an intake no less than 50 and no more than 200 µg/day should be sufficient to meet the needs of the average adult. The RDA is shown in Table 1.

VIII. IODINE

A. Overview

The essentiality of iodine has been recognized since the late 1800s. Its relationship to the production of thyroxine was not fully realized, but even the ancient medical literature recommended the consumption of seaweed or burnt sponges (both of which are rich in iodine) for the treatment of goiter. Iodine deficiency used to be endemic in all but the coastal regions of the world. Presently, it is frequently observed in Third World nations whose access to iodine is limited. With the advent and use of iodized salt and the development of means to process and distribute frozen seafoods, this once common nutritional disorder has all but disappeared.

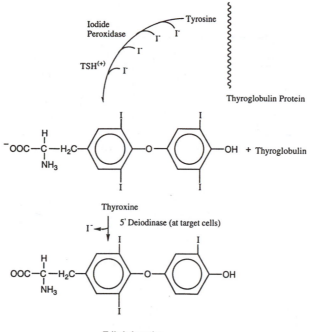

Figure 11 Schematic representation of thyroid hormone synthesis.

Iodine is a member of the halogen family which includes fluorine, chlorine, and bromine. These appear as Group VII in the fifth period of the periodic table. Iodine has an atomic number of 53 and an atomic weight of 127. There are no naturally occurring isotopes but two radioisotopes are useful in biological systems. These are ^{131}I with a half-life of 8 days and ^{125}I with a half-life of 60 days. Iodine is very labile but forms stable salts, the most common is NaI. The iodide ion has a negative one valence, I−.

B. Absorption, Metabolism, Excretion

The average human in the U.S. consumes between 170 to 250 μg/day. The iodine is converted to the iodide ion (I−) and is easily absorbed. Once absorbed, it circulates in the blood to all the tissues of the body. Salivary glands, the gastric mucosa, choroid plexus, and the lactating mammary gland as well as the thyroid gland can concentrate iodine. Of the iodine consumed, 80% is trapped by the thyroid gland which uses it for the synthesis of thyroxine. As shown in Figure 11, thyroxine is synthesized through the stepwise iodination of thyroxine. The gland produces and releases thyroxine when stimulated by the pituitary thyroid stimulating hormone (TSH). TSH acts on the tyrosine-rich thyroglobulin, serving to unravel this protein to make tyrosine available for iodination via the enzyme, iodide peroxidase. First, monoiodothyronine is produced, then diiodothyronine, triiodothyronine, and then thyroxine. TSH stimulates the thyroid to release thyroxine which is transported to its target tissues (all the cells of the body) by way of a transport protein called thyroid binding protein. Upon delivery to the target cell the thyroxine is carried into the cell and deiodinated to triiodothyronine. The enzyme catalyzing this reaction is 5′-deiodinase, a selenium-containing enzyme. Triiodothyronine is the active form of the hormone, having at least 10 times the activity of thyroxine. The iodide released by this deiodination is conserved and sent back into the bloodstream for further use by the thyroid gland. Iodide not used or sequestered is either excreted as organic iodine in the feces or as free iodine in the urine. The urinary loss is 40 times greater than the fecal loss. Figure 12 illustrates the endocrine pathway for thyroid hormone metabolism.

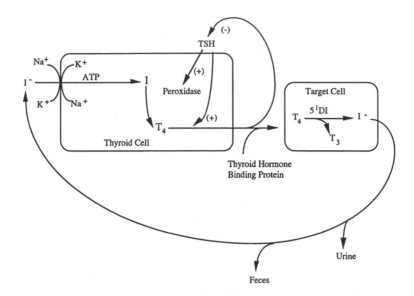

Figure 12   Overview of thyroid hormone production: TSH, thyroid stimulating hormone from pituitary; T_4, thyroxine; T_3, triiodothyronine; 5′ DI, 5′-deiodinase. The thyroid gland is stimulated to produce and release thyroxine by thyroid stimulating hormone (TSH). Thyroxine is carried by a binding hormone to all cells of the body whereupon it is deiodenated to its active form, T_3.

C. Deficiency

The enlargement of the thyroid gland (goiter) is characteristic of iodine deficiency and is marked by a hypertrophic, hyperplasic change in the gland's follicular epithelium. These epithelial cells synthesize thyroxine and their growth is stimulated by the pituitary hormone, thyroid stimulating hormone (TSH). The cells become enlarged when iodine is not available to complete the thyroxine synthetic process. A goiter is not only unsightly but may also cause obstruction of the airways and damage the laryngeal nerves. The synthesis of thyroxine is the only known function of iodine. Thyroid hormone production can be influenced not only by iodine deficiency but also by selenium deficiency. In the latter instance, the active thyroid hormone, triiodothyronine, is not produced in adequate amounts because the deiodination of thyroxine is dependent on the selenoprotein, 5′-deiodinase.

A diet deficient in iodine can cause a number of illnesses depending on the age at exposure. The developing embryo or fetus of an iodine-deficient woman will suffer a neurological deficit that is quite profound. If they survive and are born, these infants are called cretins. Infants and children consuming a deficient diet fail to grow normally and develop intellectually. Children and adults having inadequate iodine intakes develop enlarged thyroid glands and the condition is called goiter. The thyroid hormone producing cells enlarge (hypertrophy) and increase in number (hyperplasia) as a response to the pituitary hormone, TSH. The level of TSH rises as the body senses a need for thyroxine. Pregnant women may lose their pregnancies as the fetus fails to develop and dies in utero.

The deficient state can develop in instances where the population subsists on a marginal iodine intake and consumes a diet rich in vegetables of the *Brassica* genus (Cruciferae family). Although cabbage and related vegetables have been shown to contain goitrogens (compounds that inhibit thyroxine release by the thyroid gland or that inhibit iodine uptake by the gland) other vegetables contain these substances as well.

D. Recommended Dietary Allowance

Because iodine is conserved very efficiently and is not toxic even at 10 to 20 times the required intake, iodine is considered to be a benign (but essential) trace element. An intake of 1 to 2 µg/kg should be adequate for most adult humans. Pregnant females need slightly (10 to 20%) more. Thus, the Food and Nutrition Board of the National Academy of Sciences has recommended an intake of 150 µg/day for adults, 6 µg/kg/day for infants, 5 µg/kg/day for young children, 4 µg/kg/day for older children, and 175 µg/day for pregnant and lactating females. Table 1 provides the details of these RDAs.

IX. MOLYBDENUM

A. Overview

Molybdenum as an essential nutrient for humans and animals was first recognized in 1953. Its importance in relation to copper and iron was appreciated in that an excess of molybdenum interfered with copper and iron absorption. Molybdenum also interferes with the binding of copper by ceruloplasmin. In ruminants, a molybdenum excess when combined with a high sulfur intake results in a copper-deficient state. The three elements (Mo, Cu, S) combine to form cupric thiomolybdate complexes. In humans, excess molybdenum intakes occur rarely. This is because most human foods that contain molybdenum also contain copper in amounts that exceed that of molybdenum.

Molybdenum is a transition metal in the fifth period of the periodic table. It has an atomic weight of 95.94 and an atomic number of 42. There are several naturally occurring isotopes ranging in weight from 92 to 100; however, Mo^{96} is the most useful in biological research. There are 8 radioisotopes with weights ranging from 88 to 93. Molybdenum has four charged states: 3+, 4+, 5+, and 6+. The most common is the 6+ state. Where this mineral serves as a cofactor in enzymatic reactions, it vacillates between 4+ and 6+.

B. Absorption, Excretion, Function

Molybdenum is readily absorbed from most foods. Between 40 and 100% of the ingested mineral will be absorbed by the epithelial cells of the gastrointestinal system and will be found in the blood in a protein-bound complex. A plasma concentration range of 0.5 to 15 µg/dl has been reported and molybdenum may be found in very small amounts (0.1 to 1.0 µg/g) in most cell types. Some accumulation occurs in the liver, kidneys, bones, and skin. Molybdenum is readily excreted in the urine with small amounts excreted via the biliary route. The average intake of 300 µg/day is 1/3 to 1/5 that of copper.

Molybdenum's function is as a cofactor for the iron- and flavin-containing enzymes, xanthine oxidase, aldehyde oxidase, and sulfite oxidase. The molybdenum cofactor common to these enzymes is a pterin structure shown in Figure 13. This pterin is a monophosphate ester susceptible to cleavage by alkaline phosphatase. One molecule of pterin phosphatase is associated with each molybdenum atom in sulfite oxidase and xanthine dehydrogenase. Molybdenum also serves to activate adenylate cyclase in brain, cardiac, and renal tissue, and erythrocytes. It has no effect on testicular adenylate cyclase nor does it have an effect on adenylate cyclase previously stimulated with fluoride or GTP.

C. Food Sources, Recommended Intake

Molybdenum is found in very small amounts in most foods. The germ of grain is a good source of this mineral; however, much of this germ is lost when the grain is milled. No recommended

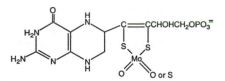

Figure 13 Pterin structure with molybdenum as part of its molecule.

dietary allowance has been set but the Food and Nutrition Board of the National Academy of Sciences has estimated that an intake of 75 to 250 µg/day for adults should be safe and adequate. For infants the recommendation is 15 to 40 µg/day, and for children an intake of 25 to 75 µg/day should suffice. Table 2 shows these recommendations.

X. MANGANESE

A. Overview

Although manganese (Mn) was recognized as an essential nutrient in 1931, its ubiquitous role as a cofactor in a variety of enzymatic reactions has only recently been appreciated. Structural abnormalities in growing birds and animals are the chief symptoms of deficiency. Depression of mucopolysaccharide synthesis and decreased mitochondrial manganese superoxide dismutase activity accompany these skeletal abnormalities, as does congenital ataxia due to abnormal inner ear development and abnormal brain function. Biochemical abnormalities were hard to document because many of the requirements for manganese as a cofactor in enzymatic reactions could be met by magnesium. Nonetheless, bone and connective tissue growth are abnormal in manganese-deficient animals. Few cases of human manganese deficiency have been reported.

Manganese, like magnesium, is a transition element. It can exist in 11 oxidation states. However, in mammalian systems it usually exists in either the 3+ or 2+ state. In the 2+ state it is less easily chelated than in the 3+ state. The 3+ state is one which interacts with the ferric ion (Fe^{3+}); it is also the state needed for service as a cofactor in the Mn superoxide dismutase enzyme.

In contrast, manganese toxicity with symptoms resembling Parkinson's disease has been reported to occur in up to 25% of miners and metal mill workers in Russia, North Africa, Chile, and the former Yugoslavia. The inhalation of mineral dust in mines and mills is the main route of excess exposure.

B. Absorption, Excretion, Function

Manganese is poorly absorbed through the gut. Between 2 and 15% of that ingested in the food appears in the blood. This has been traced using radioactive [54]Mn. As with many minerals, the route of excretion is via resecretion into the small intestine. That which is unabsorbed appears in the feces as does that which is' excreted from the body via the bile. The mechanism whereby manganese is transported from the site of absorption to the site of use is not fully known. It may share transport with iron using transferrin or another protein, notably α-2-macroglobulin. Manganese circulates throughout the body at a level of 1 to 2 µg/dl (~2 µmol/l). Widely varying blood levels of manganese have been reported. Smith et al. contend that this wide variation has to do with contamination introduced by both sampling technique and analytical technique. Contamination can double the amount of manganese in the food, blood, or tissue sample. It is for this reason that balance studies to determine apparent absorption are not useful. Actually this problem is common to many of the trace minerals. They are present in such small amounts in biological samples that extreme precautions must be taken to control contamination. Once transported from the gut to the liver almost all of the manganese is cleared from the blood. In the liver it enters one of several pools. It can be found in the bile canaliculi from which it can be exported via the bile back into the small intestine, or it can enter the hepatocytes whereupon it is used by its various organelles (lysosomes, mitochondria, nucleus) as a cofactor for several enzymes, or it can remain in the cytoplasm.

Table 9   Enzymes Requiring Manganese

Pyruvate carboxylase
Acetyl CoA carboxylase
Isocitrate dehydrogenase
Mitochondrial superoxide dismutase
Arginase
Glucokinase
Galactose transferrase
Hydroxymethyl transferase
Superoxide dismutase

Manganese is present in the bone as part of the mineral apatite, and in the lactating gland and liver to a greater extent than in other tissues. However, no tissue is free of this mineral. The turnover of manganese in the body varies depending on location. It is very short (~3 min half-life) in hepatic mitochondria, and in bone its half-life is about an hour. The pool size likewise varies from 2 mg/kg in liver to 3.5 mg/kg in bone. As mentioned, it is an essential cofactor in a wide variety of enzymatic reactions. Listed in Table 9 are some of the many enzymes shown to require manganese.

Manganese and calcium share a uniport mechanism for mitochondrial transport. It can accumulate in this organelle because it is cleared very slowly. Mitochondrial manganese efflux is not sodium dependent and in fact appears to inhibit both the sodium-dependent and -independent calcium efflux. This manganese effect on calcium is not reciprocal; calcium has no effect on manganese efflux.

It has been reported that manganese deficiency in experimental animals causes the down-regulation of the mitochondrial manganese containing superoxide dismutase (SOD) at the level of the activation of transcription of the gene which encodes this protein. Superoxide dismutases are a class of metalloproteins that catalyze the dismutation of the superoxide radical (O_2^-) to oxygen (O_2) and hydrogen peroxide (H_2O_2). These enzymes play a critical role in protecting cells against oxidative stress, particularly that produced by drugs. Most mammalian cells contain two forms of this enzyme: one in the cytosol requiring zinc and copper and the other requiring manganese. It is generally thought that the latter, present in the mitochondria, protects that organelle from potential damage by the superoxide radical that could possibly be produced through the activity of the respiratory chain. The important role of Mn SOD has been demonstrated using cell cultures. Those cultures in which the gene for this enzyme was altered, or in which the enzyme was inhibited, died. Apoptic cell death has been reported in cultured spinal neurons and in PC12 neuronal cells. Maintenance of mitochondrial manganese-dependent SOD is especially important if a drug is used that disrupts the control or function of the respiratory chain. Redox active drugs, e.g., antibiotics, tetracycline, or pesticides such as paraquat, have this effect. When these compounds are given to animals or cells in culture, the activity of the manganese superoxide dismutase increases. Interleukin-1 and tumor necrosis factor also increase the activity of this enzyme. Some tumor cells respond to chemotherapeutic agents by increasing the activity of SOD. As a result, these tumors are resistant to certain cytotoxic agents. This is particularly true for melanoma cells and may explain the resistance of this cancer to many of the therapies found successful for other tumor cell types.

C. Food Sources, Recommended Intake

Rich food sources include nuts, whole grains, and leafy vegetables. Meats, milk, seafood, and other animal products are poor sources. The germ of grains can contain up to 14 ppm. The average diet consumed in the U.S. contains about 3 to 4 mg/day, the range suggested by the National Academy of Sciences as being safe and adequate (see Table 2). A recommended dietary allowance has not been established for this nutrient.

XI. COBALT

A. Overview

The discovery of cobalt as an essential nutrient for mammals was first made in Australia by animal scientists seeking to understand the pathophysiology of a wasting disease in sheep and cattle. At first it was thought to be an iron deficiency disorder because iron supplements seemed to cure the condition. The iron supplements, however, were rather impure substances. In the mid 1930s Underwood and associates discovered that it was not the iron per se but an impurity in the supplement that cured the condition. That impurity was cobalt.

The essentiality of cobalt as a nutrient for humans was assumed based on the results of the above animal studies. Many human foods, especially green leafy vegetables, contain cobalt. Meats, including the organ meats, provide cobalt as a component of vitamin B_{12}. Of the free cobalt found in these foods, very little is used although it is absorbed by the enterocytes. The results of tracer studies have shown that almost 100% of ingested cobalt appears in the urine. Very little appears in the feces and very little is retained in the tissues. As discussed in Unit 4, Section IX, the absorption of vitamin B_{12} (and its cobalt component) is dependent on the presence of an intrinsic factor in the stomach. Whereas in ruminants the consumption of cobalt cures the wasting disease (pernicious anemia) it does this not because the ruminant can absorb and then use this metal, but because the rumen flora can synthesize vitamin B_{12} which in turn is absorbed. This then is the basis for understanding why vegetarians consuming large amounts of cobalt-rich green leafy vegetables are at risk for developing pernicious anemia. While they obtain sufficient cobalt they can not synthesize vitamin B_{12}. Cobalt has no other known function aside from its central action in vitamin B_{12} function.

B. Toxicity

Although cobalt is readily absorbed by the enterocyte, it is just as readily excreted by the kidney. Thus, toxicity in the usual sense is not a significant problem with respect to environmental exposures. Excess cobalt (1000 times normal) can be tolerated by a variety of species with little ill effect. However, cobalt does interfere with the absorption of iron and in fact can completely block iron uptake. Symptoms of iron deficiency anemia as well as symptoms of disturbed thyroid function (enlarged hyperplasic thyroid gland, myxedema) and congestive heart failure have been observed when excess cobalt was consumed accidentally as a contaminant of beer. Cobalt salts were once used in the production of beer as a foaming agent. While the occasional beer would not provide toxic amounts of cobalt, large intakes consumed regularly could and have done so. Once this was recognized, this production practice was discontinued. Actually, it was not the cobalt content of the beer alone that was responsible for the toxic response. The alcohol in the beer plus the likelihood of inadequate protein, iron, and B vitamin intake were also part of the problem.

C. Requirement

Because cobalt serves no other function than as a constituent of vitamin B_{12}, there is no requirement for this mineral. If the vitamin B_{12} requirement is met, then the cobalt need is met.

XII. OTHER MINERALS

Shown in Table 3 are a variety of minerals which have been shown to be essential to one or more species, not necessarily humans. Included in this list is fluorine, an element known to provide hardness to teeth and bones, and which also inhibits tooth decay. In excess, it is toxic. Arsenic, a known poison, has been shown to be essential to chickens, rats, pigs, and goats, but its biological function in humans is not known. It is thought to have a role in bone metabolism. Animals with arsenic deficiency exhibit depressed growth, myocardial degeneration, and premature death. Boron, likewise, is an essential nutrient for rats but its function is not known. Deficient rats have a reduced stress response which probably relates to a change in brain electrical activity. Boron-copper and boron-calcium-phosphate interactions have been reported. These interactions have to do with increased brain copper concentrations in the former and increased calcium and phosphate concentrations in the latter in boron-deprived animals.

Chromium was shown by Schwartz and Mertz to be essential for optimal peripheral insulin action with respect to glucose uptake. Studies of elderly humans with noninsulin-dependent diabetes mellitus showed an improvement in glucose tolerance in about half of the subjects following a period of chromium supplementation. The mechanism of action of chromium as a potentiator of insulin action has yet to be elucidated. Nonetheless, because a chromium supplement has been shown to be of benefit to some persons with diabetes, a safe and adequate recommendation for intake (Table 2) has been made.

Nickel is another mineral whose function has not been defined, yet animals fed nickel deficient diets fail to thrive. Nickel is a component of the urease enzyme family and although not found in mammalian urease has been found in ureases isolated from lower life forms. Similarly, nickel has been found associated with hydrogenases in lower life forms and, in these species has a role in oxidation-reduction reactions as well as in methane formation.

Silicon has been found essential to chickens and rats and appears to be involved in bone formation. Skeletal abnormalities typify silicon deficiency in these species.

Vanadium is also needed by chickens for appropriate pigmentation; however, whether this need is a true need or one induced by the particular diet ingredients used to compose the deficient diet is subject to discussion.

Aluminum, boron, tin, cadmium, lead, germanium, lithium, and rubidium have all been examined with respect to their essentiality. Data are lacking that document a need for these elements in humans.

SUPPLEMENTAL READINGS

General

Fairweather-Tait, B. 1992. Bioavailability of trace elements, *Food Chem.,* 43:213-217.

Frieden, E. 1985. New perspectives on the essential trace elements, *J. Chem. Educ.,* 62:917-923.

Lorscheider, F.L., Vimy, M.J., and Summers, A.O. 1995. Mercury exposure from silver tooth fillings: emerging evidence questions a traditional dental paradigm, *FASEB J.,* 9:504-508.

Paustenbach, D.J., Finley, B.L., and Kacew, S. 1996. Biological relevance and consequences of chemical or metal-induced DNA cross linking, *Proc. Soc. Exp. Biol. Med.,* 211:211-217.

Thompson, K.H. and Godin, D.V. 1995. Micronutrients and antioxidants in the progression of diabetes, *Nutr. Res.,* 15:1377-1410.

Iron

Bothwell, T.H. and Charlton, R.W. 1982. A general approach to the problems of iron deficiency and iron overload in the population at large, *Semin. Hematol.,* 19:54-67.

Crichton, R.R. and Charloteaux-Wauters, M. 1987. Iron transport and storage, *Eur. J. Biochem.,* 164:485-506.

Fairweather-Tait, S.J. 1987. The concept of bioavailability as it relates to iron nutrition, *Nutr. Res.,* 7:319-325.

Herbert, V., Shaw, S., Jayatilleke, E., and Stopler-Kasdan, T. 1994. Most free radical injury is iron related: it is promoted by iron, heme, holoferritin, and vitamin C and inhibited by desferoxamine and apoferritin, *Stem Cells,* 12:289-303.

Johnson, M.A. 1990. Iron: nutrition monitoring and nutrition status assessment, *J. Nutr.,* 120:1486-1491.

Kuvibidila, S., Warrier, R.P., Ode, D., and Yu, L. 1996. Serum transferrin receptor concentrations in women with mild malnutrition, *Am. J. Clin. Nutr.,* 63:596-601.

Looker, A.C., Gunter, E.W., and Johnson, C.L. 1995. Methods to assess iron status in various NHANES surveys, *Nutr. Rev.,* 53:246-254.

Morris, E.R. 1983. An overview of current information on bioavailability of dietary iron to humans, *Fed. Proc.,* 42:1716-1720.

Munro, H.N., Kikinis, Z., and Eisenstein, R.S. 1993. Iron dependent regulation of ferritin synthesis. In: *Nutrition and Gene Expression,* Berdanier, C.D. and Hargrove, J.L., Eds., CRC Press, Boca Raton, FL, pp. 525-545.

Parke, D.V., Iannides, C., and Lewis, D.F.V. 1991. The role of cytochrome P450 in the detoxification and activation of drugs and other chemicals, *Can. J. Physiol. Pharmacol.,* 69:537-549.

Proudhon, D., Wei, J., Briat, J.F., and Theil, E.C. 1996. Ferritin gene organization. Differences between plants and animals suggest possible kingdom specific selective constraints, *J. Mol. Evol.,* 42:325-336.

Rogers, J. and Munro, H. 1987. Translation of ferritin light and heavy subunit mRNAs is regulated by intracellular chelatable iron levels in rat hepatoma cells, *Proc. Natl. Acad. Sci. U.S.A.,* 84:2277-2281.

Toyokuni, S. 1996. Iron induced carcinogenesis: The role of redox regulation, *Free Radical Biol. Med.,* 20:553-566.

Zakim, M.M. 1992. Regulation of transferrin gene expression, *FASEB J.,* 6:3253-3258.

Zinc

Castro, C.E., Kaspin, L.C., Chen, S-S., and Nolker, S.G. 1992. Zinc deficiency increases the frequency of single strand DNA breaks in rat liver, *Nutr. Res.,* 12:721-736.

Conte, D., Narindrašorasak, S., and Sarkar, B. 1996. In vivo and in vitro iron replaced zinc finger generates free radicals and causes DNA damage, *J. Biol. Chem.,* 271:5125-5130.

Cousins, R.J. and Leinart, A.S. 1988. Tissue specific regulation of zinc metabolism and metallothionein genes by interleukin 1, *FASEB J.,* 2:2884-2890.

Dalton, T., Fu, K., Palmiter, R.D., and Andrews, G.K. 1996. Transgenic mice that overexpress metallothionine-I resist zinc deficiency, *J. Nutr.,* 126:825-833.

Durnam, D.M. and Palmiter, R. 1981. Transcriptional regulation of the mouse metallothionine-I gene by heavy metals, *J. Biol. Chem.,* 256:6712-6716.

Emery, M.P. and O'Dell, B.L. 1993. Low zinc status in rats impairs calcium uptake and aggregation of platelets stimulated by fluoride, *Proc. Soc. Exp. Biol. Med.,* 203:480-484.

Failla, M. and Cousins, R.J. 1978. Zinc uptake by isolated rat liver parenchymal cells, *B.B.A. Libr.,* 538:435-444.

Fosmire, G.J. 1990. Zinc toxicity, *Am. J. Clin. Nutr.,* 51:225-7.

Halsted, J.A., Smith, J.C., Jr., and Irwin, M.I. 1974. A conspectus of research on zinc requirements of man, *J. Nutr.,* 104:345-378.

Keen, C.L., Taubeneck, M.W., Daston, G.P., Rogers, J.M., and Gershwin, M.E. 1993. Primary and secondary zinc deficiency as factors underlying abnormal CNS development, *Ann. NY Acad. Sci.,* 678:37-47.

Kelly, E.J., Quaife, C.J., Froelick, G.J., and Palmiter, R.D. 1996. Metallothionein I and II protect against zinc deficiency and zinc toxicity in mice, *J. Nutr.,* 126:1782-1790.

Mahajan, S.K., Prasad, A.S., Rabbani, P., Briggs, W.A., and McDonald, F.D. 1982. Zinc deficiency: a reversible complication of uremia, *Am. J. Clin. Nutr.,* 36:1177-1183.

Masuoka, J. and Saltman, P. 1994. Zinc (II) and copper (II) binding to serum albumin, *J. Biol. Chem.,* 269:25557-25561.

McNall, A.D., Etherton, T.D., and Fosmire, G.J. 1995. The impaired growth induced by zinc deficiency in rats is associated with decreased expression of the hepatic insulin-like growth factor I and growth hormone receptor genes, *J. Nutr.,* 125:874-879.

Moser, P.B., Krebs, N.K., and Blyler, E. 1991. Zinc hair concentrations and estimated zinc intakes of functionally delayed normal sized and small for age children, *Nutr. Res.,* 2:585-590.

Oberleas, D. 1993. Understanding zinc deficiency, *J. Texas State Nutr. Counc.,* 3:3-6.

Palmiter, R.D. 1994. Regulation of metallothionein genes by heavy metals appears to be mediated by a zinc sensitive inhibitor that interacts with a constitutively active transcription factor MTF-1, *Proc. Natl. Acad. Sci. U.S.A.,* 91:1219-1223.

Prasad, A.S. 1984. Discovery and importance of zinc in human nutrition, *Fed. Proc.,* 43:2829-2834.

Price, D. and Joshi, J.G. 1982. Ferritin: a zinc detoxicant and a zinc ion donor, *Proc. Natl. Acad. Sci. U.S.A.,* 79:3116-3119.

Reeves, P.G. 1995. Adaptation responses in rats to long term feeding of high zinc diets: emphasis on intestinal metallothionein, *J. Nutr. Biochem.,* 6:48-54.

Reyes, J.G. 1996. Zinc transport in mammalian cells, *Am. J. Physiol.,* 270:C401-C410.

Shay, N.F. and Cousins, R.J. 1993. Dietary regulation of metallothionein expression. In: *Nutrition and Gene Expression,* Berdanier, C.D. and Hargrove, J.L., Eds., CRC Press, Boca Raton, FL, pp. 507-523.

Wu, H., Yang, W.-P., and Barbas, C.F. 1995. Building zinc fingers by selection: toward a therapeutic application, *Proc. Natl. Acad. Sci. U.S.A.,* 92:344-348.

Copper

Chen, Y., Saari, J. T., and Kang, Y. J. 1995. Copper deficiency increases metallothionein-I mRNA content selectively in rat liver, *J. Nutr. Biochem.,* 6:572-576.

Fields, M., Craft, N., Lewis, C., Holbrook, J., Rose, A., Reiser, S., and Smith, J.C. 1986. Contrasting effects of the stomach and small intestine of rats on copper absorption, *J. Nutr.,* 116:219-2228.

Fischer, P.W.F., Giroux, A., and L'Abbe, M.R. 1981. Effect of dietary zinc on intestinal copper absorption, *Am. J. Clin. Nutr.,* 34:1670-1675.

Frieden, E. 1983. The copper connection, *Semin. Hematol.,* 20:114-117.

Harris, E.D. 1991. Copper transport: an overview, *Proc. Soc. Exp. Biol. Med.,* 196:130-146.

Hart, E.B., Steenbock, H., Wasddell, J., and Cartwright, G. 1928. Iron in nutrition. VII. Copper as a supplement to iron for hemoglobin building in the rat, *J. Biol. Chem.,* 77:797-812.

Hopkins, R.G. and Failla, M. 1995. Chronic intake of a marginally low copper diet impairs in vitro activities of lymphocytes and neutrophils from male rats despite minimal impact on conventional indicators of copper status, *J. Nutr.,* 125:2658-2668.

Hoshi, Y., Hazeki, O., and Tamura, M. 1993. Oxygen dependence of redox state of copper in cytochrome oxidase in vitro, *J. Appl. Physiol.,* 74:1622-1627.

Johnson, M.A. and Kays, S.E. 1990. Copper: its role in human nutrition, *Nutrition Today,* Jan./Feb. 6-14.

Johnson, W.T., Dufault, S.N., and Newman, S.M. 1995. Altered nucleotide content and changes in mitochondrial energy states associated with copper deficiency in rat platelets, *J. Nutr. Biochem.,* 6:551-556.

Klevay, L.M., Inman, L., Johnson, L.K., Lawler, M., Mahalko, J.R., Milne, D.B., Lukaski, H.C., Bolonchuk, W., and Sandstead, H.H. 1984. Increased cholesterol in plasma in a young man during experimental copper deficiency, *Metabolism,* 33:1112-1118.

Lee, G.R., Cartwright, G.E., and Wintrobe, M.M. 1968. Heme biosynthesis in copper deficient swine, *Proc. Soc. Exp. Biol. Med.,* 127:977-981.

Matz, J.M., Saari, J.T., and Bode, A.M. 1995. Functional aspects of oxidative phosphorylation and electron transport in cardiac mitochondria of copper deficient rats, *J. Nutr. Biochem.,* 6:644-652.

Olivares, M. and Uauy, R. 1996. Limits of metabolic tolerance to copper and biological basis for present recommendations and regulations, *Am. J. Clin. Nutr.,* 63:846S-852S.

Reed, V., Williamson, P., Bull, P.C., Cox, D.W., and Boyd, Y. 1996. Mapping the mouse homologue of the Wilson Disease gene to mouse chromosome 6, *Genomics,* 28:573-575.

Turnlund, J.R., Keyes, W.R., Anderson, H.L., and Acord, L.L. 1989. Copper absorption and retention in young men at three levels of dietary copper by use of the stable isotope ^{65}Cu, *Am. J. Clin. Nutr.,* 49:870-878.

Wang, Y.R., Wu, J.Y.J., Reaves, S.K., and Lei, K.Y. 1996. Enhanced expression of hepatic genes in copper deficient rats detected by the messenger RNA diferential display method, *J. Nutr.,* 126:1772-1781.

Weiss, K.C. and Linder, M.C. 1985. Copper transport in rats involving a new plasma protein, *Am. J. Physiol.,* 249:E77-E88.

Wildman, R.E.C., Hopkins, R., Failla, M.L., and Medeiros, D.M. 1995. Marginal copper restricted diets produce altered cardiac ultrastructure in the rat, *Proc. Soc. Exp. Biol. Med.,* 210:43-49.

Selenium

Arthur, J.R., Nicol, F., and Beckett, G.J. 1993. Selenium deficiency, thyroid hormone metabolism and thyroid hormone deiodinases, *Am. J. Clin. Nutr.,* 57:236S-239S.

Bermano, G., Nicol, F., Dyer, J.A., Sunde, R.A., Beckett, G.J., Arthur, J.R., and Hesketh, J.E. 1996. Selenoprotein gene expression during selenium-repletion of selenium deficient rats, *Biol. Trace Element Res.,* 51:211-223.

Burk, R.F. 1989. Recent developments in trace element metabolism and function. Newer roles of selenium in nutrition, *J. Nutr.,* 119:1051-1054.

Chen, S,Y., Collipp, P.J., and Hsu, J.M. 1985. Effect of sodium selenite toxicity on tissue distribution of zinc, iron and copper in rats, *Biol. Trace Element Res.,* 7:169-179.

Chu, F.F. 1994. The human glutathione peroxidase genes GPX2, GPX3 and GPX4 map to chromosomes 14, 5 and 19 respectively, *Cytogenet. Cell Genet.,* 66:96-98.

Clark, L.C. 1985. The epidemiology of selenium and cancer, *Fed. Proc.,* 44:2584-2589.

Cohen, H.J., Brown, M.R., Hamilton, D., Lyons-Patterson, J., Avessar, N., and Liegey, P. 1989. Glutathione peroxidase and selenium deficiency in patients receiving home parenteral nutrition. Time course for development of deficiency and repletion of enzyme activity in plasma and blood cells, *Am. J. Clin. Nutr.,* 49:132-9.

Floyd, R.A. 1990. Role of oxygen free radicals in carcinogens and brain ischemia, *FASEB J.,* 4:2587-2597.

Lai, C.C., Huang, W-H., Askari, A., Klevay, L.M., and Chiu, T.H. 1995. Expression of glutathione peroxidase and catalase in copper-deficient rat liver and heart, *J. Nutr. Biochem.,* 6:256-262.

Levander, O.A., DeLoach, D.P., Moris, V.C., and Moser, P.B. 1983. Platelet glutathione peroxidase activity as an index of selenium status in rats, *J. Nutr.,* 113:55-63.

Robberecht, H. and Deelstra, H. 1994. Factors influencing blood selenium concentration values, *J. Trace Element Electrolytes Health Dis.,* 8:129-143.

Strain, J.J. 1991. Disturbances of micronutrient and antioxidant status in diabetes, *Proc. Nutr. Soc.,* 50:591-604.

Tamura, T. and Stadtman, T.C. 1996. A new selenoprotein from human lung adenocarcinoma cells: Purification, properties and thioredoxin reductase activity, *Proc. Natl. Acad. Sci. U.S.A.,* 93:1006-1011.

Thompson, K.M., Haibach, H., and Sunde, R.A. 1995. Growth and plasma triiodothyronine concentrations are modified by selenium deficiency and repletion in second generation selenium deficient rats, *J. Nutr.,* 125:864-873.

Whanger, P.D. 1989. China, a country with both selenium deficiency and toxicity. Some thoughts and impressions, *J. Nutr.,* 119:1236-1239.

Wilber, C.G. 1980. Toxicology of selenium: a review, *Clin. Toxicol.,* 17:171-230.

Yang, G.Q., Wang, S., Zhou, R., and Sun, S. 1983. Endemic selenium intoxication of humans in China, *Am. J. Clin. Nutr.,* 37:872-881.

Yeh, J-Y., Beilstein, M.A., Andrews, J.S., and Whanger, P.D. 1995. Tissue distribution and influence of selenium status on levels of selenoprotein W, *FASEB J.,* 9:392-396.

Iodine

Beckett, G.J., Nicol, F., Rae, P.W.H., Beech, S., Guo, Y., and Arthur, J.R. 1993. Effects of combined iodine and selenium deficiency on thyroid hormone metabolism in rats, *Am. J. Clin. Nutr.,* 57:240S-243S.

Boyages, S. 1993. Iodine deficiency disorders, *J. Clin. Endocrinol. Metab.,* 77:587-591.

Frieden, E. 1985. New perspectives on the essential trace elements, *J. Chem. Educ.,* 62:912-923.

Maberly, G.F. 1994. Iodine deficiency disorders: Contemporary scientific issues, *J. Nutr.,* 124:1473S-1478S.

Molybdenum

Bai, Y., Sunde, M., and Cook, M.E. 1994. Molybdenum but not copper counteracts cysteine-induced tibial dyschondroplasia in broiler chickens, *J. Nutr.,* 124:588-593.

Rajagopalan, K.V., Johnson, J.L., and Hainline, B.E. 1982. The pterin of the molybdenum factor, *Fed. Proc.,* 41:2608-2612.

Richard, J.M. and Swislocki, N.I. 1979. Activation of adenylate cyclase by molybdate, *J. Biol. Chem.,* 254:6857-6860.

Manganese

Borrello, S., DeLeo, M.E., and Galeotti, T. 1992. Transcriptional regulation of MnSOD by manganese in the liver of manganese deficient mice and during rat development, *Biochem. Int.,* 28:595-561.

Gavin, C.E., Gunter, K.K., and Gunter, T.E. 1990. Manganese and calcium efflux kinetics in brain mitochondria, *Biochem. J.,* 266:329-334.

Hirose, K., Longo, D.L., Oppenheim, J., and Matsushima, K. 1993. Overexpression of mitochondrial manganese superoxide dismutase promotes the survival of tumor cells exposed to interleukin 1, tumor necrosis factor, selected anticancer drugs and ionizing radiation, *FASEB J.,* 7:361-368.

Hurley, L.S. 1981. Roles of trace elements in fetal and neonatal development, *Philos. Trans. R. Soc. London,* 294:145-152.

Mena, I., Marin, O., Fuenzalida, S., and Cotzias, G.C. 1967. Chronic manganese poisoning and clinical pictures of manganese turnover, *Neurology,* 17:128-132.

Santiard-Baron, D., Aral, B., Ribiere, C., Nordmann, R., Sinet, P-M., and Caballos-Picot, I. 1995. Quantitation of Mn-SOD mRNAs by using a competitive reverse-transcription polymerase chain reaction, *Redox Rep.,* 1:185-189.

Smith, J.C., Anderson, R.A., Ferretti, R., Levander, O.A., Morris, E.R., Roginski, E.E., Veillon, C., Wolf, W.R., Anderson, J.B., and Mertz, W. 1981. Evaluation of published data pertaining to mineral composition of human tissue, *Red. Proc.,* 40:2120-2125.

Wolinsky, I., Klimis-Tavantzis, D.J., and Richards, L.J. 1994. Manganese and bone metabolism. In: *Manganese in Health and Disease,* Klimis-Tavantzis, D.J., Ed., CRC Press, Boca Raton, FL, pp. 115-120.

Other Minerals

Nielson, F.H. 1996. Other trace elements. In: *Present Knowledge in Nutrition,* Eckhard, E.E. and Filer, L.J., Eds., ILSI Press, Washington, D.C., pp. 353-377.

Stoecker, B.J. 1996. Chromium. In: *Present Knowledge in Nutrition,* Eckhard, E.E. and Filer, L.J., Eds., ILSI Press, Washington, D.C., pp. 344-352.

Index

W

X